Salmonella: Molecular and Clinical Aspects

Salmonella: Molecular and Clinical Aspects

Editor: Chester Edwin

FOSTER ACADEMICS
www.fosteracademics.com

www.fosteracademics.com

FOSTER ACADEMICS

Cataloging-in-Publication Data

Salmonella : molecular and clinical aspects / edited by Chester Edwin.
p. cm.
Includes bibliographical references and index.
ISBN 978-1-64646-573-6
1. Salmonella infections. 2. Salmonella infections--Treatment.
3. Salmonella infections--Diagnosis. I. Edwin, Chester.
RC182.S12 S35 2023
616.927--dc23

Foster Academics,
118-35 Queens Blvd., Suite 400,
Forest Hills, NY 11375, USA

ISBN 978-1-64646-573-6 (Hardback)

Contents

Preface VII

Chapter 1 **CdsH Contributes to the Replication of *Salmonella* Typhimurium inside Epithelial Cell in a Cysteine-Supplemented Medium** 1
Fernando Díaz-Yáñez, Ricardo Álvarez, Iván L. Calderón, Juan A. Fuentes and Fernando Gil

Chapter 2 **Validating Thermal Lethality to *Salmonella enterica* in Chicken Blood by Simulated Commercial Rendering** 16
Caleb Wong de la Rosa, Kourtney A. Daniels, Rosana G. Moreira, Chris R. Kerth and Thomas M. Taylor

Chapter 3 **Effect of a High Proportion of Rye in Compound Feed for Reduction of *Salmonella* Typhimurium in Experimentally Infected Young Pigs** 28
Bussarakam Chuppava, Volker Wilke, Clara Berenike Hartung, Amr Abd El-Wahab, Richard Grone, Andreas von Felde, Josef Kamphues and Christian Visscher

Chapter 4 **A Role for the Microbiota in the Immune Phenotype Alteration Associated with the Induction of Disease Tolerance and Persistent Asymptomatic Infection of *Salmonella* in the Chicken** 41
Annah Lee, Cristiano Bortoluzzi, Rachel Pilla and Michael H. Kogut

Chapter 5 ***Salmonella* Pathogenicity Island 1 (SPI-1): The Evolution and Stabilization of a Core Genomic type Three Secretion System** 56
Nicole A. Lerminiaux, Keith D. MacKenzie and Andrew D. S. Cameron

Chapter 6 **The not so Good, the Bad and the Ugly: Differential Bacterial Adhesion and Invasion Mediated by *Salmonella* PagN Allelic Variants** 78
Yanping Wu, Qiaoyun Hu, Ruchika Dehinwal, Alexey V. Rakov, Nicholas Grams, Erin C. Clemens, Jennifer Hofmann, Iruka N. Okeke and Dieter M. Schifferli

Chapter 7 ***Salmonella* Extracellular Polymeric Substances Modulate Innate Phagocyte Activity and Enhance Tolerance of Biofilm-Associated Bacteria to Oxidative Stress** 92
Mark M. Hahn and John S. Gunn

Chapter 8 **Genetic Markers in *S.* Paratyphi C Reveal Primary Adaptation to Pigs** 111
Satheesh Nair, Maria Fookes, Craig Corton, Nicholas R. Thomson, John Wain and Gemma C. Langridge

Chapter 9 **New Roles for Two-Component System Response Regulators of *Salmonella enterica* Serovar Typhi during Host Cell Interactions** 121
Claudie Murret-Labarthe, Maud Kerhoas, Karine Dufresne and France Daigle

Chapter 10 **The *Salmonella enterica* Plasmidome as a Reservoir of Antibiotic Resistance**......138
Jean-Guillaume Emond-Rheault, Jérémie Hamel, Julie Jeukens,
Luca Freschi Irena Kukavica-Ibrulj, Brian Boyle, Sandeep Tamber,
Danielle Malo, Eelco Franz, Elton Burnett, France Daigle, Gitanjali Arya,
Kenneth Sanderson, Martin Wiedmann, Robin M. Slawson, Joel T. Weadge,
Roger Stephan, Sadjia Bekal, Samantha Gruenheid,
Lawrence D. Goodridge and Roger C. Levesque

Chapter 11 **Iron-Uptake Systems of Chicken-Associated *Salmonella* Serovars and their Role in Colonizing the Avian Host**......156
Dinesh H. Wellawa, Brenda Allan, Aaron P. White and Wolfgang Köster

Chapter 12 **Spheres of Influence: Insights into *Salmonella* Pathogenesis from Intestinal Organoids**......180
Smriti Verma, Stefania Senger, Bobby J. Cherayil and Christina S. Faherty

Chapter 13 **Metabolic Activation of CsgD in the Regulation of *Salmonella* Biofilms**......203
Akosiererem S. Sokaribo, Elizabeth G. Hansen, Madeline McCarthy,
Taseen S. Desin, Landon L. Waldner, Keith D. MacKenzie, George Mutwiri Jr.,
Nancy J. Herman, Dakoda J. Herman, Yejun Wang and Aaron P. White

Permissions

List of Contributors

Index

Preface

Salmonella infection, also called salmonellosis is a common bacterial disease that causes gastrointestinal illness and fever. It is caused by salmonella bacteria. Some common signs and symptoms of salmonella infection are diarrhea, fever, vomiting, nausea, headache and abdominal cramps. Contaminated food and water, improperly handled food, infected surfaces, infected pets or other infected animals can cause salmonellosis. There are several complications associated with salmonella infection such as dehydration, bacteremia, and reactive arthritis. The transfer of salmonella bacteria can be prevented by adopting certain lifestyle changes such as washing hands regularly, cooking and storing food properly, and avoiding consumption of raw eggs. The presence of salmonella bacteria can be diagnosed through a stool sample test and blood test. Treatment of dehydration caused by salmonella infection is based on replacing lost fluids and electrolytes by minerals that balance the amount of water in the body. Medications such as anti-diarrheals and antibiotics are also used to relieve the symptoms of infection. This book outlines the molecular and clinical aspects of salmonella infection in detail. It will prove to be immensely beneficial to medical students and researchers.

The information shared in this book is based on empirical researches made by veterans in this field of study. The elaborative information provided in this book will help the readers further their scope of knowledge leading to advancements in this field.

Finally, I would like to thank my fellow researchers who gave constructive feedback and my family members who supported me at every step of my research.

Editor

CdsH Contributes to the Replication of *Salmonella* Typhimurium inside Epithelial Cells in a Cysteine-Supplemented Medium

Fernando Díaz-Yáñez [1,2], Ricardo Álvarez [1], Iván L. Calderón [3], Juan A. Fuentes [4,*] and Fernando Gil [1,2,*]

1 Microbiota-Host Interactions and Clostridia Research Group, Departamento de Ciencias Biológicas, Facultad de Ciencias de la Vida, Universidad Andres Bello, 8370186 Santiago, Chile; f.diazyanez@outlook.com (F.D.-Y.); rh.alvareze@gmail.com (R.Á.)
2 ANID-Millennium Science Initiative Program-Millennium Nucleus in the Biology of the Intestinal Microbiota, 8370186 Santiago, Chile
3 Laboratorio de RNAs Bacterianos, Departamento de Ciencias Biológicas, Facultad de Ciencias de la Vida, Universidad Andres Bello, 8370186 Santiago, Chile; lcalderon@unab.cl
4 Laboratorio de Genética y Patogénesis Bacteriana, Departamento de Ciencias Biológicas, Facultad de Ciencias de la Vida, Universidad Andres Bello, 8370186 Santiago, Chile
* Correspondence: jfuentes@unab.cl (J.A.F.); fernandogil@unab.cl (F.G.)

Abstract: *Salmonella* Typhimurium is a facultative, intracellular pathogen whose products range from self-limited gastroenteritis to systemic diseases. Food ingestion increases biomolecules' concentration in the intestinal lumen, including amino acids such as cysteine, which is toxic in a concentration-dependent manner. When cysteine's intracellular concentration reaches toxic levels, *S.* Typhimurium expresses a cysteine-inducible enzyme (CdsH), which converts cysteine into pyruvate, sulfide, and ammonia. Despite this evidence, the biological context of *cdsH*'s role is not completely clear, especially in the infective cycle. Since inside epithelial cells both *cdsH* and its positive regulator, *ybaO*, are overexpressed, we hypothesized a possible role of *cdsH* in the intestinal phase of the infection. To test this hypothesis, we used an in vitro model of HT-29 cell infection, adding extra cysteine to the culture medium during the infective process. We observed that, at 6 h post-invasion, the wild type *S.* Typhimurium proliferated 30% more than the Δ*cdsH* strain in the presence of extra cysteine. This result shows that *cdsH* contributes to the bacterial replication in the intracellular environment in increased concentrations of extracellular cysteine, strongly suggesting that *cdsH* participates by increasing the bacterial fitness in the intestinal phase of the *S.* Typhimurium infection.

Keywords: *cdsH* expression; cysteine toxicity; epithelial cell infection

1. Introduction

Salmonellosis corresponds to one of the most common food diseases, affecting an estimated ten million people annually, with more than 100.000 deaths worldwide. The disease symptoms are noticeable between 6 and 72 h after consuming *Salmonella*, with a duration of 2–7 days [1].

Salmonella enterica serovar Typhimurium (*S.* Typhimurium) is one of the most relevant etiologic agents of salmonellosis. The infection begins with the consumption of contaminated food or water, where bacteria reach the distal ileum and induce their internalization into epithelial cells and M cells, among others, in the so-called intestinal phase of the infection [2]. *S.* Typhimurium produces self-limited gastroenteritis in healthy humans at this phase, whereas, in immunosuppressed individuals, children, and older adults, it can cause bacteriemia, or even a systemic infection in certain particular cases [3].

The small intestine epithelium's primary function is to absorb nutrients from the lumen, since 80% of the total cells in this epithelium correspond to absorptive cells known as enterocytes [4]. Carbohydrates, fatty acids and proteins are biomolecules that can be uptaken by these cells. For their part, proteins are broken down into amino acids, capable of entering by active or secondary active transport, either as monomers or small peptides. The latter can be hydrolyzed inside the epithelial cells to become monomers [5,6].

Cysteine is a semi-essential amino acid for humans, belonging to the group of neutral polar amino acids. There are transporters for cysteine and cystine, an oxidized dimer form of cysteine, in the intestine epithelial cells. However, different systems are used for the absorption of these molecules from the intestinal lumen. For cysteine, the neutral transporter systems are used, such as the sodium-dependent ASC (alanine-serine-cysteine) system and symport or antiport mechanisms; for cystine, the transporters belong to the basic system, which transports cationic amino acids and cystine by means of an antiport mechanism independent of ions [7].

To our knowledge, the concentration of cysteine has not been reported for enterocytes. However, the intracellular cysteine levels reported for other cells were around 0.1–0.25 mM in eukaryotes [8]. The intracellular concentration of other amino acids in the jejunum's epithelial cells is approximately 0.2–5 mM, with methionine having the lowest concentration [9]. On the other hand, the luminal concentration of amino acids (excluding cysteine) before food intake is 0.05–0.32 mM in the jejunum and between 0.6 and 0.86 μM in the ileum. In both cases, methionine has the lowest concentration [9]. Since methionine and cysteine have a similar presence in proteins, i.e., 2.3 and 1.9%, respectively [10], it is possible to infer that the increase in the concentration of these amino acids after consuming a diet rich in proteins should be similar in the intestinal lumen. A protein-rich diet increases methionine concentration from 0.05 to 0.6 mM in the jejunum and from 0.06 to 0.29 mM in the ileum [9], concentrations that plausibly are similar for cysteine.

In 2008, the gene encoding the inducible cysteine desulfhydrase enzyme, CdsH, was described, which produces pyruvate, ammonia and sulfide from cysteine degradation [11]. Under anaerobic conditions, a YbaO-dependent increase in *cdsH* expression has been shown in response to high cysteine concentrations (>0.2 mM). YbaO corresponds to a positive transcriptional regulator belonging to the Lrp family [11]. The range of cysteine concentrations in which CdsH would function in *Salmonella* (0.1–0.2 mM) suggests that this amino acid's physiological concentration should be within these same limits, similar to what was described for *Escherichia coli* [12]. Interestingly, this cysteine concentration range allows bacteria to synthesize glutathione, a tripeptide that participates in defense against oxidative stress [13]. Besides, glutathione also generates hydrogen sulfide, which decreases the oxidative stress produced by certain antibiotics [14]. The synthesis of these defense compounds is explained by the fact that, at higher concentrations than physiological, cysteine is toxic in various microorganisms [12,15–17]. In *Salmonella*, excess cysteine induces a temporary toxic effect, causing a decreased growth in minimal media [18]. Many mechanisms explain the toxic effect of higher levels of cysteine. In both *E. coli* and *Salmonella*, the addition of cysteine has been shown to promote the Fenton reaction, with the consequent increase in the hydroxyl radical (·OH) in the presence of hydrogen peroxide, causing breaks in the DNA strands [12,17]. Another toxicity mechanism is related to the hindrance of obtaining or synthesizing branched-chain amino acids (BCAAs), such as valine, leucine, and isoleucine. In *E. coli*, cysteine has been shown to inhibit enzymes related to BCAA biosynthesis [19–23]. This mechanism is similar to that observed in some *Streptococcus mutans* strains, where the inhibitory effect on the bacterial growth under higher concentrations of cysteine is reversed by the addition of BCAA to the culture medium [16].

At present, the role of *csdH* in *S.* Typhumiurium's infective cycle is not clear. A transcriptomic study of *S.* Typhimurium inside epithelial cells found that both *cdsH* and *ybaO* were overexpressed at different times post-infection. This evidence suggests that both genes play a role at this stage of the infection [24]. Due to the induction of *cdsH* expression inside epithelial cells and considering that this gene is overexpressed under high-cysteine concentrations, we wondered whether *cdsH* contributes to the *S.* Typhimurium replication inside epithelial cell lines in the presence of exogenous cysteine in vitro. We found that, at 6 h post-invasion, the wild type *S.* Typhimurium strain proliferates 30% more when extra cysteine is added to the medium, compared with the Δ*cdsH* strain in HT-29 cells. The contribution of *cdsH* to the replication of *S.* Typhimurium inside epithelial cells in response to cysteine is discussed.

2. Materials and Methods

Bacterial growth. Bacteria were grown at 37 °C in Luria–Bertani medium (tryptone, 10 g/L; yeast extract, 5 g/L; NaCl, 5 g/L) or glucose-supplemented M9 minimal medium (M9-glu) ($Na_2HPO_4 \times 7H_2O$, 12.8 g/L; KH_2PO_4, 3 g/L; NaCl, 0.5 g/L; NH_4Cl, 1 g/L; $MgSO_4$, 0.24 g/L; $CaCl_2$, 0.011 g/L; glucose, 4 g/L, Merck® KGaA, Darmstadt, Germany), and for solid medium agar-agar was added (15 g/L, Becton Dickinson®, Franklin Lakes, NJ, USA). When needed, antibiotics (Sigma-Aldrich®, Merck® KGaA, Darmstadt, Germany) were added at the following concentrations: Ampicillin (Amp) 100 μg/mL, chloramphenicol (Cam) 20 μg/mL or kanamycin (Kan) 50 μg/mL.

Cell line culture. The HT-29 cell line was cultured in Dulbecco's Modified Eagle Medium (DMEM) (Gibco®, ThermoFischer, Pittsburgh, PA, USA) supplemented with fetal bovine serum (Gibco®, ThermoFischer, Pittsburgh, PA, USA) (10%). Culture conditions were maintained at 37 °C in a humified atmosphere containing 5% CO_2.

The construction of mutants and complemented strains of *S.* Typhimurium LT2. *S.* Typhimurium Δ*cdsH*::FRT or Δ*ybaO*::FRT were constructed as described by Datsenko and Wanner (2000) [25]. *S.* Typhimurium *cdsH*-3×FLAG and *ybaO*-3×FLAG mutants were constructed as described by Uzzau et al. (2001) [26]. The respective primers and strains are listed in Tables 1 and 2, respectively. For complemented strains, primers were designed to amplify the promoter and coding regions of *cdsH* or *ybaO* (Table 1). Amplicons were cloned into the pBAD-TOPO (Invitrogen®, ThermoFischer, Pittsburgh, USA) vector following the manufacturer's instructions, and then electrotransformed into *E. coli* DH5α. Then, the insert was released (EcoRI, New England Biolabs®, Ipswich, MA, USA) and subcloned into pACYCDuet (pACYC, Novagen®, Merck® KGaA, Darmstadt, Germany, Cam^R, P15A *ori*, intermediate/medium copy number) or pMCL210 (Cam^R, P15A *ori*, intermediate/medium copy number). The resulting plasmids (pACYC::*cdsH* or pMCL210::*ybaO*) were used to complement the respective deletion (Table 2).

Cysteine minimum inhibitory concentration (MIC). An overnight culture of each strain was used to generate a new culture with approximately 1×10^4 CFU/mL (the equivalent of a 0.5 McFarland standard). Bacterial cultures were disposed in 96-well microtiter plates and treated with decreasing concentrations of freshly prepared cysteine solutions. Microtiter plates were incubated in a Thermo shaker incubator (HILAB® MSC-100, Curitiba, Brazil) at 37 °C with shaking for 16 h, and OD_{600} was measured in a microtiter plate reader. The MIC was defined as the lowest concentration that completely inhibited visible growth compared with the cysteine-free control. In other words, a lower MIC is interpreted as an increased susceptibility.

Cysteine toxicity assay (Kirby–Bauer Assay). To qualitatively assess the toxic effect of cysteine under aerobic conditions, both LB and M9-glucose plates were used. Overnight cultures were used to generate a 3 mL bacterial suspension in M9-glucose with agar-agar (0.7%) with approximately 10^6 CFU. This bacterial suspension was added over an M9-glucose plate (agar-agar 1.5%) to generate a bacterial suspension layer. A filter-paper disc was then placed in the center of each bacterial layer before being loaded with 15 μL of a fresh solution of cysteine (0.5 M). The inhibition zone diameter was measured after 16 h incubation at 37 °C.

Table 1. Primers used in this study.

Primers	Comment	Sequence (5′-3′)
cdsHwannerF	Generation of Δ*cdsH*	GGCACAAAATGATAAATGGATATTAATGATGAGTAGCAATGTAGGCTGGAGCTGCTTCGA
cdsHwannerR	Generation of Δ*cdsH*	ATTCAGTCTGGCTTTTTTTTGGTTTCTAGTCGCCGGTAAGATATGAATATCCTCCTTAG
ybaOwannerF	Generation of Δ*ybaO*	GAAAAATATTCTCTATGGAGTGGGTATGTTAGATAAAATTGTAGGCTGGAGCTGCTTCGA
ybaOwannerR	Generation of Δ*ybaO*	ATTTCCGGCAATACCGGGAGAATTATTCAATGGGCAGAGACATATGAATATCCTCCTTAG
cdsHextF	Test the generation of Δ*cdsH*	AATAAGCAAAGCAGCTTACGGTCAA
cdsHextR	Test the generation of Δ*cdsH*	CACACCTTTCGGTTATCGGACATTG
ybaOextF	Test the generation of Δ*ybaO*	ATCCATTTATCATTTTGTGCCAAGA
ybaOextR	Test the generation of Δ*ybaO*	GCCAAGATAGCGACGCCATT
cdsH3×FLAGF	Generation of *cdsH*-3×FLAG	GCCGTGGTCAGCGGCCATCGCAAAATTACTTACCGGCGACGACTACAAAGACCATGACGG GACTACAAAGACCATGACGG
cdsH3×FLAGR	Generation of *cdsH*-3×FLAG	ATTGGCTGGACAATCCGCATCTACCTTATTCCCCCGAATGCATATGAATATCCTCCTTAG
ybaO3×FLAGF	Generation of *ybaO*-3×FLAG	GATGGAACAGATTAAGTACACCACCTCTCTGCCCATTGAAGACTACAAAGACCATGACGG
ybaO3×FLAGR	Generation of *ybaO*-3×FLAG	CGACGCCATTCCCGGCGAAAGTACCAGCTTAATTGAGCAACATATGAATATCCTCCTTAG
cdsHpMCL210F	Cloning of *cdsH*	GAATTCTCAGATTAACGGCATCCGCC
cdsHpMCL210R	Cloning of *cdsH*	AAGCTTCTAGTCGCCGGTAAGTAATTTTGC
ybaOpMCL210F	Cloning of *ybaO*	GAATTCAGGGGCAAACGAATAAGATGCG
ybaOpMCL210R	Cloning of *ybaO*	AAGCTTTTATTCAATGGGCAGAGAGGTGG
cdsHRTF	RT–PCR	CGGCTGGCGCATGAACTGAA
cdsHRTR	RT–PCR	TTCCGGCGCTCATGACGATAA
ybaORTF	RT–PCR	TGGAAGATGACGGTATCCTGCTTGG
ybaORTR	RT–PCR	CCAAGCACTTCCGGCATCTCAGAG
16SF	RT–PCR	GTAGAATTCCAGGTGTAGCG
16SR	RT–PCR	TTATCACTGGCAGTCTCCTT

Table 2. Strains used in this study.

Genotype	Antibiotic Resistance	Source
S. Typhimurium LT2	-	ATCC®700720
S. Typhimurium LT2 Δ*cdsH*::FRT *	-	This study
S. Typhimurium LT2 Δ*cdsH*::FRT/pACYC	Cam^R	This study
S. Typhimurium LT2 Δ*cdsH*::FRT/pACYC::*cdsH* **	Cam^R	This study
S. Typhimurium LT2 Δ*ybaO*::FRT ***	-	This study
S. Typhimurium LT2 Δ*ybaO*::FRT/pMCL210	Cam^R	This study
S. Typhimurium LT2 Δ*ybaO*::FRT/pMCL210::*ybaO* ****	Cam^R	This study
S. Typhimurium LT2 *cdsH*-3×FLAG	Kan^R	This study
S. Typhimurium LT2 *ybaO*-3×FLAG	Kan^R	This study

* This strain is also called Δ*cdsH*. ** This plasmid is also called pCdsH. *** This strain is also called Δ*ybaO*. **** This plasmid is called pYbaO.

Growth curves. Growth curves were performed in LB and M9-glucose media with or without cysteine supplementation (0.2 mM). Bacteria were grown aerobically until the stationary phase, and optical density at 600 nM (OD_{600}) was measured in a microtiter plate reader (Guangzhou Jet Bio-Filtration Co®, Guangzhou, China) every hour.

RNA isolation and mRNA detection. Total RNA extraction and RT–qPCR analyses were performed as previously described by Álvarez et al. (2015) [14]. Cultures of *S.* Typhimurium LT2 wild type and Δ*ybaO* mutant strain were grown in M9-glucose broth and incubated with shaking at 37 °C until OD_{600} = ~0.4. When necessary, bacterial cultures were exposed to 0.2 mM cysteine for 20 min. RNA was obtained by the acid–phenol method. Briefly, RNA was precipitated with isopropanol for 10 min at room temperature, washed with ice-cold 70% *v/v* ethanol and resuspended in DEPC-treated water before treating with 2U DNase I (Promega) to remove any DNA trace. The purity of the extracted RNA was determined by spectrometry (Absorbance 260/280). cDNA synthesis was carried out at 37 °C for 1 h in 25 µL of a mixture that contained 2.5 pmol of the specific reverse primers, 1 µg of template RNA, 0.2 mM dNTPs, 1 mL of nuclease-free water, 4 µL of M-MLV Reverse Transcriptase 5× Reaction Buffer (250 mM Tris-HCl pH 8.3, 375 mM KCl, 15 mM MgCl2, 10 mM 1,4-dithiothreitol (DTT), 40 U of RNasin) and 100 U of M-MLV reverse transcriptase (Promega®, Madison, WI, USA). The relative quantification of transcript levels was performed by RT–qPCR using the Brilliant II SYBR Green QPCR master reagent kit and the Mx3000P detection system (Stratagene®, San Diego, CA, USA). The 16s rRNA levels were used for normalization. The RT–qPCR mixture (20 µL) contained 50 ng of cDNA template, 120 nM each primer (cdsHRTF-cdsHRTR for *cdsH*, ybaORTF-ybaORTR for *ybaO*, and 16SF–16SR for 16s gene, see Table 1) and 1 µL of ROX reference dye (1:200). RT–qPCR was performed under the following conditions: 10 min at 95 °C followed by 40 cycles of 15 s at 95 °C, 15 s at 60 °C, and 25 s at 72 °C, followed by a melting cycle from 65 to 95 °C to check for amplification specificity. A previous standard quantification curve with serial dilutions of RT–qPCR products was constructed for each gene to calculate the amplification efficiency. These values were used to obtain the ratio between the gene of interest and the 16s rRNA gene expression. The experiment was performed for three biological and technical replicates. These data were analyzed with the MxPRO software (Agilent Technologies®, Santa Clara, CA, USA).

Western blot. Total protein extraction was performed as previously described by Nevermann et al. (2019) [27]. Briefly, cultures of *S.* Typhimurium LT2 wild type and Δ*ybaO* mutant strain were grown in M9-glucose broth and incubated with shaking at 37 °C until OD_{600} = ~0.4. When necessary, bacterial cultures were exposed to cysteine 200 µM for 1 h before centrifugation, and the pellet was resuspended in Tris-HCl 100 mM buffer. Total proteins were extracted by sonication on ice (30 s pulses, amplitude 70%) with sonicator Vibra-Cell. Protein quantification was performed with the classical Bradford method [28].

Western blot was performed as previously described by Jofre et al. (2014) [29]. Briefly, 100 μg of protein extracts of each sample were loaded by SDS-PAGE (12% acrylamide). Proteins were transferred to a nitrocellulose membrane (Bio-Rad) and blocked overnight at 4 °C with milk in TBS (1.4% NaCl, 0.6% glycine pH 7.4). The membrane was washed three times with TBS-Tween (NaCl 1.4%, glycine 0.6%, Tween 0.1%). The western blots were probed with a 1:5000 dilution of primary antibody anti-FLAG for 12 h at 4 °C. The membrane was rewashed with TBS-Tween and then probed with a mix of 1:10,000 dilution of secondary antibody anti-mouse-horseradish peroxidase (HRP) conjugate (Promega) and 1:25,000 dilution anti-mouse-HSP for 2 h with shaking at room temperature. Finally, the membrane was washed with TBS-Tween prior to being revealed by the BCIP/NTB (Invitrogen®) kit according to the manufacturer's instructions. Hsp60 was used as a control load, as described [30]. The Western blot was repeated at least three independent times and analyzed by densitometry to quantify the relative amounts of protein by ImageJ Software.

Deoxycholate survival assay. A 25 mL OD_{600} ~0.5 culture of each strain growing on LB broth was washed three times with phosphate saline buffer (PBS) and finally resuspended in 5 mL of PBS. Then, 20 μL of each bacterial suspension was resuspended in a 96-well microplate with 180 μL of deoxycholate (Sigma-Aldrich®, Merck® KGaA, Darmstadt, Germany) 0.5% or PBS (control) before incubating them for 2 h. Finally, each well was serially diluted in PBS and seeded in LB plates for CFU counting.

Bacterial viability in the HT-29 cell line with extra supplementation of cysteine. Cell viability was determined by neutral red uptake assay, as previously described by Repetto et al. (2008) [31]. Briefly, HT-29 cell cultures (DMEM) were washed with PBS and refilled with DMEM alone or supplemented with cysteine. This procedure was repeated at 1 h and 3 h of incubation. After 24 h of incubation, cells were washed with PBS, and a neutral red solution diluted in DMEM (Sigma-Aldrich®, Merck® KGaA, Darmstadt, Germany) (60 μg/mL) was added before incubation at 37 °C for 2 h. Next, each well was washed twice with PBS, and a destaining solution (50% ethanol (Merck® KGaA, Darmstadt, Germany) 49% deionized water, 1% glacial acetic acid (Merck® KGaA, Darmstadt, Germany)) was used to remove the neutral red solution from cells. Finally, OD_{540} was measured for each well. A well was treated with deoxycholate 0.5% for 5 min before neutral red was added as a control.

Epithelial cell line replication assay. *S.* Typhimurium LT2 invasion and replication were determined using the gentamycin-protection assay described by Fuentes et al. (2008) with some modifications [32]. Briefly, the *S.* Typhimurium strains used to infect HT-29 monolayer were grown in microaerophilic conditions to an OD_{600} = 0.2 at 37 °C. Then, bacteria were washed three times with PBS and finally resuspended in DMEM with or without cysteine (0.2 mM). This suspension was immediately used for HT-29 monolayer infection in 96-well plates using a multiplicity of infection of 100:1. One hour after infection, cells were washed three times with PBS and a DMEM solution supplemented with gentamycin (200 μg/mL), with or without cysteine, was added to each well. The previous procedure was repeated three hours after infection but without gentamycin, and infected cells were incubated for 3, 6 or 24 h post-infection (p.i.). To assess bacterial invasion and replication, the CFU were determined in each time and condition. Bacteria were recovered from HT-29 cells at 3 (invasion), 6 and 24 h (replication) p.i. using a deoxycholate solution (0.5% in PBS) and mechanical disruption. The bacterial suspension was seeded in LB plates, and CFU were counted after 16 h of incubation at 37 °C.

Statistical analysis. All analyses were performed using IBM SPSS and GraphPad Prism 8 software. ANOVA with Tuckey's test as post hoc and Mann–Whitney tests were performed in the cysteine Kirby–Bauer and mRNA expression experiments, respectively. Two-way ANOVA with post hoc Tukey's multiple comparisons test was performed for the replication experiment analysis.

3. Results

3.1. The cdsH and ybaO Genes Participate in the Response of S. Typhimurium against High Concentrations of Cysteine in Minimal Medium

Since CdsH responds to an excess of cysteine and YbaO controls the expression of CdsH under anaerobic conditions [11], we wondered whether *S.* Typhimurium Δ*cdsH* exhibited increased susceptibility to exogenous cysteine under aerobic growth. For this aim, a Kirby–Bauer test was carried out in M9-glucose minimal medium, a culture medium that does include cysteine. A cysteine solution of 0.5 M was added to a filter-paper disc placed on the M9-glucose minimal medium plates, previously seeded with the tested bacteria, before incubation for 16 h at 37 °C to obtain growth inhibition haloes. Growth inhibition haloes of approximately 40 mM diameter were observed for the mutant strains, while the wild type exhibited no growth inhibition. The mutant phenotype was fully complemented by the corresponding plasmid (Figure 1). This result argues for the role of *cdsH* in the resistance to high cysteine concentrations.

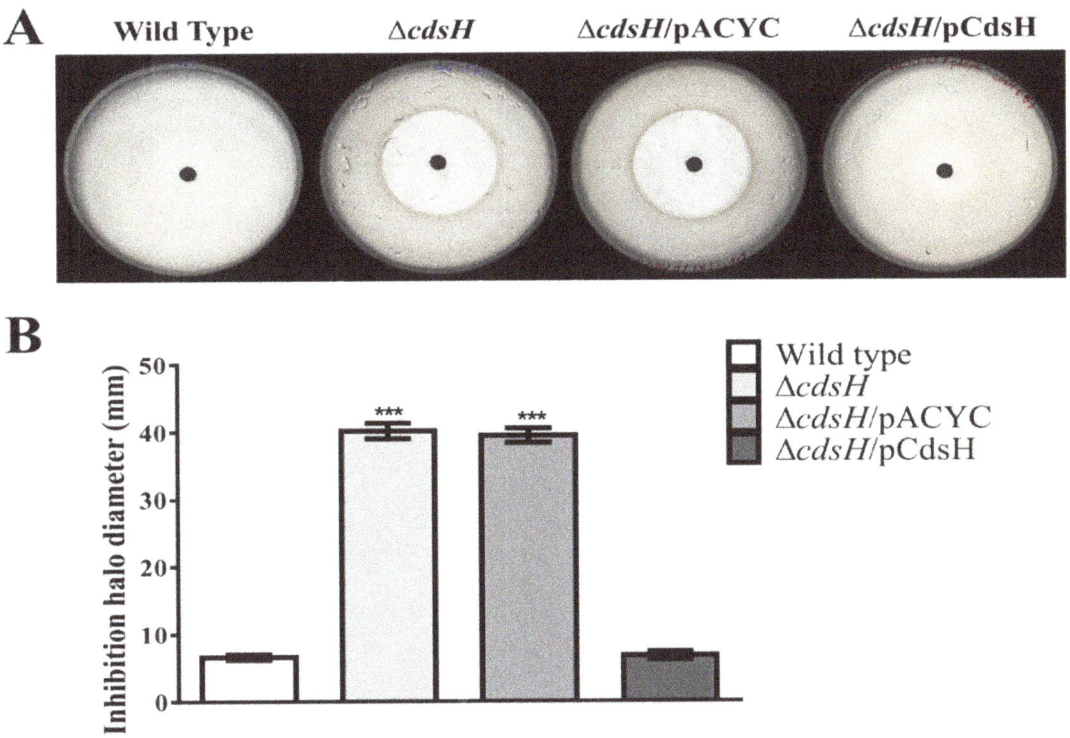

Figure 1. Inhibitory effect of cysteine in minimal medium (M9-glucose) under aerobic conditions. Overnight cultures in M9-glucose of *S.* Typhimurium strains were used to generate an agar-agar (0.7%) layer with approximately 10^6 CFU. A filter-paper disc was placed over the layer and loaded with 15 μL of 0.5 M cysteine solution. (**A**) Inhibition haloes generated by cysteine on wild type, Δ*cdsH* mutant, Δ*cdsH*/pACYC (empty vector), and Δ*cdsH*/pCdsH (complemented strain). (**B**) Graphic representation of inhibition haloes generated by cysteine in A). ANOVA test (post hoc: Tuckey's test) was performed (error bars represent standard error of the mean, $n = 7$; ***, $p < 0.001$ in comparison with the wild type strain).

In order to set the sublethal concentration of cysteine for the following experiments, the MIC of cysteine was determined for the *S.* Typhimurium wild type strain and the mutant derivatives (Table 3). Compared to the wild type strain, mutant strains (and mutants harboring the empty vector) showed a 16-fold lower MIC. On the other hand, the respective complemented mutants showed MICs even higher than those presented by the WT, plausibly due to the increased gene dosage provided by the respective cloning vector (Table 3). All these results support the participation of both *cdsH* and *ybaO* in cysteine susceptibility under the tested conditions. Based on these results, we set the work concentration of cysteine to 0.2 mM, half of the MIC regarding *S.* Typhimurium Δ*csdH* and Δ*ybaO* (Table 3). This concentration is similar to the higher concentration inferred for cysteine in the ileum (as extrapolated from the methionine concentration, see above) [9]. As a control, and to determine any additional detrimental effects of cysteine, we analyzed the growth curve of *S.* Typhimurium wild type and mutant derivatives, either in M9-glucose supplemented with 0.2 mM cysteine or in LB (rich medium) supplemented with 0.2 mM cysteine (37 °C with shaking). As shown in Figure S1, we found no differences in the growth curves of the wild types and mutants in LB, despite the presence of cysteine. In the case of M9, we observed a slightly extended lag phase, although no differences in the growth rate (μ) were observed. No differences were observed when bacteria were cultured in the absence of supplemented cysteine (Figure S2). These results show that the addition of 0.2 mM of exogenous cysteine exerts no detrimental effects in the *S.* Typhimurium Δ*cdsH* or Δ*ybaO* in a rich medium (LB). By contrast, in a poorer environment (i.e., minimal medium M9), the lack of either *cdsH* or *ybaO* seems to slightly delay the adaptation of strains, although no significant effects in the growth rate were observed under the tested conditions (Table S1).

Table 3. MIC for cysteine in M9-glucose medium.

Strain	MIC (mM)
S. Typhimurium LT2	6.4
S. Typhimurium LT2 Δ*cdsH*	0.4
S. Typhimurium LT2 Δ*cdsH*/pACYC	0.4
S. Typhimurium LT2 Δ*cdsH*/pCdsH	>12.8
S. Typhimurium LT2 Δ*ybaO*	0.4
S. Typhimurium LT2 Δ*ybaO*/pMCL210	0.4
S. Typhimurium LT2 Δ*ybaO*/pYbaO	12.8

3.2. The Expression of the cdsH Gene is Induced in the Presence of Cysteine

Since our results show that *cdsH* and *ybaO* participate in the adaptation to the presence of exogenous cysteine, we explored whether this amino acid induces the expression of these genes. For this purpose, RT–qPCR and Western blot assays were carried out from cultures in M9-glucose medium alone (control) or M9-glucose supplemented with 0.2 mM cysteine. As shown in Figure 2, the addition of cysteine induced the expression of *cdsH* only when the *ybaO* gene was present (Figure 2), corroborating the previous work of Oguri et al. (2012) [11]. By contrast, in a Δ*ybaO* context, this induction was not observed (Figure 2C). Regarding the expression of *ybaO*, we found that, under the tested condition, the addition of cysteine produced no effect compared with the M9-glucose alone (Figure 2B), which can be explained by the negative self-regulation of the LRP regulator family [33].

The *S.* Typhimurium *ybaO*-3×FLAG strain was also used to assess the *ybaO* expression at the protein level. Nevertheless, the Western blot assay could not detect this protein, even in the presence of cysteine (data not shown), strongly suggesting that the amount of YbaO is too low to be detected by the performed procedure. All these results agree with that previously described by Oguri et al. (2012) [11], who assessed the *cdsH* expression with a nutrient-deficient medium but under anaerobic conditions.

Altogether, these results show that *cdsH* increased its expression in the presence of cysteine in a YbaO-dependent manner, even under aerobic conditions. Since *ybaO* showed no increase in its transcription or translation in the presence of cysteine, unlike what was observed for *cdsH*, we decided to continue assessing only the participation of *cdsH*.

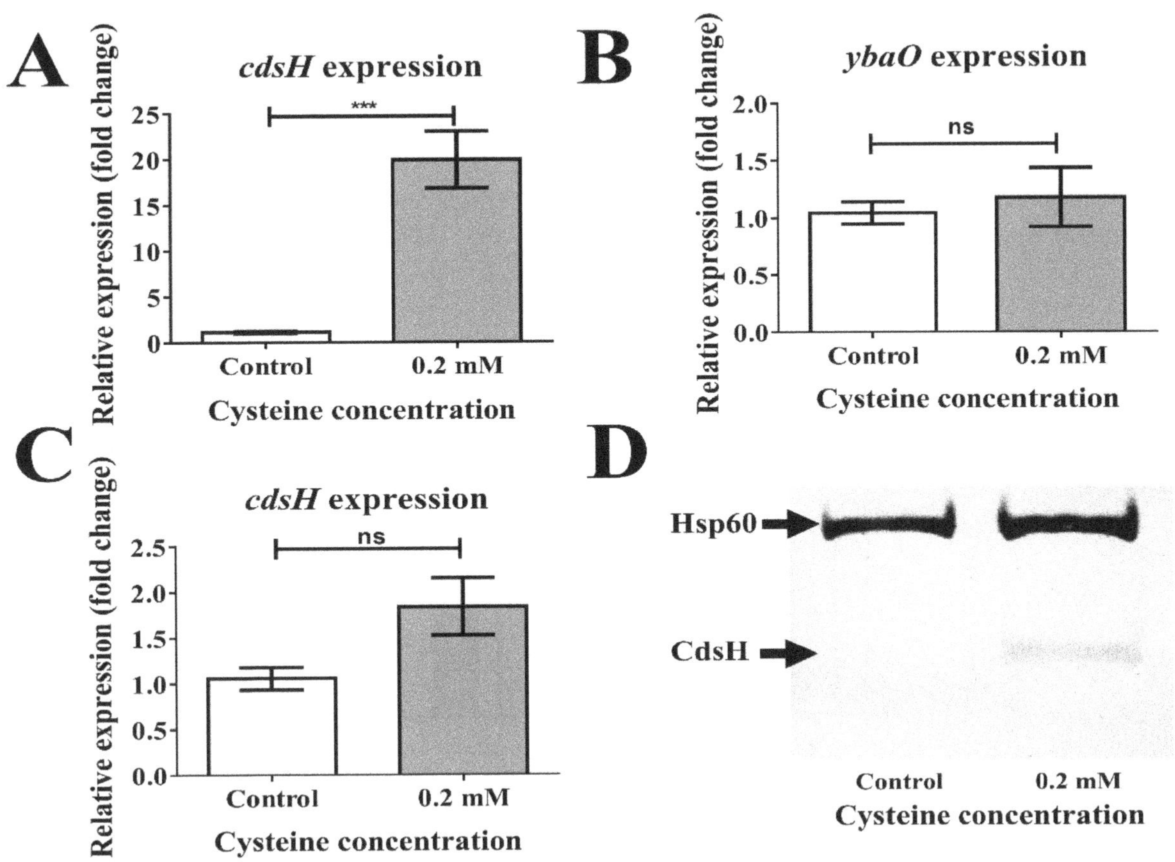

Figure 2. Aerobic *cdsH* and *ybaO* expression in response to cysteine. *S.* Typhimurium strains were grown in M9-glucose to OD_{600} 0.4–0.5 prior to supplementing with cysteine (0.2 mM, final concentration) or water (control). After 20 min incubation, bacteria were harvested, and an RT–PCR assay was performed as described in Materials and Methods (**A**–**C**). (**A**) *cdsH* expression in the WT context. (**B**) *ybaO* expression in the WT context. (**C**) *cdsH* expression in the Δ*ybaO* context. A-C, Mann–Whitney test (error bars represent standard error of the mean, $n = 4$, ns, no significative; ***, $p < 0.001$). For the Western blot assay (**D**), the *S.* Typhimurium *cdsH*-3×FLAG was cultured in M9-glucose to OD_{600} 0.4–0.5 prior to supplementing with cysteine (0.2 mM, final concentration) or water (control). Hsp60 was used as a control load, as described [30]. After 1 min incubation, bacteria were harvested, and the Westen blot assay was performed as described in Materials and Methods (a representative result of $n = 3$).

3.3. Cysteine Promotes Replication of S. Typhimurium inside Epithelial Cells in a cdsH-Dependent Manner

According to the transcriptomic analysis carried out by Hautefort et al. (2008), *cdsH* is overexpressed when *Salmonella* is inside epithelial cells. Since this gene is induced in response to the presence of harmful cysteine concentrations, we wondered whether the increased *cdsH* expression is related to a bacterial defense response inside epithelial cells. To this end, both the invasion and the replication of *S.* Typhimurium strains were assessed in the HT-29 cell line, comparing the standard DMEM medium with DMEM supplemented with extra cysteine (0.2 mM).

Since HT-29 cells are typically cultured in standard DMEM medium, we first assessed whether the supplementation with additional cysteine (0.2 mM) affects cell viability. To that aim, we performed a neutral red uptake [31]. As shown in Figure S3A, extra cysteine in the DMEM medium produced no effects on the HT-29's viability. Similarly, we found that the DMEM supplemented with additional cysteine exerted no detrimental effects on the growth of *S.* Typhimurium and derivatives, even after an incubation of 3, 6, 12, or 24 h (Figure S3B), in agreement with what was found with LB supplemented with cysteine (Figure S1). Having ruled out possible artifactual results, we tested the invasion and replication of *S.* Typhimurium and mutant derivatives in either DMEM or DMEM supplemented with cysteine by the gentamicin protection assays with HT-29. As shown in Figure 3A, we found indistinguishable invasions between the *S.* Typhimurium wild type and Δ*cdsH*, with or without additional cysteine. By contrast, the addition of extra cysteine to the DMEM medium slightly decreased the replication of Δ*cdsH* bacteria, while it increased the wild type strain replication up to 30% at 6 h, but not at 24 h, where the number of intracellular bacteria similarly increased for all the strains, even with the addition of extra cysteine cultures (Figure 3B). As shown in Table 4, the generational time of intracellular bacteria was longer in the Δ*cdsH* strain only when extra cysteine was added, supporting our results.

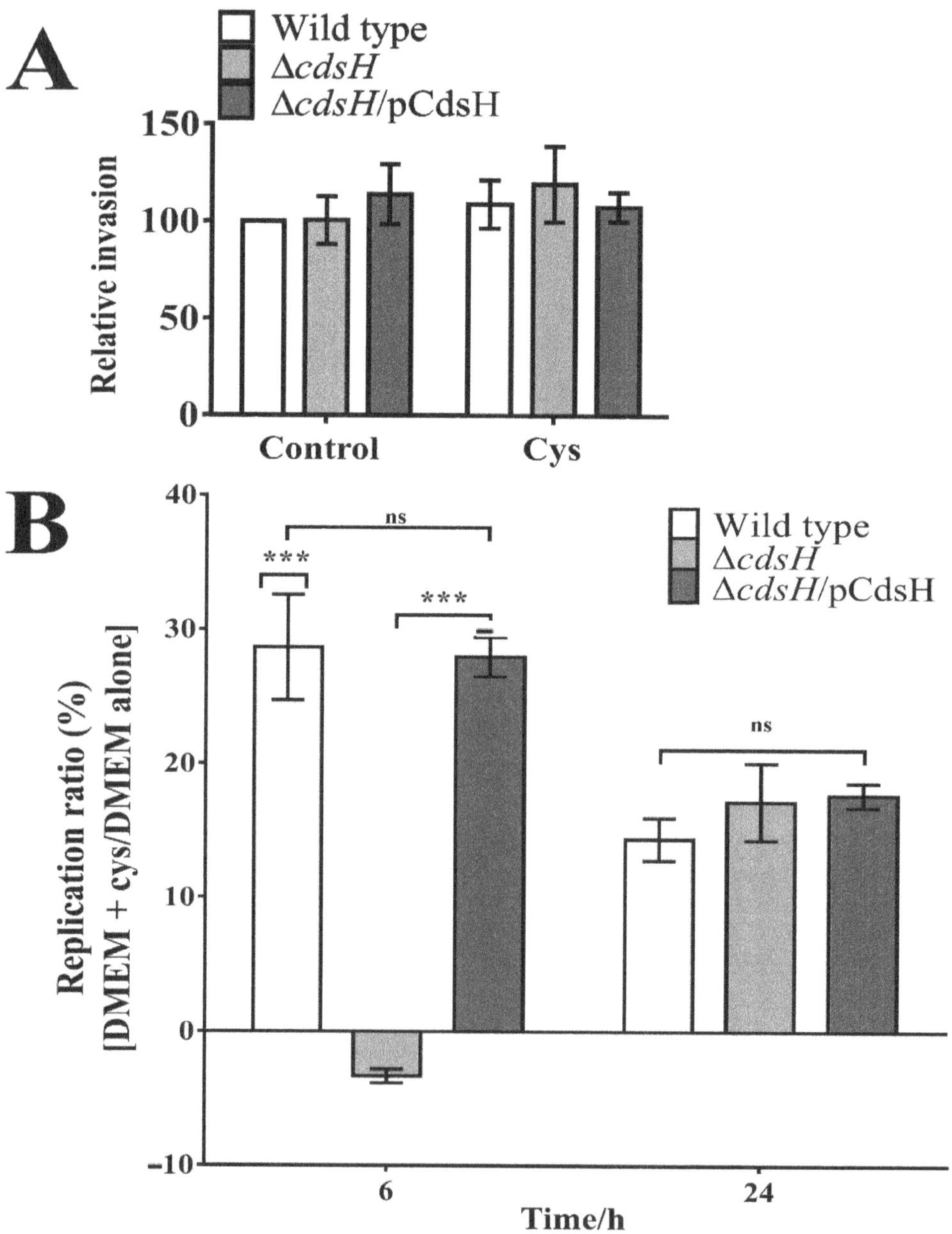

Figure 3. *S.* Typhimurium replication in HT-29 cell line with and without cysteine. HT-29 cell line cultures in 96-well plates were infected with wild type, Δ*cdsH*, or Δ*cdsH*/pCdsH strains in DMEM medium alone or supplemented with 0.2 mM cysteine. (**A**) Three hours post-infection (relative invasion related to the wild type strain); (**B**) Six and twenty-four hours post-infection (early and late replication). The Figure Shows the percentage replication ratio of DMEM + cys:DMEM alone. Bacteria were recovered from the intracellular environment by disrupting cells with 0.5% sodium deoxycholate prior to plating on LB agar to count CFU. Two-way ANOVA (post hoc: Tukey) was performed for analysis (error bars represent standard error of the mean, $n = 5$; ns, no significance; ***, $p < 0.001$).

Table 4. Generation time at 24 h of the strains within the HT-29 line under normal conditions and with the addition of exogenous cysteine.

Strain	Generation Time without Cysteine (h)	Generation Time with 0.2 mM Cysteine (h)
S. Typhimurium LT2	12.64	10.01
S. Typhimurium LT2 Δ*cdsH*	16.90	28.46
S. Typhimurium LT2 Δ*cdsH*/pCdsH	16.84	16.56

All these results together argue for the participation of *cdsH* in *S.* Typhimurium replication within epithelial cells in high cysteine concentrations. Thus, *cdsH* contributes to improving the bacterial fitness inside epithelial cells.

4. Discussion

Salmonella is an enteric pathogen that produces a wide variety of diseases, from self-limited gastroenteritis to systemic infections and death. During the infective process, before the internalization into epithelial cells, *Salmonella* overcomes different stressful conditions such as acid pH, bile salts, high osmolarity, and low oxygen tension [2]. Inside epithelial cells, *Salmonella* responds to the intracellular environment to achieve a successful replication, which is an essential process for the bacteria's virulence and develops a successful infection [34]. Since intestinal epithelial cells are continually absorbing nutrients from the lumen, the intracellular amino acid concentration increases [9]. Under these conditions, intracellular bacteria could use these high amino acid concentrations for their own purpose. In this context, *S.* Typhimurium has a cysteine desulfhydrase enzyme, CdsH, that responds to high cysteine concentrations to avoid the toxicity of this amino acid. As *cdsH* increases its expression inside epithelial cells [24], *S.* Typhimurium may use this enzyme to prevent the toxic effect, or use cysteine to increase its fitness.

4.1. Cysteine Susceptibility Occurs only in Minimal Medium

It has been shown that cysteine affects the growth of multiple bacteria in minimal media, and *S.* Typhimurium is not an exception. *S.* Typhimurium is also susceptible to the toxic effect of excess cysteine in minimal media, although this is not the case in a rich medium (Figures S1 and S3). The cysteine susceptibility increases when the CdsH enzyme cannot be synthesized in the Δ*cdsH* mutant, or as a result of the absence of its positive regulator YbaO in the Δ*ybaO* context (Figure 2 and Table 3). When *S.* Typhimurium grows in minimal media, the expression of the genes involved in the transport of molecules is increased [35]. Accordingly, under sulfur-limited conditions, bacteria respond by synthesizing CysB-regulated sulfide transporters [36]. Thus, cysteine can enter bacteria in multiple ways, including derivatives such as cystine. For instance, in *E. coli*, extracellular cystine increases the intracellular cysteine concentration, exerting a toxic effect [12,17]. Therefore, the addition of both exogenous cysteine and cystine to the culture medium increases the concentration of intracellular cysteine when *Salmonella* is in a nutrient-deficient environment, and would cause the toxic effect produced by this amino acid. This could be explained by the differences in the global expression patterns when bacteria grow in nutrient-rich media versus nutrient-deficient media. For example, in *E. coli*, the number of transport genes overexpressed in minimal media is higher than the number of transport genes overexpressed in a rich medium when the expression is compared between both media [35]. Considering that cysteine enters the cell by specific transporters, the overexpression of these transporters could explain why, in minimal media, cysteine is toxic in lower concentration than in rich media.

Under aerobic conditions, we observed similar results to those previously reported in anaerobic conditions by Oguri et al. (2012) [11], i.e., *S.* Typhimurium is susceptible to excess cysteine only in minimal medium (Figure S2), and *cdsH* is overexpressed in response to the addition of exogenous cysteine to the medium in a YbaO-dependent manner, this being an Lrp family regulator that does not change its expression in response to cysteine.

4.2. CdsH Contributes to the Replication of S. Typhimurium in the HT-29 Line, against the Addition of Exogenous Cysteine

As mentioned before, during the invasion of the intestine, *Salmonella* is exposed to different conditions [37]. These conditions produce changes in bacterial genetic profile, promoting the invasion and subsequent replication inside epithelial cells [38,39]. In both processes, the effector and regulatory genes from *Salmonella* pathogenicity island I and II are important, since mutation on these genes produces non-invasive phenotypes [40]. In the replication assay, at 3 h post-infection, no differences between wild type and Δ*cdsH* strains were observed in both DMEM and DMEM + cysteine media (Figure 3A). Since the replication of *Salmonella* inside epithelial cells begins between 3 and 4 h after the invasion [41,42], this process was not affected by *cdsH* deletion in both conditions; therefore, *cdsH* does not contribute to the invasion of epithelial cells. This result is in accordance with the function of CdsH, which participates in the elimination of cysteine, and its expression is regulated in that context, unlike the expression of genes such as *invA* and *sipA*, among others, whose expression is directly related to the *Salmonella*-invasion of epithelial cells. Therefore, according to our results, CdsH does not participate in the invasion process.

Even though replication within epithelial cells mainly depends on the genes present in SPI-1 and SPI-2 [43,44], genes involved in other processes can also contribute to bacterial replication within this cell type. An example of this was reported in *S.* Typhi, where the mutation in genes related to anaerobic respiration causes lower bacterial replication inside epithelial cells, possibly because these genes would allow bacteria to perform more energy-efficient metabolic processes [45]. Other genes could also be indirectly related to the replication process, such as *trxA* and *trxB*, components of the thioredoxin pathway (a protein that acts as an antioxidant), where a mutation in these genes slightly decreases replication inside of epithelial cells [46].

In other cell types, non-classical factors that contribute to *Salmonella* replication have also been seen. The Tsx porin participates in nucleoside uptake, where a mutation in this gene has been shown to decrease *Salmonella*'s replicative capacity inside a line of macrophages [47]. Likewise, the *S.* Typhimurium Δ*cdsH* strain's replication does not respond to the addition of cysteine to the medium as the wild type strain at 6 h (Figure 3B). Since this gene is overexpressed in the presence of exogenous cysteine [11,48,49] and cystine [50], overexpression within epithelial cells [24] can be attributed to the entry of cysteine or cystine into bacteria. Although culture media do not have cysteine, they do have cystine. In this sense, the increased *cdsH* expression may be due to cystine uptake by bacteria. Related to this, YdjN, one of the primary transporters for cystine, was also found to have an increased expression within epithelial cells [24]. When comparing the replication of each strain in the supplemented versus the non-supplemented medium at different times, we found that the wild type strain exhibits an advantage in replication at 6 h p.i. when cysteine is added to the medium, increasing the replication. An explanation could be the pyruvate synthesis from cysteine by CdsH [11], which contributes to bacteria's energy production. In addition, it has been shown that *Salmonella* can use CdsH to synthesize thiamine, in a different way from the conventional, which is transformed into thiamine pyrophosphate, a coenzyme required for enzymes of the central metabolism [51]. In fact, in *Listeria monocytogenes*, it has been shown that replication inside epithelial cells requires the uptake and biosynthesis of thiamine precursors [52]. Thus, this could represent an advantage of the wild type over the Δ*cdsH* strain. On the other hand, at 24 h p.i., the mutant strain was able to use cysteine, reaching a replication ratio comparable to that of the wild strain, thus suggesting the existence of another redundant system that can fulfill this function. In this sense, it is known that other enzymes such as CysK or CysM also have cysteine desulfhydrase activity, although these are not cysteine-inducible [11].

Cysteine can exert its toxic activity mainly by producing oxidative stress through the reduction of Fe(III) to Fe(II) and the subsequent stimulation of the Fenton reaction, as well as hydroxyl radical production [12]. In this context, CdsH has been described as the major cysteine-degrading and sulfide-producing enzyme [11]. The degradation of cysteine could be the more immediate response in order to prevent the cysteine-dependent ROS. Nevertheless, in the absence of CdsH and ROS's eventual appearance, other mechanisms to circumvent the insult are plausibly triggered [53]. Besides, cysteine concentration might decrease over time due to its consumption in anabolic processes. In this context, the role of CdsH could be circumscribed to more early stages, providing a possible explanation of why the lack of CdsH does not affect bacterial replication at 24 h post-infection (Figure 3).

In addition to classic virulence factors, other factors related to various bacterial processes, such as molecule transport, protein synthesis, and metabolism under certain conditions, contribute to bacterial replication inside the host cells and thus favor the virulence. In this context, CdsH promotes bacterial replication, at least in an in vitro assay, when it is internalized in epithelial cells in a medium with extra cysteine, which could partially simulate the intestinal environment after consumption of a high-protein meal.

Supplementary Materials
Figure S1: Growth curve in LB and M9-glucose; Figure S2. Growth curve with cysteine in LB and M9-glucose; Figure S3. Controls for cysteine supplemented replication assay; Table S1. Growth rate μ (h-1) in different culture media.

Author Contributions: Conceptualization, F.D.-Y., J.A.F., and F.G.; methodology, F.D.-Y., and R.Á.; software, F.D.-Y.; validation, F.D.-Y., and F.G.; formal analysis, J.A.F., and F.G.; investigation, F.D.-Y. and R.Á.; resources, F.G.; data curation, I.L.C., J.A.F., and F.G.; writing—original draft preparation, F.D.-Y., I.L.C., J.A.F., and F.G.; writing—review and editing, F.D.-Y., I.L.C., J.A.F., and F.G.; visualization, F.G.; supervision, F.G.; project administration, F.G.; funding acquisition, F.G. All authors have read and agreed to the published version of the manuscript.

References

1. World Health Organization. Salmonella (non-typhoidal), who.int. 2018. Available online: https://www.who.int/news-room/fact-sheets/detail/salmonella-(non-typhoidal) (accessed on 12 November 2020).
2. Haraga, A.; Ohlson, M.B.; Miller, S.I. Salmonellae interplay with host cells. *Nat. Rev. Microbiol.* **2008**, *6*, 53–66. [CrossRef]
3. LaRock, D.L.; Chaudhary, A.; Miller, S.I. Salmonellae interactions with host processes. *Nat. Rev. Microbiol.* **2015**, *13*, 191–205. [CrossRef] [PubMed]
4. Snoeck, V.; Goddeeris, B.; Cox, E. The role of enterocytes in the intestinal barrier function and antigen uptake. *Microbes Infect.* **2005**, *7*, 997–1004. [CrossRef] [PubMed]
5. Tortora, G.J.; Derrickson, B. *Principles of Anatomy and Physiology*, 12th ed.; Wiley: Hoboken, NJ, USA, 2008.
6. Muthayya, N.M. *Human Physiology*, 3rd ed.; Jaypee Brothers Medical Publishers: Delhi, India, 2002.
7. Bröer, S. Amino Acid Transport Across Mammalian Intestinal and Renal Epithelia. *Physiol. Rev.* **2008**, *88*, 249–286. [CrossRef] [PubMed]
8. Kwaik, Y.A.; Bumann, D. Microbial quest for food in vivo: "Nutritional virulence" as an emerging paradigm. *Cell. Microbiol.* **2013**, *15*, 882–890. [CrossRef]
9. Adibi, S.A.; Mercer, D.W. Protein digestion in human intestine as reflected in luminal, mucosal, and plasma amino acid concentrations after meals. *J. Clin. Investig.* **1973**, *52*, 1586–1594. [CrossRef]
10. Nelson, D.L.; Cox, M.M. *Lehninger Principios de Bioquímica*, 5th ed.; Omega: Barcelona, Spain, 2009.
11. Oguri, T.; Schneider, B.; Reitzer, L. Cysteine catabolism and cysteine desulfhydrase (CdsH/STM0458) in *Salmonella enterica* serovar typhimurium. *J. Bacteriol.* **2012**, *194*, 4366–4376. [CrossRef]
12. Park, S.; Imlay, J.A. High levels of intracellular cysteine promote oxidative DNA damage by driving the fenton reaction. *J. Bacteriol.* **2003**, *185*, 1942–1950. [CrossRef]

13. Farr, S.B.; Kogoma, T. Oxidative stress responses in *Escherichia coli* and *Salmonella typhimurium*. *Microbiol. Rev.* **1991**, *55*, 561–585. [CrossRef]
14. Alvarez, R.; Neumann, G.; Fravega, J.; Díaz, F.; Tejías, C.; Fuentes, J.A.; Paredes-Sabja, D.; Calderón, I.L.; Gil, F. Biochemical and Biophysical Research Communications CysB-dependent upregulation of the *Salmonella typhimurium* cysJIH operon in response to antimicrobial compounds that induce oxidative stress. *Biochem. Biophys. Res. Commun.* **2015**, 1–6. [CrossRef]
15. Allen, H.; Hussey, G. Inhibition of the growth of *Helminthospovium cavbonum* by Lcysteine. *Can. J. Microbiol.* **1971**, *17*, 101–103. [CrossRef] [PubMed]
16. Cowman, R.A.; Baron, S.S.; Fitzgerald, R.J. Cysteine toxicity for oral streptococci and effect of branched-chain amino acids. *Infect. Immun.* **1983**, *39*, 1107–1113. [CrossRef] [PubMed]
17. Gomez, R.F.; Montville, T.; Blais, K. Toxic effect of cysteine against Salmonella typhimurium. *Appl. Environ. Microbiol.* **1980**, *39*, 1081–1083. [CrossRef] [PubMed]
18. Collins, J.M.; Wallenstein, A.; Monty, K.J. Regulatory Features of the Cysteine Desulfhydrase of Salmonella Typhimurium. *Growth (Lakel.)* **1973**, *313*, 156–162. [CrossRef]
19. Harris, C.L.; Lui, L. Cysteine and growth inhibition of Escherichia coli: Derepression of the ilvGEDA operon. *Biochem. Biophys. Res. Commun.* **1981**, *101*, 1145–1151. [CrossRef]
20. Kari, C.; Nagy, Z.; Kovacs, P.; Hernadi, F. Mechanism of the growth inhibitory effect of cysteine on Escherichia coli. *J. Gen. Microbiol.* **1971**, *68*, 349–356. [CrossRef]
21. Fiorucci, S.; Distrutti, E.; Cirino, G.; Wallace, J.L. The Emerging Roles of Hydrogen Sulfide in the Gastrointestinal Tract and Liver. *Gastroenterology* **2006**, *131*, 259–271. [CrossRef]
22. Kovács, P.; Kari, C.; Nagy, Z.; Hernádi, F.; Kovacs, P.; Hernadi, F. Possible Explanation for the Metabolic Radioprotective Effect of Cysteine on Escherichia coli B. *Radiat. Res.* **1968**, *36*, 217. [CrossRef]
23. Sorensen, M.A.; Pedersen, S. Cysteine, even in low concentrations, induces transient amino acid starvation in Escherichia coli. *J. Bacteriol.* **1991**, *173*, 5244–5246. [CrossRef]
24. Hautefort, I.; Thompson, A.; Eriksson-Ygberg, S.; Parker, M.L.; Lucchini, S.; Danino, V.; Bongaerts, R.J.M.; Ahmad, N.; Rhen, M.; Hinton, J.C.D. During infection of epithelial cells *Salmonella enterica* serovar Typhimurium undergoes a time-dependent transcriptional adaptation that results in simultaneous expression of three type 3 secretion systems. *Cell. Microbiol.* **2008**, *10*, 958–984. [CrossRef]
25. Datsenko, K.A.; Wanner, B.L. One-step inactivation of chromosomal genes in Escherichia coli K-12 using PCR products. *Proc. Natl. Acad. Sci. USA* **2000**, *97*, 6640–6645. [CrossRef] [PubMed]
26. Uzzau, S.; Figueroa-Bossi, N.; Rubino, S.; Bossi, L. Epitope tagging of chromosomal genes in *Salmonella*. *Proc. Natl. Acad. Sci. USA* **2001**, *98*, 15264–15269. [CrossRef] [PubMed]
27. Nevermann, J.; Silva, A.; Otero, C.; Oyarzún, D.P.; Barrera, B.; Gil, F.; Calderón, I.L.; Fuentes, J.A. Identification of Genes Involved in Biogenesis of Outer Membrane Vesicles (OMVs) in *Salmonella enterica* Serovar Typhi. *Front. Microbiol.* **2019**, *10*, 104. [CrossRef] [PubMed]
28. Bradford, M.M. A Rapid and Sensitive Method for the Quantitation of Microgram Quantities of Protein Utilizing the Principle of Protein-Dye Binding. *Anal. Biochem.* **1976**, *72*, 248–254. [CrossRef]
29. Jofré, M.R.; Rodríguez, L.M.; Villagra, N.A.; Hidalgo, A.A.; Mora, G.C.; Fuentes, J.A. RpoS integrates CRP, Fis, and PhoP signaling pathways to control Salmonella Typhi hlyE expression. *BMC Microbiol.* **2014**, *14*, 139. [CrossRef]
30. Ortega, A.P.; Villagra, N.A.; Urrutia, I.M.; Valenzuela, L.M.; Talamilla-Espinoza, A.; Hidalgo, A.A.; Rodas, P.I.; Gil, F.; Calderón, I.L.; Paredes-Sabja, D.; et al. Lose to win: MarT pseudogenization in *Salmonella enterica* serovar Typhi contributed to the surV -dependent survival to H_2O_2, and inside human macrophage-like cells. *Infect. Genet. Evol.* **2016**, *45*, 111–121. [CrossRef]
31. Repetto, G.; Del Peso, A.; Zurita, J.L. Neutral red uptake assay for the estimation of cell viability/cytotoxicity. *Nat. Protoc.* **2008**, *3*, 125. [CrossRef]
32. Fuentes, J.A.; Villagra, N.; Castillo-Ruiz, M.; Mora, G.C. The Salmonella Typhi hlyE gene plays a role in invasion of cultured epithelial cells and its functional transfer to *S. Typhimurium* promotes deep organ infection in mice. *Res. Microbiol.* **2008**, *159*, 279–287. [CrossRef]
33. Wang, Q.; Wu, J.; Friedberg, D.; Plakto, J.; Calvo, J.M. Regulation of the *Escherichia coli* lrp gene. *J. Bacteriol.* **1994**, *176*, 1831–1839. [CrossRef]
34. Leung, K.Y.; Finlay, B.B. Intracellular replication is essential for the virulence of *Salmonella typhimurium*. *Proc. Natl. Acad. Sci. USA* **1991**, *88*, 11470–11474. [CrossRef]

35. Tao, H.A.N.; Bausch, C.; Richmond, C.; Blattner, F.R.; Conway, T.; Acteriol, J.B. Functional Genomics: Expression Analysis of Escherichia coli Growing on Minimal and Rich Media. *J. Bacteriol.* **1999**, *181*, 6425–6440. [CrossRef] [PubMed]
36. Imlay, K.R.C.; Korshunov, S.; Imlay, J.A. The physiological roles and adverse effects of the two cystine importers of *Escherichia coli*. *J. Bacteriol.* **2015**, *197*, 3629–3644. [CrossRef] [PubMed]
37. Carter, P.B.; Collins, F.M. The route of enteric infection in normal mice. *J. Exp. Med.* **1974**, *139*, 1189–1203. [CrossRef] [PubMed]
38. Lee, C.A.; Falkow, S. The ability of *Salmonella* to enter mammalian cells is affected by bacterial growth state. *Proc. Natl. Acad. Sci. USA* **1990**, *87*, 4304–4308. [CrossRef] [PubMed]
39. Ernst, R.K.; Dombroski, D.M.; Merrick, J.M. Anaerobiosis, type 1 fimbriae, and growth phase are factors that affect invasion of HEp-2 cells by *Salmonella typhimurium*. *Infect. Immun.* **1990**, *58*, 2014–2016. [CrossRef]
40. Raffatellu, M.; Wilson, R.P.; Chessa, D.; Andrews-Polymenis, H.; Tran, Q.T.; Lawhon, S.; Khare, S.; Adams, L.G.; Bäumler, A.J. SipA, SopA, SopB, SopD, and SopE2 Contribute to *Salmonella enterica* Serotype Typhimurium Invasion of Epithelial Cells. *IAI* **2005**, *73*, 146–154. [CrossRef]
41. Gahring, L.C.; Heffron, F.; Finlay, B.B.; Falkow, S. Invasion and replication of *Salmonella typhimurium* in animal cells. *Infect. Immun.* **1990**, *58*, 443–448. [CrossRef]
42. Knodler, L.A.; Steele-Mortimer, O. Taking possession: Biogenesis of the Salmonella-containing vacuole. *Traffic* **2003**, *4*, 587–599. [CrossRef]
43. Hensel, M.; Bakteriologie, L.; Von Pettenkofer-Institut, M. Salmonella pathogenicity island 2. *Mol. Microbiol.* **2000**, *36*, 1015–1023. [CrossRef]
44. Steele-Mortimer, O.; Brumell, J.H.; Knodler, L.A.; Méresse, S.; Lopez, A.; Finlay, B.B. The invasion-associated type III secretion system of *Salmonella enterica* serovar Typhimurium is necessary for intracellular proliferation and vacuole biogenesis in epithelial cells. *Cell. Microbiol.* **2002**, *4*, 43–54. [CrossRef]
45. Contreras, I.; Toro, C.S.; Troncoso, G.; Mora, G.C. Salmonella typhi mutants defective in anaerobic respiration are impaired in their ability to replicate within epithelial cells. *Microbiology* **1997**, *143*, 2665–2672. [CrossRef] [PubMed]
46. Bjur, E.; Eriksson-Ygberg, S.; Åslund, F.; Rhen, M. Thioredoxin 1 Promotes Intracellular Replication and Virulence of Salmonella enterica *Serovar typhimurium*. *IAI* **2006**, *74*, 5140–5151. [CrossRef] [PubMed]
47. Bucarey, S.A.; Martinic, M.P.; Trombert, A.N.; Santiviago, C.A.; Maule, N.P.; Mora, G.C. The Salmonella enterica Serovar Typhi tsx Gene, Encoding a Nucleoside-Specific Porin, Is Essential for Prototrophic Growth in the Absence of Nucleosides. *Infect. Immun.* **2005**, *73*, 6210–6219. [CrossRef] [PubMed]
48. Collins, J.M.; Monty, K.J. The cysteine Desulfhydrase of Salmonella typhimurium. *J. Biol. Chem.* **1972**, *248*, 5943–5949.
49. Kredich, N.M.; Keenan, B.S.; Foote, L.J. The Purification and Subunit Structure of Cysteine Desulfhydrase from *Salmonella typhimurium*. *J. Biol. Chem.* **1972**, *247*, 7157–7163. [PubMed]
50. Baptist, E.W.; Kredich, N.M. Regulation of L-cystine transport in *Salmonella typhimurium*. *J. Bacteriol.* **1977**, *131*, 111–118. [CrossRef] [PubMed]
51. Palmer, L.D.; Leung, M.H.; Downs, D.M. The Cysteine Desulfhydrase CdsH Is Conditionally Required for Sulfur Mobilization to the Thiamine Thiazole in *Salmonella enterica*. *J. Bacteriol.* **2014**, *196*, 3964–3970. [CrossRef]
52. Schauer, K.; Stolz, J.; Scherer, S.; Fuchs, T.M. Both Thiamine Uptake and Biosynthesis of Thiamine Precursors Are Required for Intracellular Replication of *Listeria monocytogenes*. *J. Bacteriol.* **2009**, *191*, 2218–2227. [CrossRef]
53. Rhen, M. *Salmonella* and Reactive Oxygen Species: A Love-Hate Relationship. *J. Innate Immun.* **2019**, *11*, 216–226. [CrossRef]

2

Validating Thermal Lethality to *Salmonella enterica* in Chicken Blood by Simulated Commercial Rendering

Caleb Wong de la Rosa [1], Kourtney A. Daniels [2], Rosana G. Moreira [3], Chris R. Kerth [1] and Thomas M. Taylor [1,*]

1 Department of Animal Science, Texas A&M AgriLife Research, College Station, TX 77843-2471, USA; calebwong19@gmail.com (C.W.d.l.R.); c-kerth@tamu.edu (C.R.K.)
2 Department of Food Science and Technology, Texas A&M AgriLife Research, College Station, TX 77843-2253, USA; kdaniel5@tamu.edu
3 Department of Biological and Agricultural Engineering, Texas A&M AgriLife Research, College Station, TX 77843-2117, USA; rmoreira@tamu.edu
* Correspondence: matt_taylor@tamu.edu

Abstract: The U.S. rendering industry produces materials for use in further processed animal foods and feeds and is required to scientifically validate food safety hazard control. This study aimed to provide lethality validation for *Salmonella enterica* during simulated commercial rendering of whole chicken blood. Chicken blood was inoculated with a blend of multiple serovars of the pathogen (*S.* Heidelberg, Typhimurium, Senftenberg) and subjected to heating at 82.2, 87.8, or 93.3 °C; surviving cells were enumerated incrementally up to 5.0 min. Survivor data were modeled using the GInaFiT 1.7 freeware package. *D*-values and t_{7D} (time to a 7.0 log_{10}-cycle inactivation) values were generated from best-fit model parameters. Predictive modeling analysis revealed that the survival curves of *Salmonella* possessed log-linear components but also possessed shoulder and/or tail components. Mean *D*-values declined from 0.61 to 0.12 min as heating temperature was raised from 82.2 to 93.3 °F, respectively, differing by heating temperature ($p = 0.023$). t_{7D} values differed significantly by heating temperature ($p = 0.001$), as was also the case for shoulder length (S_L) ($p = <0.0001$), where, at lower temperatures, a shoulder was observed versus heating at 93.3 °F. These data aid scientific validation of *Salmonella enterica* inactivation during thermal rendering of poultry blood for use in further processed animal foods.

Keywords: *Salmonella*; rendering; chicken blood; validation; lethality; blood meal

---

1. Introduction

Rendering of animal carcass components and materials for subsequent conversion into animal and/or human food or feed provides sustainable recycling of resources and a nutritious feed/food stream for consumers, livestock, and companion animals [1]. Nevertheless, raw carcass materials, including blood, present a food safety hazard risk through contamination with microbial human and/or animal pathogens, including *Salmonella enterica* subsp. *enterica*. Multiple studies in recent years have reported the presence of biological food safety hazards such as *Salmonella* on animal carcass components as well as finished rendered products, including blood meal, in the U.S. and in other countries [2–4]. Jiang [5] reported that rendered blood meal products contained salmonellae at numbers as high as 240 MPN/g meal. Others reported that *Salmonella* prevalence ranged from 8.7 to 31.3% throughout various rendered products, including poultry meal and blood meal [6,7].

The U.S. Food and Drug Administration Food Safety Modernization Act (FDA-FSMA) and its implementing final rule mandating food safety preventive controls during the manufacture of animal foods (Title 21, U.S. Code of Federal Regulations Section 507) requires covered establishments to scientifically validate process-type preventive controls for identified food safety hazards [8]. Scientific validation of food safety hazard control may be accomplished by various means, including scientific experiments that simulate critical aspects of the antimicrobial process, as well as through other means such as in-plant inoculated product challenge trials that utilize pathogen surrogates exhibiting similar sensitivity to the process as the pathogen of concern [9]. In past research, determination of decimal reduction times (*D*-values) and other thermal inactivation kinetic parameters from testing of pathogen-inoculated products have been developed to assist the validation of effective lethality for commercial food processing. Ceylan and Bautista [10] reported that *S. enterica* *D*-values ranged from 0.48 to 17.30 min on dried pet food kibble products in a temperature- and moisture content-dependent manner. Bianchini et al. [11] determined that a 5.0 $\log_{10}$ CFU/g reduction in *Salmonella enterica* was achieved by heating commercially produced pet food meals to at least 60.6 °C. Our group previously produced *D*-values for multiple serovars of human and avian pathogenic *Salmonella* in poultry offal at 60 °C, reporting the $D_{60°C}$ = 0.89 min for a poultry animal-recovered *S.* Enteritidis [12].

Despite these and other studies reporting the prevalence of *Salmonella* in rendered animal food components or products, or validating thermal lethality to microbial pathogens during rendering, data validating *Salmonella* lethality during rendering of whole blood by for manufacture of blood meal are lacking. Thus, the main objective of this study was to characterize the thermal lethality during simulated commercial rendering of whole chicken blood to human pathogenic *S. enterica*.

2. Materials and Methods

2.1. Microorganisms and Inoculum Preparation

Isolates belonging to *Salmonella enterica* serovars Senftenberg, Heidelberg, and Typhimurium, recovered from U.S. Department of Agriculture Food Safety and Inspection Service (USDA-FSIS)-inspected chicken harvesting environments (*S.* Typhimurium, *S.* Heidelberg) or procured from American Type Culture Collection (ATCC, Manassas, VA, USA; *S.* Senftenberg 775W ATCC #43845), were chosen from the Food Microbiology Laboratory culture collection (Department of Animal Science, Texas A&M University, College Station, TX, USA). Cultures were revived from −80 °C cryo-storage by inoculating each isolate individually into 10.0 mL sterile brain heart infusion broth (BHIB; Becton, Dickinson and Co., Sparks, MD, USA)—containing tubes and then incubating tubes for 24 h at 35 °C. Following the initial revival, cells from each isolate were aseptically transferred to new, sterile BHI-containing tubes and then incubated in identical fashion (35 °C, 24 h) in order to prepare isolates for subsequent inoculum preparation. Following revival, an inoculum of *Salmonella* isolates (i.e., cocktail) of *S.* Senftenberg 775W, Heidelberg, and Typhimurium was prepared by blending 10.0 mL of each culture into a sterile 50.0 mL conical tube and centrifuging (2191× *g*, 25 ± 2 °C, 15 min) to pelletize cells. After centrifuging the cocktail preparation, the resulting supernatant was discarded and 30.0 mL 0.1% (*w/v*) peptone water (Becton, Dickinson and Co.) was added to wash cells. The resulting suspension of cells was centrifuged again identically, the resulting supernatant was poured off, and the remaining pellet was hydrated with 3.0 mL of 0.1% peptone water. This was completed to yield a 9.0–10.0 $\log_{10}$ CFU/mL inoculum in the cocktail.

2.1.1. Preliminary Enumeration of Salmonellae from Non-Inoculated Chicken Blood

In order to verify whether the final inoculum preparation for *S. enterica* was capable of overwhelming any naturally occurring pathogen cells by at least 2 to 3 orders of magnitude, samples of chicken blood were obtained from a cooperating U.S. commercial renderer. Samples were aseptically transported to the Food Microbiology Laboratory in insulated coolers packed with sealed ice packs and serially diluted in 0.1% peptone diluent. Serial dilutions were then inoculated onto Petri dishes containing bismuth sulfite agar (BSA; Becton, Dickinson and Co.) to selectively enumerate salmonellae. Inoculated plates were incubated for 24 to 48 h at 36 ± 1 °C prior to colony counting.

2.1.2. Preliminary Experiment to Verify *Salmonella* Growth for Subsequent Inoculum Preparation

An experiment was conducted to verify that counts of overnight cultures of individual *Salmonella* isolates utilized for the cocktail did not differ from one another, and approximated 9.0 $\log_{10}$ CFU/mL, allowing researchers to produce a cocktail with non-differing numbers of each *Salmonella* strain. Revived *Salmonella* strains were aseptically inoculated (10.0 μL each) into sterile 10.0 mL volumes of BHIB and then aerobically incubated without shaking at 36 ± 1 °C for 24 h before enumerating strains individually on tryptic soy agar (TSA; Becton, Dickinson and Co.) poured into Petri dishes. Inoculated Petri plates were incubated for 24 h at 36 ± 1 °C prior to colony enumeration.

2.1.3. Preliminary Experiment to Identify Optimal Medium for Selective Recovery of Non-Injured and Injured Salmonella Cells from Heat-Treated Chicken Blood

An experiment was conducted to identify a chemical supplement to BSA providing effective repair and recovery of sub-lethally injured salmonellae following heating. *Salmonella* cells were revived as described (Section 2.1) and then heated at 93.3 °C for 3.0 min in re-sealable metal vessels (1″ × 6″ galvanized steel by 1″ iron screwcap; SouthLand, Memphis, TN, USA). Immediately after heating, vessels were placed in ice-cold water for 1.0 min to halt further heat-induced inactivation or injury, and samples were extracted thereafter. Surviving *Salmonella* cells were serially diluted in 0.1% (*w/v*) peptone diluent (Becton, Dickinson and Co.) and plated on Petri plates containing TSA (control), BSA without any supplement, BSA ± 0.1% (*w/v*) sodium pyruvate (Sigma-Aldrich Co, St. Louis, MO, USA), BSA ± 0.1% (*w/v*), 3,3′-thiodipropionic acid (TDP; Sigma-Aldrich Co.), or BSA with TSA overlay. Reagents selected were chosen based on the report of Gurtler and Kornacki [13]. Following 24 h incubation at 36 ± 1 °C, counts of *Salmonella*-typical colonies were recorded for determination of the optimal medium for later use in inoculated thermal lethality trials.

2.2. *Sample Inoculation with Salmonella Cocktail*

Raw chicken blood, visually free of carcass tissue, bone, and foreign material, was obtained from the aforementioned commercial rendering establishment (Section 2.1.1). Sample inoculation was achieved by pipetting 0.1 mL of prepared *Salmonella* inoculum into 50.0 mL conical tubes containing 25.0 mL chicken blood and then vortexing for 1 min to homogenize the inoculum in the sample. Following homogenization, serial dilutions of inoculated chicken blood were inoculated on BSA-containing Petri dishes and incubated for 24 h at 36 ± 1 °C to quantify the efficiency of inoculation of microbial cells prior to thermal lethality testing.

2.3. *Lethality to Salmonella Inoculated into Chicken Blood*

Inoculated chicken blood samples were heated to 93.3 °C for 5.0 min to determine total lethality achieved against the pathogen during a simulated commercial rendering process. Inoculation was achieved by pipetting 0.5 mL of *Salmonella* inoculum (Section 2.1) into a 50.0 mL sterile conical tube containing 50 mL chicken blood. Inoculated sample vials were then vortexed for 1.0 min to homogenize the inoculum throughout blood. Samples were then loaded into metal vessels (1″ × 6″ galvanized steel by 1″ iron screwcap; SouthLand) that were then closed and partially submerged in sterile distilled water in a stainless-steel cookpot on an induction-type cooktop. Following heating, vessels were immediately placed in ice-cold water (0 °C) to halt further microbial inactivation. Sample material was aseptically extracted from metal vessels and placed in sterile stomacher pouches, serially diluted with 0.1% peptone diluent, and surviving cells were inoculated on Petri plates. Surviving *Salmonella* were enumerated on Petri plates containing BSA ± 0.1% (*w/v*) sodium pyruvate and then incubated at 36 ± 1 °C for 24 to 48 h prior to colony enumeration.

2.4. Temperature-Dependent Thermal Lethality to Salmonella in Chicken Blood

Figure 1 depicts the simple flow of work for the determination of *Salmonella* survival during lethality experiments. Metal vessels (described in Section 2.1.3) were used to help simulate rendering conditions within the commercial rendering establishment with respect to material contacting rendered material during commercial processing. A VWR™ Enviro-Safe® K 50,531 thermometer (VWR Int., Radnor, PA, USA) was set inside an open metallic vessel control filled with 50.0 mL distilled water to monitor temperature readings within sample vessels. Metal vessels were partially submerged in sterile distilled water in a stainless-steel cookpot on an induction cooking device tuned to produce final cook temperatures in the metal vessels of 82.2, 87.8, or 93.3 °C. Vessels were heated to one of the three targeted processing temperatures prior to loading in inoculated blood to pre-heat the vessel but avoid an extended temperature come-up period. This was designed to determine the thermal lethality resulting solely from the simulated commercial rendering process (5 min of heat exposure at one of the three targeted cook temperatures assuming continuous processing in a pre-heated cooking apparatus). Any additional lethality that would be expected to be achieved during commercial rendering come-up periods would thus add to observed lethality.

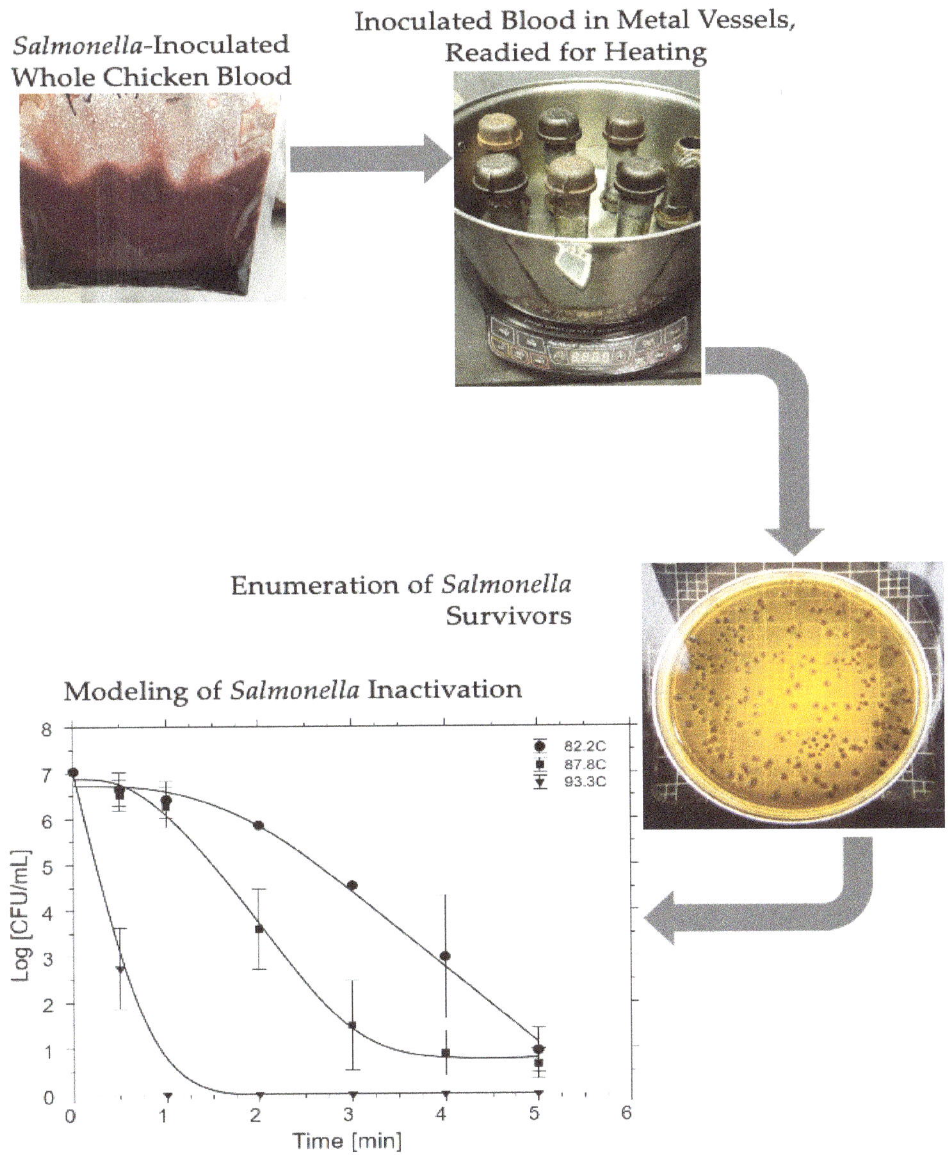

Figure 1. Flow process depiction of *Salmonella* lethality determination from heating of pathogen-inoculated whole chicken blood.

Once the metal vessel reached the targeted cook temperature, inoculated chicken blood samples were poured immediately into metal vessels, and vessels were sealed with screw-cap closure and replaced in the heated distilled water bath as quickly as possible. One vessel was left unsealed after filling with non-inoculated blood to allow for temperature monitoring. After loading sample vessels into the heating water bath, vessels were removed after 0.0, 0.5, 1.0, 2.0, 3.0, 4.0, or 5.0 min of heat exposure at the experimental temperature. Once removed from heat, metal vessels were immediately placed in ice-cold water (0 °C) to halt further microbial inactivation. Vessels were allowed to cool for at least 1.0 min to ensure complete cooling and allow researcher handling for survivor enumeration. Sample material was thereafter subjected to serial dilution in 0.1% peptone diluent and surviving *Salmonella* were enumerated on BSA supplemented with 1.0 g/L sodium pyruvate to allow recovery and detection of sub-lethally injured salmonellae. Inoculated plates were incubated at 36 ± 1 °C for 24 to 48 h before colony counting. The limit of detection of the assay was 1 CFU/mL (0.0 $\log_{10}$ CFU/mL).

2.5. Data Analysis

All preliminary and research experiments were replicated three times in identical fashion; experiments for *D*-value determination were designed as a full factorial, randomly assigning samples by three targeted heating temperatures (82.2, 87.8, or 93.3 °C) and seven heating periods (0.0, 0.5, 1.0, 2.0, 3.0, 4.0, and 5.0 min). Plate counts of *Salmonella* were $\log_{10}$-transformed prior to data analysis. Survivor data generated from replicates of thermal lethality experiments (Section 2.4) were then fit to non-log-linear models using the freeware Microsoft, Inc. (Redmond, WA, USA) Excel® add-in GInaFiT v.1.7 [14], identifying the best fitting model(s) by use of adjusted R^2 and root mean square error (RMSE) outputs as indices of a model's goodness of fit to data. GInaFiT-returned parameters of the fitted model:

$$\log(N) = \log\left[10^{\log(N_o)-\log(N_{res})} e^{-k_{max}t}\left(\frac{e^{k_{max}S_L}}{1 \pm (e^{k_{max}S_L}-1)e^{-k_{max}t}}\right) \pm 10^{\log(N_{res})}\right] \quad (1)$$

where N is microbial cell count (CFU/mL); N_0 is initial microbial cell count (CFU/mL); k_{max} is the first order microbial inactivation constant (1/min); S_L is the shoulder length (min), and N_{res} is the residual microbial cell population (CFU/mL). Additionally, the times required for a 4.0 $\log_{10}$-cycle inactivation (t_{4D}) at each heating temperature were recorded and used for purposes of determining *D*-values and t_{7D} times (time required for a 7.0 $\log_{10}$-cycle reduction in *Salmonella* counts).

Statistical analysis of microbiological plate counts ($\log_{10}$-transformed) calculated *D*-values, t_{7D} values, and GInaFiT-returned S_L values were completed by one- or two-way analysis of variance (AOV), as appropriate. Statistically significant differences between least squares means of main effects and/or their interactions ($p < 0.05$) were separated using Dunnett's test in the case of the preliminary experiment comparing TSA-recovered *Salmonella* counts against other recovery/plating media (Section 2.1.3), or by Fisher's least squares differences (LSD) test (all others). For all analyses, $p < 0.05$ was set as the significance level. Finally, a *z*-value providing the temperature change required to achieve a 10-fold change in the *D*-value for the process was determined by linear regression analysis of the plot of heating temperatures (*x*-axis) against $\log_{10}$-transforms of mean *D*-values (*y*-axis). Data analyses were completed using Prism v9.0 for MacOS (GraphPad Software, LLC, San Diego, CA, USA).

3. Results and Discussion

3.1. Results of Preliminary Experiments Enumerating Salmonellae from Non-Inoculated Chicken Blood and Overnight Growth of Salmonella Isolates for Inoculum Preparation

Whole chicken blood samples were tested for the presence of contaminating non-typhoidal salmonellae to ascertain the organism's presence prior to inoculation. The mean number of salmonellae was 4.9 ± 0.6 $\log_{10}$ CFU/mL of non-rendered blood; this was significantly higher than previous reports of *Salmonella* numbers on inedible offal, where *Salmonella* loads were reported at 3.7 MPN/100 g [15]. *Salmonella enterica* isolates grew reliably during overnight growth, achieving means of 8.8 ± 0.1, 9.0 ± 0.1, and 9.0 ± 0.1 log_{10} CFU/mL for isolates belonging to serovars *S.* Senftenberg, *S.* Typhimurium, and *S.* Heidelberg, respectively. Results of statistical analysis indicated that mean counts of *Salmonella* isolates did not differ from one another ($p = 0.069$).

3.2. Identification of Suitable Medium for Use in Selective Plating and Recovery of Non-Injured and Injured Salmonella Cells from Heated Chicken Blood

Results of preliminary testing to determine which chemical supplement to BSA best facilitated the repair and recovery of injured *S. enterica* inoculated into chicken blood during lethality trials are presented in Figure 2. While statistical analysis indicated no differences between means of recovered *Salmonella* cells based on medium ($p = 0.130$), BSA ± 0.1% pyruvate produced counts of *S. enterica* which numerically differed the least from TSA control counts while also maintaining the selectivity of BSA and was used throughout subsequent experiments.

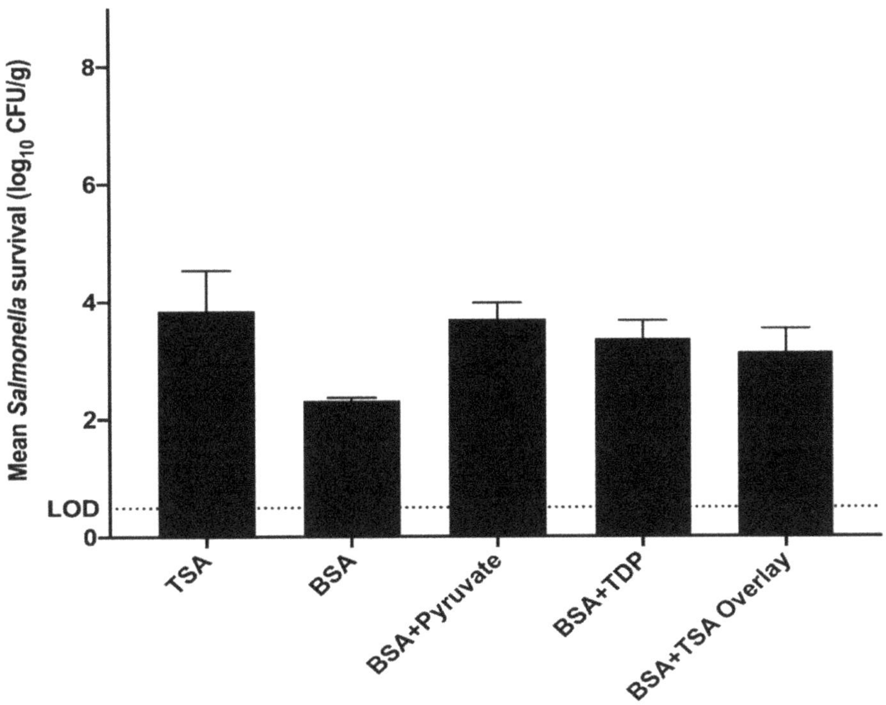

Figure 2. Mean numbers of survivors of *Salmonella enterica* recovered from whole chicken blood subjected to heating for 3.0 min at 93.3 °C ($p = 0.130$; pooled standard error = 0.565). Bars depict means from three identically completed replicates ($N = 3$); error bars present one standard error. *Salmonella* cells were enumerated on tryptic soy agar (TSA), bismuth sulfite agar (BSA), BSA supplemented with 0.1% (*w/v*) sodium pyruvate (BSA ± Pyruvate), BSA supplemented with 0.1% (*w/v*) 3,3′-thiodipropionic acid (BSA ± TDP), or BSA with TSA overlay. *Salmonella* colonies were enumerated after plates were incubated at 36 ± 1 °C for 24–48 h.

3.3. Total Lethality Achieved in Chicken Blood against Salmonella

Experiments determining the lethality achieved against the *S. enterica* inoculum in chicken blood following 5.0 min continuous heating at 93.3 °C confirmed the ability of commercial rendering to substantially reduce the pathogen, aiding in the manufacture of products not adulterated by *S. enterica*. Numbers of *Salmonella* were reduced to non-detectable counts (detection limit: 0.0 log_{10} CFU/mL) from initial mean counts of 7.4 ± 0.1 log_{10} CFU/mL. Jiang [5] discussed how recent U.S. rendering industry changes have apparently resulted in a decreased prevalence of *Salmonella* presence and transmission than in years past, potentially the result of federal food safety rules requiring industry members to adopt and monitor validated food safety process preventive controls. The U.S. Department of Agriculture Food Safety and Inspection Service (USDA-FSIS) [16] mandates a minimum 7.0 $\log_{10}$-cycle lethality for *Salmonella* on human foods derived from poultry, including edible offal. Achieved lethality for *Salmonella* would therefore likely be effective for reducing the pathogen to non-detectable counts in whole blood during rendering, a regulatory requirement for the production of non-adulterated animal food/feeds [17].

3.4. Inactivation of S. enterica in Chicken Blood as a Function of Thermal Processing

Figure 3 depicts the inactivation of inoculated *Salmonella* in chicken blood as a function of heating temperature and period. *Salmonella* cells inoculated into blood demonstrated an initial shoulder to survival curve for samples heated at 82.2 and 87.8 °C, with increases in the rates of cell death only observed after approximately 1.0 min of heating. Thereafter, death rates for the pathogen at both temperatures increased, with a characteristic log-linear *Salmonella* count decline for 87.8 °C-heated cells until 3.0 min of heating, after which a tailing effect was observed to occur with a consequent slowing of the death rate. Conversely, 82.2 °C-heated *S. enterica* cells in blood displayed a more rapid inactivation rate after 1.0–1.5 min of heating, presumably due to the *S.* Senftenberg displaying enhanced survival at the lower heating temperature, and from 2.0 min until the 5.0 min mark, the curve was generally log-linear.

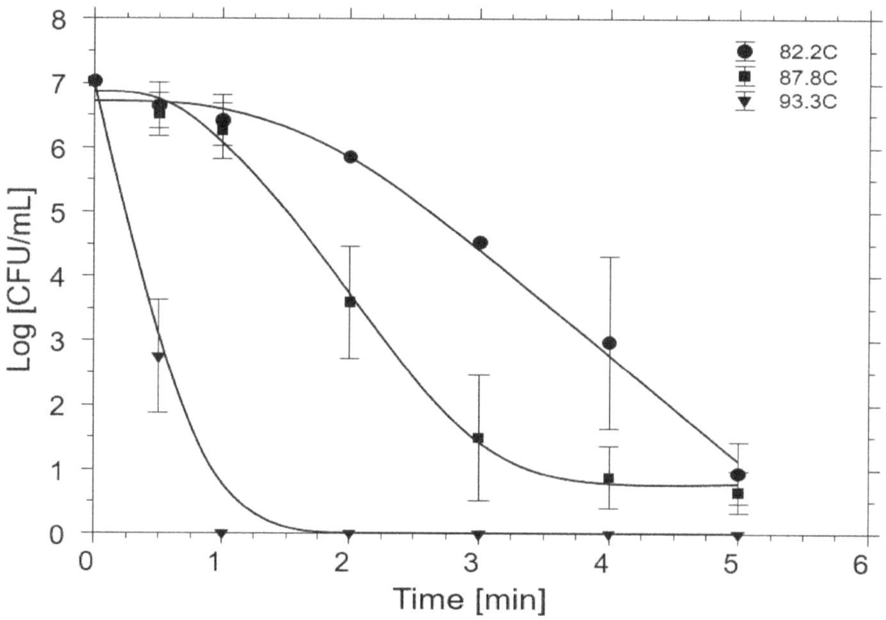

Figure 3. Mean numbers of surviving *Salmonella enterica* in whole chicken blood subjected to heating at 82.2, 87.8, or 93.3 °C. Values depict means from three identically completed replicates (N = 3); error bars present one standard error. *Salmonella* cells were enumerated on bismuth sulfite agar supplemented with 0.1% (*w/v*) sodium pyruvate, after plates were incubated at 36 ± 1 °C for 24–48 h.

Two-way AOV indicated that the interaction of heating temperature by period was highly significant for the survival of *Salmonella* in whole chicken blood (p = <0.0001). Counts of the pathogen differed at 0.5 min between samples subjected to the differing heating temperatures, with 82.2 °C- and 87.8 °C-heated cell populations each differing from the count of *Salmonella* cells heated to 93.3 °C ($p < 0.0001$), but not from one another. A similar trend was also observed at 1.0 min of heating, where the counts of 93.3 °C-heated cells (0.0 $\log_{10}$ CFU/mL) were significantly lower than either of the populations of *Salmonella* heated to the two lower experimental temperatures (p = <0.0001). From 2.0 to 4.0 min of heating, statistical differences became even more pronounced between samples heated to differing target temperatures, where mean populations at each of the three temperatures differed from one another ($p = 0.043$). However, after 5 min of heating, the counts of surviving inoculated salmonellae declined to no more than 0.94 $\log_{10}$ CFU/mL, and counts did not differ from one another as a function of heating temperature ($p = 0.193$).

3.5. *Thermal Death Kinetics for Microorganisms in Chicken Blood as a Function of Heating Temperature*

The application of the GInaFiT 1.7 program for the modeling of microbial inactivation allows the user to apply multiple log-linear and non-linear models for the purposes of obtaining predicted inactivation kinetic parameters for a process [14]. In the current study, *D*-values were calculated by re-arrangement of Equation (5) by Valdramidis et al. [18] to:

$$D = (t_{4D} - S_L)/4 \quad (2)$$

using t_{4D} and S_L values returned from GInaFiT. Statistical comparison of means of calculated *D*-values and GInaFiT-returned t_{4D} values indicated differences occurring between both *D* and t_{4D} values as a function of heating temperature (Table 1).

Table 1. Least squares means of *D*- (min) and t_{4D} values (min) for *Salmonella* inoculated into whole chicken blood and heated to differing target temperatures.

	Heating Temperature (°C)			
	82.2	**87.8**	**93.3**	**$p > F$; Pooled SE** [2]
D-value [1]	0.61 ± 0.18 ^{A} (0.22, 1.06)	0.41 ± 0.19 ^{A,B} (0.00, 0.88)	0.12 ± 0.02 ^{B,C} (0.04, 0.21)	0.023; 0.13
t_{4D}	4.12 ± 0.19 ^{A} (3.32, 4.92)	2.42 ± 0.38 ^{B} (0.80, 4.04)	0.50 ± 0.08 ^{C} (0.17, 0.83)	0.0001; 0.35

[1] Means are determined from three identically completed replicates ± one standard error. Values in parentheses present the lower and upper 95% confidence limits. Means within a row not sharing common letters (^{A}, ^{B}, ^{C}) differ by Fisher's least squares differences test at $p = 0.05$. [2] SE: standard error about mean.

Table 2 reports the model parameters returned by GInaFiT v1.7 for *Salmonella* lethality by heating target temperature. Shoulder lengths for inoculated *Salmonella* cells statistically differed in blood as a function of heating temperature ($p = <0.0001$), with each shoulder length at a specific heating temperature differing from shoulder lengths at the other two temperatures. Observed differences in residual S_L values may have resulted from the inclusion of the high heat-resistant *S.* Senftenberg 775W isolate in the current study and its impacts on apparent inactivation kinetics, especially at the lower heating temperatures. Jones-Ibarra et al. [12] previously reported that the $D_{140°F}$ for *S.* Senftenberg 775W in chicken offal was approximately 6× higher than those for *S.* Enteritidis, *S.* Heidelberg, and *S.* Gallinarum isolates. Vaddella et al. [19] reported *S.* Typhimurium lethality in ground whole chicken carcasses when heated at 78 °C, equivalent to one of the heating temperatures used in the current study. The presence of a shoulder was observed in their data, as was the case in the current study, with accelerated lethality occurring after the initial shoulder. However, multiple $\log_{10}$-cycles' inactivation of the organism required a much longer exposure period for the whole carcass versus that reported here, presumably due to the increased content of fat and bone material providing enhanced thermal insulation as compared to blood. Peleg [20] noted that the existence and duration of a shoulder would be expected to diminish as the intensity of the process intervention, in this heating temperature, was increased, as is the case in the present study.

Table 2. Least squares means of lethality model parameters for *Salmonella* inoculated into and heated in whole chicken blood.

Model Parameter [1]	82.2 °C	87.8 °C	93.3 °C	p > F; Pooled SE [2]
S_L (min)	1.62 ± 0.12 [A]	0.71 ± 0.09 [B]	0.0 ± 0.0 [C]	<0.0001; 0.125
k_{max} (1/min)	3.80 ± 0.29	5.59 ± 0.47	19.71 ± 0.04	
N_{res} (log CFU/mL)	– [3]	0.77 ± 0.17	–	
N_0 (log CFU/mL)	6.71 ± 0.16	6.87 ± 0.19	7.03 ± 0.01	0.089; 0.117
RMSE	0.26	0.23	0.01	
Adjusted R^2	0.99	0.99	1.00	

[1] Means are determined from three identically completed replicates ± one standard error. Values not sharing common letters ([A], [B], [C]) within a row differ by Fisher's least squares differences test at $p = 0.05$. [2] Values depict main effect-specific p-value; Pooled SE: standard error about mean. [3] – Indicates no N_{res} determined from modeling of *Salmonella* survivor data.

Goodness of fit parameters (RMSE, adjusted R^2) both indicated that the fitted models were suitable for the prediction of *Salmonella* lethality during commercial rendering of blood, wherein RMSE declined as heating temperature increased, with a shift to log-linear ± tail being observed at the highest temperature of processing along with a disappearance of the shoulder, and adjusted R^2 remaining near 1.0 for all experimental heating data. This would indicate that the experimental data did not deviate substantially from model-predicted values, fitting with a high degree of precision (Table 2).

The determination of the z-value affords the processor the opportunity to alter a process with a predictable outcome in microbial lethality; the z-value for the rendering of chicken blood was 15.68 °C (Figure 4). Cautious application of this value is recommended; z-values (much like D-values) rely on log-linear death kinetics for their determination and do not easily accommodate non-linearity in microbial inactivation. This would not likely be problematic were a commercial renderer desiring to increase the processing temperature in order to increase production throughput but would become increasingly unreliable were the processing temperature decreased, given the presence of non-zero S_L values at lower heating temperatures (Table 2; Figure 3). The z-value determined in the current study aligns well with those previously reported (14.1–27.8 °C) against *Escherichia coli* O157:H7 and *Salmonella* in rendered oils [21]. Nevertheless, it is substantially lower than was reported by others testing *Salmonella* lethality in beef-derived carcass materials of 42.8 °C [22]. Nonetheless, those authors reported incorporation of 20% or 50% fat as well as lean meat and connective tissue, much different than the liquid chicken blood free of solid tissue used in the current study.

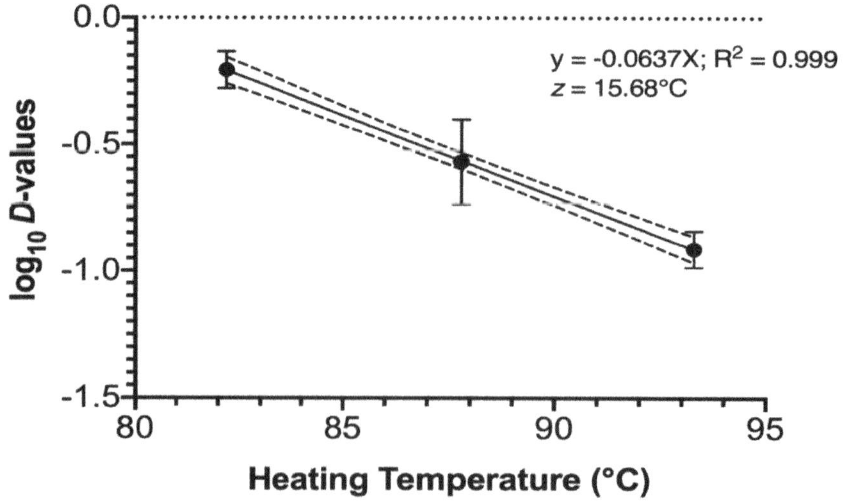

Figure 4. Thermal process constant (z-value) for *Salmonella enterica* inoculated and heated in whole chicken blood. Symbols depict mean calculated from three identically completed replicates ($N = 3$); error bars depict one standard error. Dashed lines present the 95% confidence limit boundaries.

Buchanan et al. [23] previously recommended the use of a desired cumulative lethality process, arbitrarily set at t_{4D}, as compared to designing a process strictly according to a multiple of the *D*-value. Jackson et al. [24] followed this approach for producing a predicted 5.0 $\log_{10}$ CFU/g inactivation of *E. coli* O157:H7 cells in ground beef patties during cooking. This method bears a distinct advantage in designing and validating thermal processes when microbial death kinetics are known or suspected to not follow a strictly log-linear kinetic, such as in the current report. The t_{xD} metric facilitates the processor accounting for the existence of a shoulder and/or tail in the identification of processing time needed for desired lethality and should produce a more conservative estimate of the needed processing conditions to achieve desired food safety hazard reduction. As was stated above (Section 3.3), the USDA-FSIS [16] mandates a performance objective of a 7.0 $\log_{10}$-cycle inactivation of *Salmonella* in poultry-derived human food. In the current study, t_{7D} values for *Salmonella* differed by targeted heating temperature, with each t_{7D} at a specific heating temperature differing from those of the other two ($p = 0.001$; Figure 5). Juneja et al. [25] previously recommended that food processors apply a t_{xD} for achieving a desired lethality performance objective, even recommending the application of the upper limit of a 95% confidence limit for the sake of producing conservative processing schedules for pathogen control. In the present study, mean t_{7D} values declined from 6.04 at 82.2 °C, to 3.37 min at 87.8 °C, and to 0.88 min at 93.3 °C. Processing at 82.2 °C or 93.3 °C, each with incorporation of the 95% confidence limit, would require processing periods of 8.09 or 1.45 min at 93.3 °C, respectively (Figure 5). These would represent conservative processes for the rendering of chicken blood, with a high degree of *Salmonella* lethality generally assured.

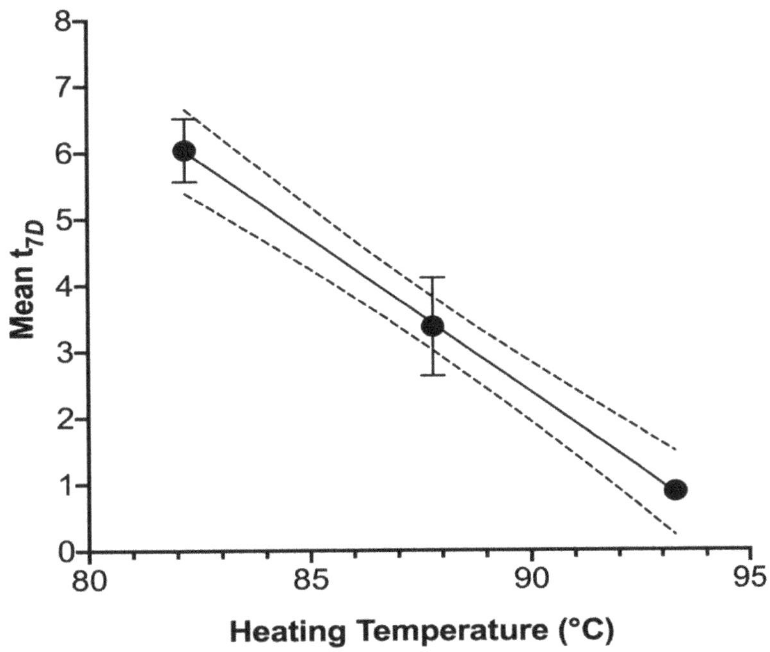

Figure 5. Least squares means of time required to achieve a 7.0 $\log_{10}$-cycle inactivation (t_{7D}) for *Salmonella enterica* heated in whole chicken blood to differing target temperatures. Symbols depict means from three identically completed replicates ($N = 3$); error bars depict one standard error ($p = 0.001$; pooled standard error = 0.73). Dashed lines depict 95% confidence limit boundaries.

4. Conclusions

The U.S. rendering industry remains in need of scientific validation of the thermal processing systems applied to the manufacturing of components of further processed animal foods and feeds, in order to assist in complying with federal regulations. *Salmonella enterica* was effectively inactivated in whole chicken blood heated to differing endpoint temperatures, yielding *D*-values that differed by heating temperature, as might be expected. Survival curves tended to possess log-linear portions with or without shoulder and/or tail components, overall yielding non-linear survival curves. Time requirements for a 7.0 $\log_{10}$ CFU/mL inactivation of *Salmonella* also differed between the three heating temperatures. Finally, a *z*-value of 15.68 °C was produced, giving the temperature change in the process producing a 10-fold change in the *Salmonella* *D*-value. Data presented demonstrate that the commercial process simulated in this report is effective for achieving significant *Salmonella* inactivation in whole chicken blood for the safe manufacture of blood meal and other derived products not adulterated by the microbial pathogen.

Author Contributions: Conceptualization, T.M.T.; methodology, T.M.T., C.W.d.l.R., K.A.D.; formal analysis, R.G.M., C.R.K., T.M.T.; writing—original draft preparation, T.M.T.; writing—review and editing, T.M.T., R.G.M., C.R.K., C.W.d.l.R., K.A.D.; project administration, T.M.T.; funding acquisition, T.M.T. All authors have read and agreed to the published version of the manuscript.

References

1. Meeker, D.L.; Hamilton, C.R. *An overview of the rendering industry In Essential Rendering: All about the Animal by-Products Industry*; Meeker, D.L., Ed.; National Renderers Association: Alexandria, VA, USA, 2006; pp. 1–16.
2. Pepe, T.; De Dominicis, R.; Esposito, G.; Ventrone, I.; Fratamico, P.M.; Cortesi, M.L. Detection of *Campylobacter* from poultry carcass skin samples at slaughter in southern Italy. *J. Food Prot.* **2009**, *72*, 1718–1721. [CrossRef]
3. Narvaez-Bravo, C.; Miller, M.F.; Jackson, T.; Jackson, S.; Rodas-Gonzalez, A.; Pond, K.; Echeverry, A.; Brashears, M.M. *Salmonella* and *Escherichia coli* O157:H7 prevalence in cattle and on carcasses in a vertically integrated feedlot and harvest plant in Mexico. *J. Food Prot.* **2013**, *76*, 786–795. [CrossRef]
4. Bacon, R.T.; Sofos, J.N.; Belk, K.E.; Hyatt, D.R.; Smith, G.C. Prevalence and antibiotic susceptibility of *Salmonella* isolated from beef animal hides and carcasses. *J. Food Prot.* **2002**, *65*, 284–290. [CrossRef]
5. Jiang, X. Prevalence and characterization of *Salmonella* in animal meals collected from rendering operations. *J. Food Prot.* **2016**, *79*, 1026–1031. [CrossRef]
6. Kinley, B.; Rieck, J.; Dawson, P.; Jiang, X. Analysis of *Salmonella* and enterococci isolated from rendered animal products. *Can. J. Microbiol.* **2010**, *56*, 65–73. [CrossRef]
7. Ge, B.; Lafon, P.C.; Carter, P.J.; McDermott, S.D.; Abbott, J.; Glenn, A.; Ayers, S.L.; Friedman, S.L.; Paige, J.C.; Wagner, D.D.; et al. Retrospective analysis of *Salmonella*, *Campylobacter*, *Escherichia coli*, and *Enterococcus* in animal feed ingredients. *FoodBorne Pathog. Dis.* **2013**, *10*, 684–691. [CrossRef]
8. U.S. Food and Drug Administration. Title 21: Food and Drugs, Part 507: Current Good Manufacturing Practice, Hazard Analysis, and Risk-Based Preventive Controls for Food for Animals. Available online: https://www.ecfr.gov/cgi-bin/text-idx?SID=b4e880ff425c66edad94b50e64f286a3&mc=true&node=pt21.6.507&rgn=div5 (accessed on 23 September 2020).
9. Consortium of Food Process Validation Experts. Validation of antimicrobial interventions for small and very small processors: A how-to guide to develop and conduct validations. *Food Prot. Trends* **2013**, *33*, 95–104.
10. Ceylan, E.; Bautista, D.A. Evaluating *Pediococcus acidilactici* and *Enterococcus faecium* NRRL B-2354 as a thermal surrogate microorganisms for *Salmonella* for in-plant validation studies of low-moisture pet food products. *J. Food Prot.* **2015**, *78*, 934–939. [CrossRef]
11. Bianchini, A.; Stratton, J.; Weier, S.; Hartter, T.; Plattner, B.; Rokey, G.; Hertzel, G.; Gompa, L.; Martinez, B.; Eskridge, K.M. Use of *Enterococcus faecium* as a surrogate for *Salmonella enterica* during extrusion of a balanced carbohydrate-protein meal. *J. Food Prot.* **2014**, *77*, 75–82. [CrossRef]
12. Jones-Ibarra, A.M.; Acuff, G.R.; Alvarado, C.Z.; Taylor, T.M. Validation of thermal lethality against *Salmonella enterica* in poultry offal during rendering. *J. Food Prot.* **2017**, *80*, 1422–1428. [CrossRef]
13. Gurtler, J.B.; Kornacki, J.R. Comparison of supplements to enhance recovery of heat-injured *Salmonella* from egg albumen. *Lett. Appl. Microbiol.* **2009**, *49*, 503–509. [CrossRef]
14. Geeraerd, A.H.; Valdramidis, V.P.; van Impe, J.F. GInaFiT, a freeware tool to assess non-log-linear microbial survivor curves. *Int. J. Food Microbiol.* **2005**, *102*, 95–105. [CrossRef]
15. Russell, S.M.; Fletcher, D.L.; Pancorbo, O.C.; Merka, W.C. Effect of lactic acid fermentation on bacterial pathogens and indicator organisms in broiler processing waste. *Poult. Sci.* **1993**, *72*, 1573–1576. [CrossRef]
16. USDA-FSIS. Performance standards for the production of certain meat and poultry products. *Fed. Regist.* **1999**, *64*, 732–749.

17. FDA. Compliance Policy Guide, Section 690.800: *Salmonella* in food for animals. *Fed. Regist.* **2013**, *78*, 42526–42527.
18. Valdramidis, V.P.; Bernaerts, K.; Van Impe, J.F.; Geeraerd, A.H. An alternative approach to non-log-linear thermal microbial inactivation: Modelling the number of log cycles reduction with respect to temperature. *Food Technol. Biotechnol.* **2005**, *43*, 321–327.
19. Vaddella, V.; Pitesky, M.; Cao, W.; Govinthasamy, V.; Shi, J.; Pandey, P. Assessing *Salmonella typhimurium* persistence in poultry carcasses under multiple thermal conditions consistent with composting and wet rendering. *Poult. Sci.* **2016**, *95*, 705–714. [CrossRef]
20. Peleg, M. Microbial survivor curves—The reality of flat "shoulders" and absolute thermal death times. *Food Res. Int.* **2000**, *33*, 531–538. [CrossRef]
21. Murphy, R.L.; Woerner, D.R.; Geornaras, I.; Martin, J.N.; Yang, H.; Sofos, J.N.; Delmore, R.J.; Belk, K.E. Determining process lethality of *Escherichia coli* O157:H7 and *Salmonella* in heat treated, rendered oil. *Meat Muscle Biol.* **2016**, *1*, 124. [CrossRef]
22. Ramirez-Hernandez, A.; Inestroza, B.; Parks, A.; Brashears, M.M.; Sanchez-Plata, M.X.; Echeverry, A. Thermal inactivation of *Salmonella* in high-fat rendering meat products. *J. Food Prot.* **2018**, *81*, 54–58. [CrossRef]
23. Buchanan, R.L.; Golden, M.H.; Whiting, R.C. Differentiation of the effects of pH and lactic or acetic acid concentration on the kinetics of *Listeria monocytogenes* inactivation. *J. Food Prot.* **1993**, *56*, 474–478. [CrossRef]
24. Jackson, T.C.; Hardin, M.D.; Acuff, G.R. Heat resistance of *Escherichia coli* O157:H7 in a nutrient medium and in ground beef patties as influenced by storage and holding temperatures. *J. Food Prot.* **1996**, *59*, 230–237. [CrossRef]
25. Juneja, V.K.; Eblen, B.S.; Marks, H.M. Modeling non-linear survival curves to calculate thermal inactivation of *Salmonella* in poultry of different fat levels. *Int. J. Food Microbiol.* **2001**, *70*, 37–51. [CrossRef]

3

Effect of a High Proportion of Rye in Compound Feed for Reduction of *Salmonella* Typhimurium in Experimentally Infected Young Pigs

Bussarakam Chuppava [1,†], Volker Wilke [1,†], Clara Berenike Hartung [1], Amr Abd El-Wahab [2], Richard Grone [3], Andreas von Felde [3], Josef Kamphues [1] and Christian Visscher [1,*]

[1] Institute for Animal Nutrition, University of Veterinary Medicine Hannover, Foundation, Bischofsholer Damm 15, D-30173 Hanover, Germany; bussarakam.chuppava@tiho-hannover.de (B.C.); volker.wilke@tiho-hannover.de (V.W.); clara.berenike.hartung@tiho-hannover.de (C.B.H.); josef.kamphues@tiho-hannover.de (J.K.)

[2] Department of Nutrition and Nutritional Deficiency Diseases, Faculty of Veterinary Medicine, Mansoura University, Mansoura 35516, Egypt; amrwahab5@mans.edu.eg

[3] KWS LOCHOW GmbH, Ferdinand von Lochowstrasse 5, D-29303 Bergen, Germany; richard.grone@kws.com (R.G.); andreas.vonfelde@kws.com (A.v.F.)

* Correspondence: christian.visscher@tiho-hannover.de

† These authors contributed equally to this study.

Abstract: Public health concerns and the potential for food-borne zoonotic transmission have made *Salmonella* a subject of surveillance programs in food-producing animals. Forty-two piglets (25 d of age and initially 7.48 kg) were used in a 28 d infection period to evaluate the effects of a high proportion of rye on reducing *Salmonella* Typhimurium. Piglets were divided into two diet groups: control diet (wheat 69%) and experimental diet (rye 69%). After a one-week adaptation period, all piglets were orally infected with *Salmonella* Typhimurium (10^7 log CFU/mL; 2mL/pig). *Salmonella* in fecal shedding were evaluated at day 1, 3, 5, 7 and then weekly after infection. At the end of the experimental period (at day 28 after infection), the piglets were euthanized to sample feces, cecal digesta contents and ileocecal lymph nodes to determine the bacterial counts of *Salmonella*. The results suggest that the bacterial counts in the experimental group fed rye diets showed evidence of reducing *Salmonella* fecal shedding from day 14 onwards and decreasing the number of *Salmonella* in cecal digesta. However, the translocation of *Salmonella* in ileocecal lymph nodes was not affected. Furthermore, feed intake, weight gain and feed conversion did not differ between the groups ($p >$ 0.05).

Keywords: rye; wheat; *Salmonella*; foodborne pathogen; zoonosis; public health; swine; pig

1. Introduction

Salmonellosis is primarily a zoonosis and interventions are possible at any stage from farm to fork [1]. *Salmonella enterica* serovar Typhimurium is strongly associated with pigs, with infections in humans caused by contaminated pork and meat products, causing an impact on public health [2,3]. In Germany, 33% of acquired infections or 13,529 cases of salmonellosis were reported in 2018 [4], making salmonellosis the second most commonly reported bacterial gastrointestinal disease in Germany after *Campylobacter* enteritis [4].

With regard to reducing the number of *Salmonella* cases in the feed-to-food chain, it has frequently been demonstrated that the use of antimicrobial agents in food animals favors the development of resistance among foodborne pathogens like *Salmonella* spp. [5]. Since antimicrobial resistance is on the rise, therefore, there is an urgent need for new strategies to focus on the reduction of *Salmonella* in the intestinal tract by competitive binding of bacteria and support of intestinal function to reduce colonization [6]. Due to their bacteriostatic and bacteriolytic properties, short-chain fatty acids such as formic or butyric acid and their derivatives were reported in previous studies, these being widely used to control *Salmonella* in the pork production chain already at the farm level [7–9].

Feeding concepts for fattening pigs are often based on wheat, triticale and maize [10]. However, due to the improvements attained through rye, the concentrations of anti-nutritional factors such as alkylresorcinols and trypsin inhibitors, as well as ergot poisoning, have been reduced [11,12]. In recent years, intensive studies on rye focused on the use of high proportions of rye in rations with high dietary fiber contents, which had various positive effects [13–16]. The effects of rye in pig feeding, which are of particular interest, are induced by the fraction of non-starch polysaccharides (NSPs) [17]. Rye is by far the most fiber-rich grain [16], with high levels of arabinoxylans and fructans, which can only be broken down by microorganisms of the large intestine, opening up opportunities for a targeted influence on the fermentation pattern in the direction of forced butyrate formation in the cecum [16,18]. Consequently, butyrate is the main metabolic product of anaerobic bacteria fermentation in the intestine, which can contribute to intestinal health [19]. It is tempting to speculate that modifying the gut microbiota to produce more butyrate could reduce invasive *Salmonella* infections in animals [7–9,19]. Butyrate can interact with *Salmonella* proteins and, as a result, the invasion capacity decreases. Furthermore, it can reduce the penetration of *Salmonella* into intestinal epithelial cells and thus reduce the exposure of pigs to *Salmonella* [9,19–21].

In the present study, the focus of interest was the question of whether the effects of a new concept, especially high rye content in the feed mixture of young pigs, could reduce the prevalence of *Salmonella* in fecal shedding. In addition, cecal contents of pigs were examined because the invasion of *Salmonella* takes place primarily in this location [22]. Furthermore, possible translocation of the pathogen from the intestine into the animal body by detecting of *Salmonella* in the lymph nodes was investigated. This is of crucial importance due to the risk of *Salmonella* entering the food chain. The issue of animal health on growing performance is also of great concern.

2. Materials and Methods

2.1. Ethical Statement

The experiments took place in the biosafety level 2 infection stable (S2) of the Institute for Animal Nutrition, University of Veterinary Medicine Hannover, Foundation, Germany in accordance with German regulations and were approved by the Ethics Committee of Lower Saxony for the Care and Use of Laboratory Animals, LAVES (Niedersächsisches Landesamt für Verbraucherschutz und Lebensmittelsicherheit; reference: 33.8-42502-04-19/3257; announcement dated 27.11.2019).

2.2. Animal and Housing

A total of forty-two weaned pigs came from piglet production from the Farm for Education and Research in Ruthe, University of Veterinary Medicine Hannover, Foundation (N = 42). The piglets were divided into three consecutive trials (T) with fourteen animals each (n = 14 per trial), at the age of 24.9 ± 0.7 days. The animals were selected for the formation of two comparable groups in each trial (control: n = 7 and experimental: n = 7) on the basis of the following criteria: weight (control: 7.48 ± 1.11 kg and experimental: 7.48 ± 1.20 kg), sex ratio (female/male castrated) and sow (siblings distributed to both groups). At the time of grouping, the animals were weighed and marked with an individual ear tag.

The stable was divided into fourteen compartments, the piglets were housed individually. The pen dimensions measured 1.1 m × 2.2 m per animal. Each animal pen was equipped with a nipple drinker, a tiltable feeding trough, a 1 m^2 rubber mat as a lying surface and an infrared lamp hanging above the animal. Room temperature was recorded with a data logger (EBI 20-T1, Xylem Analytics

Germany Sales GmbH & Co. KG, Weilheim, Germany) during the respective trial period (24.5 ± 0.8 °C) and the lighting program in the stable was set at a twelve-hour day and night rhythm, so that the light was switched on from 07:00 to 19:00.

Before beginning the trials, the stable and all materials were disinfected and tests were carried out to confirm that they were free of *Salmonella* species contamination. To rule out *Salmonella* contamination of the feed and thus entry thereof via the feed into the infection stable, the feed batches were examined in advance for *Salmonella*. To prevent cross-contamination between the individual pens, each pen was equipped with its own utensils (brooms, trays, spatulas). Protective clothing, disposable boot covers and gloves could be changed before entering the corresponding area of the stable. The positions of the groups in the stable were changed between the trials.

2.3. Diets

The composition of diets is described in Table 1. The piglets were allocated to two groups (control: N = 21, n = 7 and experimental: N = 21, n = 7) and fed ad libitum with the complete pelleted feed depending on whether wheat served as the control group (contained 69% wheat) or rye (experimental group; contained 69% rye, Table 1), according to the previous result from Wilke [14].

Table 1. Composition of diets during the experiment as percentages.

Feedstuffs	Control	Experimental
Wheat	69.0	
Rye	-	69.0
Soybean meal *	11.5	11.5
Barley	10.0	10.0
Potato protein	5.10	4.90
Calcium carbonate	1.00	0.90
Monocalcium phosphate	0.90	1.00
Fat (soybean oil) *	0.50	0.50
Sodium chloride	0.35	0.40
Feed additives **	1.65	1.80

* Soybean meal (steam heated, with soapstock) made from genetically modified soybeans. ** Additives (per kg as fed); nutritional additives: vitamin A (12,000 IU), vitamin D3 (2000 IU), vitamin E (150 mg), copper from copper-(II)-glycinate chelate hydrate (4 mg), copper from copper-(II)-sulfate pentahydrate (110 mg), manganese from manganese glycine manganese chelate hydrate (35 mg), manganese from manganese-(II)-oxide (45 mg), zinc from glycine zinc chelate hydrate (40 mg), zinc from zinc oxide (80 mg), iron from iron-(II)-sulfate monohydrate (200 mg), iodine from calcium iodate anhydrous (2.0 mg), and selenium from sodium selenite (0.40 mg); zootechnical additives: 5.0×10^9 CFU *Saccharomyces cerevisiae*.

Feed chemical composition as well as particle size distribution of the diets are summarized in Table 2. Diets were analyzed by standard procedures in accordance with the official methods of the Verband Landwirtschaftlicher Untersuchungs- und Forschungsanstalten (VDLUFA [23]). The standardized methods of the Department of Animal Science, Aarhus University, Denmark were used to evaluate the NSP and arabinoxylans levels. Feed particle size distribution was assessed by a wet-sieve method of Wolf et al. [24].

Table 2. Feed chemical composition of control and experimental diets (g/kg dry matter).

Item	Control	Experimental
Dry matter (g/kg as fed)	897	903
Crude ash	51.4	54.2
Crude protein	205	213
Ether extract	28.0	23.6

Table 2. *Cont.*

Item	Control	Experimental
Crude fiber	28.7	28.2
Starch	516	461
Sugar	41.0	61.0
Nitrogen-free extract (NfE) [1]	584	681
Metabolizable energy (ME) [2](MJ/kg DM)	15.6	15.5
Calcium	9.21	9.26
Phosphorus	5.74	6.42
Arginine	10.4	10.8
Cysteine	3.73	4.01
Isoleucine	7.98	8.01
Leucine	14.5	14.3
Lysine	14.4	15.1
Methionine	4.64	5.71
Phenylalanine	9.89	9.72
Threonine	7.97	9.60
Valine	9.62	10.0
Non-starch polysaccharides (NSPs) *	123	140
Arabinoxylans *	63.0	74.0
Particle size (in%)		
>2 mm	3.55	2.83
>1–≤2 mm	28.1	25.3
≥0.2–≤1 mm	30.5	30.4
<0.2 mm	37.9	41.5

[1] Nitrogen-free extract (NfE) = dry matter—(crude ash + ether extract + crude fiber + crude protein). [2] Metabolizable energy (ME) calculated from the specified raw nutrient content. * NSPs and arabinoxylans were analyzed by the Department of Animal Science, Aarhus University, Denmark.

2.4. Experimental Design

The *Salmonella* Typhimurium strain in this study was obtained from the field study [25]: *S.* Typhimurium (antigenic formula: 1,4,5,12:i:1,2, Phage type DT 193). Three consecutive trials of the infection experiment followed in accordance with the same investigation scheme (Figure 1). For the experiment carried out after a one-week adaptation period, all piglets were orally infected (day 0) with 2 mL of a broth containing ~ 1×10^7 colony-forming units (CFU) *S.* Typhimurium/animal directly into the throat using a drencher as already described [26].

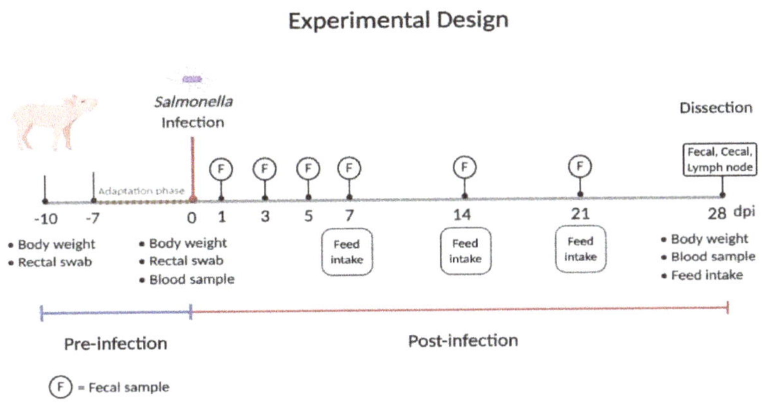

Figure 1. Overview concerning the time and sample plan for *Salmonella* diagnostics.

After the infection, animals were used in a 28-day experiment to determine the effects of control (69% wheat) or experimental group (69% rye) in complete pelleted feed, and to determine a possible effect of the diets on the duration of and level of *Salmonella* excretion. Fecal samples of the piglets were examined microbiologically for *Salmonella* species at defined time points (at 1, 3, 5, 7, 14, 21 and 28 days post-infection (dpi), as shown in Figure 1) to evaluate the status of the *Salmonella* infection. At the end of the experimental period (28 dpi), cecal chyme and lymph nodes were tested for *Salmonella*.

During the experimental phase, performance parameters, i.e., feed intake, were recorded on a weekly basis (Figure 1). To prevent cross-contamination between the animals during the infection, animals were weighed before the infection (0 dpi) and again at the end of the experiment (28 dpi; Figure 1). Corresponding parameters, average body weight gain (BWG) and feed conversion ratio (FCR) were determined.

In accordance with standardized *Salmonella* diagnostics, a blood sample was taken from each animal on the day of the experimental infection and at the end of the experiment (Figure 1). Serum was examined serologically for specific antibodies against *Salmonella*; *Salmonella* antibody ELISA (IDEXX Swine *Salmonella* antibody Test, IDEXX Europe B.V., Hoofddorp, the Netherlands) was used. The cut-off value was ≥10% optical density (OD).

2.5. Bacteriological Analyses and Salmonella Detection

Samples were taken for bacteriological analysis, and bacterial counts were determined for *Salmonella* detection. All test sections were carried out following the DIN EN ISO 6579-1 and 6579-2 guidelines [27,28]. Briefly, all collected samples were first placed for pre-enrichment in buffered peptone water (BPW; Oxoid Deutschland GmbH, Wesel, Germany), the ratio of which was 1:10, based on the volume of fecal or cecal chyme sample or the mass of the lymph node. For the next process of qualitative analysis, an incubation overnight at 37 °C took place. Each BPW-inoculated sample was placed with three drops (100 µL/drop) on modified semisolid Rappaport–Vassiliadis agar (MSRV; Oxoid Deutschland GmbH, Wesel, Germany) and incubated for a further 24 h (h) at 41 °C. After the incubation period, the evaluation was carried out macroscopically. If the result was positive, a white-grayish cloudy swarming zone spread over the entire agar resulting from the drops. Suspected *Salmonella* samples were also spread on the second selective nutrient media, xylose lysine deoxycholate agar (XLD; Oxoid Deutschland GmbH, Wesel, Germany) and Brilliance Salmonella agar (Oxoid Deutschland GmbH, Wesel, Germany) so that a confirmed result could be read after a 24 h incubation period.

In addition, *Salmonella* quantitative analysis of the fecal and cecal contents was performed as previously described [28,29]. Due to the high number of samples, a most probable number (MPN) method was used. One gram of the homogenized fecal or cecal content and 9 mL of BPW were vortexed. The bacterial count of the sample material was determined by a serial dilution with BPW in a deep well block (Sarstedt AG & Co, Nümbrecht, Germany). Quantitative proof of the dilution steps in a microtiter plate (Sarstedt AG & Co, Nümbrecht, Germany) was carried out in triplicate, as already described in detail [26]. After a 24 h incubation at 37 °C, the total volume of each well was transferred to another deep well block filled with MSRV agar and incubated for 24 h at 41 °C. The results were confirmed by cultural cultivation on Brilliance Salmonella agar, and subsequently the number of bacteria was calculated by an MPN software program [30]. To confirm the experimentally used *Salmonella* strain, salmonella-like colonies on Brilliance Salmonella agar were finally excluded by serotyping.

2.6. Statistical Analysis

The SAS software package version 7.1 (SAS Institute, Cary, NC, USA) was used for the statistical evaluation. The evaluation was carried out in cooperation with the Institute for Biometry, Epidemiology and Information Processing of the University of Veterinary Medicine Hannover, Foundation. Measurements such as mean values and standard deviations were calculated for the descriptive statistics. *Salmonella* results and performance parameters, i.e., body weight and feed intake, were analyzed at the level of the individual animal.

For evaluating the quantitative parameters between the control and experimental groups, two-way analysis of variance (ANOVA) with group and trial as independent factors was conducted. For analysis differences concerning distribution in qualitative parameters (*Salmonella* detection in cecal content, etc.), the chi-squared homogeneity test was used. Differences with a significant level of $p < 0.05$ were considered significant.

3. Results

3.1. Salmonella Prevalence

The results of this study demonstrated that at the beginning of the post-infection period (1, 3, 5, 7 dpi), all the pigs were colonized. There were no significant differences in mean bacterial counts ($\log_{10}$ ± SD) of *Salmonella* in the feces between the wheat and rye groups. A peak in *Salmonella* shedding occurred at day 5 after infection in our study. However, at day 14 onwards after infection, feeding a pellet diet containing 69% rye was associated with a significantly lower bacterial count of *Salmonella* in fecal samples than in those taken from the group fed with 69% wheat in the diet, as shown in Figure 2 and in detail in Table S1 (control and experimental, 14 dpi: $3.30^{a} \pm 0.50$ and $2.62^{b} \pm 0.18$ ($p < 0.001$), 21 dpi: $3.11^{a} \pm 0.36$ and $2.40^{b} \pm 0.65$ ($p < 0.001$), 28 dpi: $3.02^{a} \pm 0.45$ and $2.36^{b} \pm 0.57$ ($p = 0.001$), respectively).

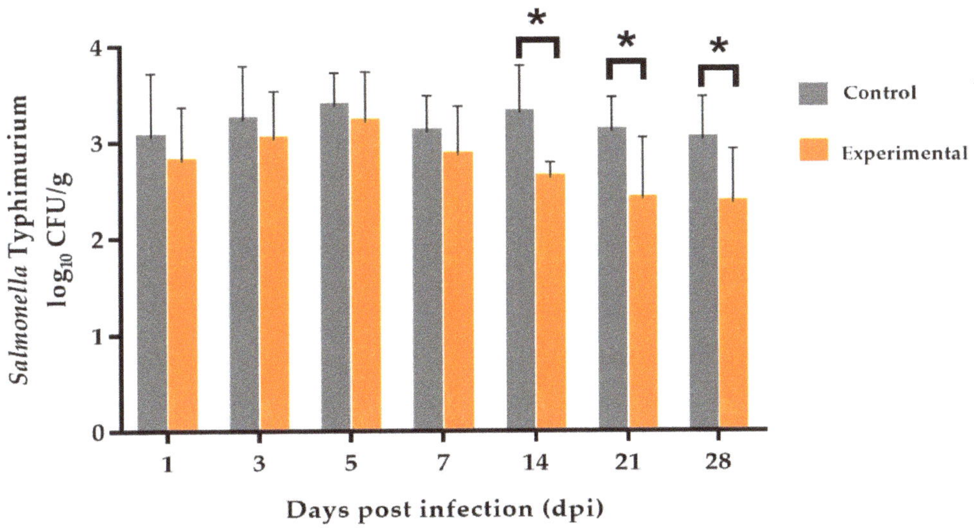

Figure 2. Counts of *Salmonella* ($\log_{10}$ CFU/g fecal sample) of piglets after an experimental oral infection with *S.* Typhimurium in different diets. Means of bacterial counts between the control (69% wheat) and experimental (69% rye) groups differ significantly (* $p < 0.05$).

After oral infection with *S.* Typhimurium, different diets had significant influence on the counts of *Salmonella* in the cecal content (Table 3). The bacterial counts in the cecal content also differed significantly ($\log_{10}$ CFU/g; control group: 3.34 ± 0.50, experimental: 3.08 ± 0.56; $p = 0.038$; Table 3).

However, cecal content and ileocecal lymph node samples were qualitatively *Salmonella* positive (control: 100% and 61.9% and experimental: 100% and 66.7%, respectively; Table 3), but no differences could be seen between the two groups.

Table 3. Number of *Salmonella*-positive samples from cecal content and ileocecal lymph nodes at dissection after oral infection with *S.* Typhimurium.

Sample	*Salmonella* Test	Control	Experimental
Cecal content	Quantitative $\log_{10}$ CFU/g	$3.34^{a} \pm 0.50$	$3.08^{b} \pm 0.56$
	Qualitative (n_{pos}/n_{total})	$21^{a}/21$	$21^{a}/21$
Lymph nodes	Qualitative (n_{pos}/n_{total})	$13^{a}/21$	$14^{a}/21$

^{a,b} Means in a row with different superscripts differ significantly between groups ($p < 0.05$). n_{pos} = number of positive samples, n_{total} = number of total samples.

Three consecutive experiments were conducted using piglets from different sows. The results of the counts of *Salmonella* ($\log_{10}$ CFU/g fecal sample) for different trials and different diets are shown in Table 4. After initial statistical evaluations, a marked effect for the factor trial was shown, with significant effects at 1 dpi ($p < 0.001$), 7 dpi ($p = 0.036$), 21 dpi ($p = 0.001$) and 28 dpi ($p < 0.001$). An effect of diet seems to be present for days 14 ($p < 0.001$), 21 ($p < 0.001$) and 28 ($p < 0.001$) after infection. In addition, a bacterial count for *Salmonella* in cecal content was significantly affected by the diet ($p = 0.035$). Interestingly, the two-way analysis of variance (ANOVA) showed significant interactions between the factors diet and trial, which were observed for days 5 and 7 ($p = 0.011$ and $p = 0.041$, respectively; Table 4). On the other hand, there was not a significant effect of the type of diet by the trial interaction at day 3 after infection ($p = 0.188$; Table 4).

Table 4. Counts of *Salmonella* ($\log_{10}$ CFU/g fecal sample) of piglets after an experimental oral infection with *Salmonella* Typhimurium for different trials and different diets.

Time Point	Trial						*p*-Value		
	Trial 1		Trial 2		Trial 3				
	Diet								
	Con	Exp	Con	Exp	Con	Exp	Trial	Diet	Trial x Diet
1 dpi	2.46 ^{b} ± 0.40	2.46 ^{b} ± 0.50	2.97 ^{b} ± 0.53	2.46 ^{b} ± 0.10	3.71 ^{a} ± 0.36	3.49 ^{a} ± 0.11	**<0.001**	0.089	0.206
3 dpi	3.00 ^{a} ± 0.58	3.14 ^{a} ± 0.73	3.20 ^{a} ± 0.77	2.63 ^{a} ± 0.18	3.49 ^{a} ± 0.11	3.29 ^{a} ± 0.20	0.054	0.187	0.188
5 dpi	3.29 ^{ab} ± 0.23	3.66 ^{a} ± 0.55	3.51 ^{ab} ± 0.43	2.94 ^{b} ± 0.36	3.31 ^{ab} ± 0.38	3.00 ^{b} ± 0.40	0.111	0.176	**0.011**
7 dpi	3.01 ^{ab} ± 0.39	3.23 ^{a} ± 0.64	2.94 ^{b} ± 0.41	2.54 ^{b} ± 0.10	3.34 ^{a} ± 0.25	2.80 ^{b} ± 0.42	**0.036**	0.059	**0.041**
14 dpi	3.40 ^{a} ± 0.85	2.71 ^{b} ± 0.28	3.23 ^{a} ± 0.21	2.57 ^{b} ± 0.08	3.29 ^{a} ± 0.20	2.57 ^{b} ± 0.08	0.524	**<0.001**	0.981
21 dpi	2.71 ^{ab} ± 0.28	2.00 ^{c} ± 1.05	3.40 ^{a} ± 0.00	2.57 ^{b} ± 0.08	3.23 ^{ab} ± 0.21	2.63 ^{b} ± 0.18	**0.001**	**<0.001**	0.807
28 dpi (Dissection)	2.43 ^{b} ± 0.08	1.97 ^{c} ± 0.90	3.34 ^{a} ± 0.15	2.54 ^{b} ± 0.10	3.29 ^{a} ± 0.20	2.57 ^{b} ± 0.08	**<0.001**	**<0.001**	0.478
Cecal content	3.48 ^{a} ± 0.86	3.09 ^{b} ± 0.97	3.43 ^{a} ± 0.08	2.99 ^{b} ± 0.23	3.43 ^{a} ± 0.08	3.17 ^{b} ± 0.21	0.883	**0.035**	0.888

^{a,b,c} Different subscripts within a row mark significant differences ($p < 0.05$). Con (control): animals fed with 69% wheat compound pelleted diet; Exp (experimental): animals fed with 69% rye compound pelleted diet.

3.2. Serological Test for Specific Antibodies Against Salmonella

Optical density (OD)% was used to determine the *Salmonella* antibody status in blood samples from piglets. In both groups, on the day before infection, all of the pigs were seronegative. At day 28 after infection, regarding the number of positive blood samples from piglets, there was no significant difference in seroprevalence detected between the groups ($p > 0.05$; Table S2).

3.3. Animal Performance

As a result of the evaluations carried out, there were no significant differences in the performance parameters between the groups. During the experimental period, before and after infection, there were no significant differences in the body weight (BW), as shown in Figure 3 and in detail in Table 5 and Supplementary Table S3. Furthermore, feed intake was measured individually for the entire trial period. Differences between the groups regarding the mean weekly feed intake (FI) were not statistically significant (control and experimental; mean FI at week 5 (21–28 dpi, in kg): 9.78 ^{a} ± 1.52 and 9.40 ^{a} ± 1.48; $p = 0.136$; Figure 3 and Table S3).

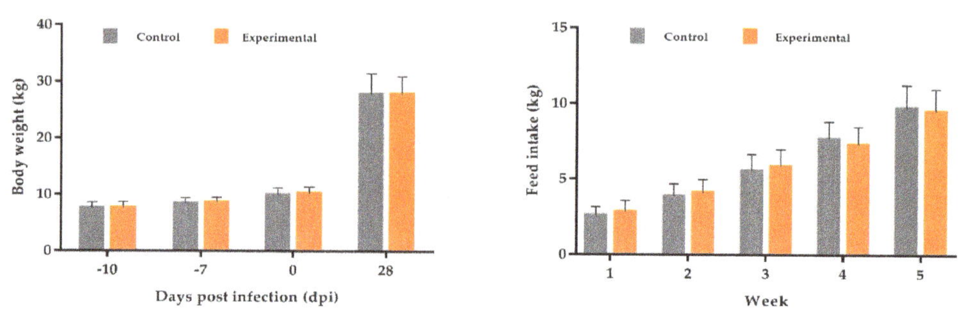

Figure 3. Performance data during the entire experimental period.

Table 5. Performance data during the experiments with experimental *Salmonella* infection, in kg.

Parameter	Group		p-Value
	Control (n = 21)	Experimental (n = 21)	
Body weight (0 dpi)	9.89 [a] ± 1.28	10.1 [a] ± 1.31	0.085
Body weight (28 dpi)	27.8 [a] ± 3.72	27.7 [a] ± 3.28	0.980
BWG/piglet (0–28 dpi)	17.9 [a] ± 2.54	17.6 [a] ± 2.29	0.847
BWG/group (0–28 dpi)	376 [a] ± 2.54	370 [a] ± 2.29	0.229
ADG (g/d)	639 [a] ± 3.12	629 [a] ± 2.75	0.079
Total feed intake (0–28 dpi)	564 [a] ± 3.93	560 [a] ± 4.11	0.126
FCR (kg/kg)	1.50 [a] ± 0.07	1.51 [a] ± 0.13	0.786

[a] Means ± SD within the same row with same superscripts do not differ significantly ($p > 0.05$). Control: animals fed with 69% wheat compound pelleted diet; Experimental: animals fed with 69% rye compound pelleted diet. dpi = day after infection; BWG = body weight gain, ADG = average daily weight gain, FCR = feed conversion ratio.

Table 5 summarizes the performance data during the experiments with experimental *Salmonella* infection from the day before infection (0 dpi) to the day of dissection (28 dpi). No significant differences were noted between the groups for BW at each time point (0 dpi (p = 0.085) and 28 dpi (p = 0.980)) and body weight gain (BWG; Table 5). The average daily weight gain (ADG) in the control group was about 639 g and in the experimental group, 629 g (Table 5). Similarly, the feed conversion ratio (FCR = feed requirement in kg per kg BWG) was not significantly affected between the wheat and rye diet groups (1.50 and 1.51, respectively).

4. Discussion

In recent years, the interest in rye has increased in terms of its good sustainability [31]. However, the use of rye in large amounts in diets for pig production is not typical because it can be associated with ergot poisoning [32]. On the other hand, rye has a high dietary fiber content [17], the fraction of NSPs in rye being more fermentable for monogastric animals than is the case for other cereals [13]. Nowadays, varieties of rye have been developed which reduce its susceptibility to ergot contamination; therefore, we can include rye in diets for swine [11,33].

The present study shows results of a feeding concept in young pigs fed with a high proportion of rye, and its effects on *Salmonella* prevalence, along with analyzing its effects on performance. In terms of *Salmonella* shedding, a significant reduction in the number of bacterial counts of *Salmonella* was seen in feces from 14 day onwards when considering the entire infection period for the experimental group. Feeding a diet containing 69% rye to young pigs may play a significant role in reducing *Salmonella* shedding after infection. In addition, the prevalence of *Salmonella* was found to be significantly lower in the cecal chyme of pigs fed with rye diets. Hence, if there was a reduction in the incidence of *Salmonella* in feces of pigs, which is the most likely source of contamination in the pig production chain, then it may help to reduce the risk of human salmonellosis.

To our knowledge, fermented rye has been previously studied to control *Salmonella* in nursery pigs [34]. Fabà et al. [34] reported that pigs fed with organic acids combined with fermented rye had reduced *S.* Typhimurium shedding compared to pigs fed with organic acids plus coated butyrate (3.11 and 3.87 $\log_{10}$ CFU/g, respectively) over the 21 d period post-challenge with 10^9 CFU/mL. However, the pigs in our study were infected with 10^7 CFU of *S.* Typhimurium, so comparison across infection studies is difficult. In this respect, an infection dosage in the present study could provide more opportunities to determine the effects of diet, which corroborates with other studies [8,35,36]. The *S.* Typhimurium oral challenge resulted in an effective infection in our study. At the beginning of the trial, all the pigs in the study showed a *Salmonella*-negative result. Then, after oral infection, nearly all infected animals excreted *Salmonella* until the end of the study. In addition, it is assumed that the challenge dose in practice or natural infection is often established with low or moderate numbers of *Salmonella* when compared with our study [36]. However, the scientific literature on the usefulness of a high proportion of rye in diets in a dry and pelleted form for *Salmonella* reduction in livestock animals, specifically young pigs, is scarce.

A reduction in *Salmonella* shedding in pigs in this study was possibly related to the components in rye such as dietary fiber, including NSPs. Compared to the total concentration of NSPs and arabinoxylans between groups, the mean concentration was higher in rye in the present study. The concentration of total NSPs was 123 g/kg dry matter (DM) in wheat and 140 g/kg DM in rye. In addition, the mean concentration of arabinoxylans was 63 g/kg DM and 74 g/kg DM in wheat and rye diets, respectively (Table 2). The concentrations of carbohydrate fractions in wheat and rye were in general agreement with those values of previous studies [17,18]. The NSP content of rye has traditionally been put forward to explain the effects on gut health benefits for pigs, especially arabinoxylans (8–9%) and fructans (approximately 3% and range up to about 6%) [33,37]. Rye has greater concentrations of arabinoxylans and fructans than other cereal grains [38,39] that can be changed by microorganisms to butyrate in the digestive tract [10,17].

According to Wilke [14], the effects in terms of nutritional physiology have been evaluated. In the group with 69% rye in the diet, significantly higher concentrations of lactate in the anterior digestive tract were found, as well as an increased entry of fermentable organic substances in the large intestine (approx. 35% higher butyrate concentrations) in the ingesta of cecum and colon, the preferred colonization area of *Salmonella*, in comparison to those animals given a wheat-based diet [22]. How rye affects *Salmonella* colonization is unclear. Consequently, the antimicrobial effects of lactate and butyrate seem to play an important role against *Salmonella* [14]. High butyrate concentrations in the hindgut have been found when a high amount of rye in diets is given to young pigs [14]. The focus on the mechanism of action of butyrate in reducing *Salmonella* has been explained in various studies [7,9,19,40,41]; similar mechanisms possibly play a role in our study. Further investigations are needed to better elucidate the *Salmonella* shedding reduction and other health-promoting mechanisms potentially associated with rye on the physiological processes in the gastrointestinal tract and the stability of the intestinal microbiota of pigs.

Less fecal *Salmonella* excretion indicates less colonization of *Salmonella* in the intestine and reduced severity of the infection [42,43]. In addition, in our study, the lymph node was used to confirm colonization. A translocation of *Salmonella* from the intestine into the adjacent ileocecal lymph nodes was investigated in all experimental runs. The piglets were totally *Salmonella* positive at the time of dissection (in cecal chyme), but positive evidence in lymph nodes was found in twenty-seven of a total of forty-two animals (control: n = 13; experimental: n = 14). Less is known about the role of rye in the translocation effect of *Salmonella* in the pig model. However, in previous experiments with poultry, this was determined with other pathogens such as *Escherichia coli* and *Clostridium perfringens* [44,45]. When observing the elevated bacteria translocation while feeding a diet rich in NSPs [44], the prolonged transit time of the intestinal contents possibly induces proliferation of pathogenic bacteria. Moreover, Tellez et al. [45] also reported that a rye diet negatively influences bacterial translocation and intestinal viscosity in poultry. Nevertheless, the viscosity does not pose a large problem in swine as much as in poultry [46].

The outcome of the current study showed that the use of compound feeds with higher dietary proportions of rye in young pigs caused no significant differences in performance, i.e., average body weight gain, feed intake and feed conversion ratio compared with those of animals fed with generally high amounts of wheat. Similar results were obtained by Grone [15] and Wilke [14], who observed no negative impact on growth performance when young pigs were fed diets containing a high proportion of rye. Previous studies have shown positive effects of feeding rye on performance data [46–48]. Among the beneficial effects of the dietary fiber components in rye, it can provide energy to the pig mostly via the digestion of starch and fermentation of fiber in the hindgut. Moreover, the NSPs in rye may promote greater butyrate production and improve intestinal health [33]. Furthermore, scientific studies have evaluated the feed digestibility in pigs concerning diets containing rye [48]. The rye-based diets had higher digestibility coefficients for dry matter, crude protein and gross energy than barley when rye was included in a young growing pig diet at 60% [49]. Thacker et al. [46] suggest that rye may have much more potential in pig performance when administered in pellet form. Furthermore, to improve feed efficiency and average daily gain, the NSP enzyme would be recommended for diets containing high rye levels [47]. Contrary to the present results, a previous study on the use of rye in pig feeding reported that if more than 50% of the barley or wheat in a swine diet was replaced with rye, a significant reduction in pig performance was observed [50]. The reason for rye being less palatable is that it is more bitter than other small grains such as wheat [51]. Alkylresorcinols in rye may be responsible for the unpleasant taste, but reduced levels of alkylresorcinols are found in hybrid rye [11].

5. Conclusions

The results of this study support the view that a high proportion of rye might contribute to reducing *Salmonella* shedding via feces in young pigs. In addition, overall, the animal performance was good, so that no relevant differences could be observed between the rye and wheat diets. It can be suggested that up to 70% rye in compound pelleted feed poses no problem for animal health and welfare, additionally decreasing possible contamination with *Salmonella*. Another advantage that puts rye in a better light today than in the past is its sustainable benefits, namely, it needs less fertilizer, demands substantially less water, can reduce CO_2 emissions in pork production in comparison with wheat [52] and its price, as it is an inexpensive raw feed material compared to other cereals [11].

Nonetheless, to our knowledge, this is the first time that high amounts of rye were used in a *Salmonella* challenge in a young pig model. Furthermore, our results can provide useful information, prompting further studies of a field trial on a commercial pig farm or large-scale farming study over a longer period, not only in young pigs, but also in all phases of pig production. However, we cannot consider all factors when only a small group of pigs are observed. Therefore, research is needed to better understand the gut and fecal microbiota composition underlying the effects observed when a high proportion of rye is fed to pigs.

Supplementary Materials
Table S1: Counts of *Salmonella* (log_{10} CFU/g fecal sample) of piglets after an experimental oral infection with *Salmonella* Typhimurium for different diets. Table S2: *Salmonella* antibody status in serum of piglets in control and experimental groups. Table S3: Performance data during the entire experimental period.

Author Contributions: Conceptualization, R.G., A.v.F., J.K. and C.V.; Methodology, B.C., V.W., C.B.H., A.A.E.-W., J.K. and C.V.; Validation, B.C., V.W. and C.V.; Formal analysis, B.C. and C.V.; Investigation, B.C., V.W. and C.V.; Resources, C.V.; Data curation, B.C., V.W. and C.V.; Writing—original draft preparation, B.C., V.W. and C.V.; Writing—review and editing, B.C., V.W., C.B.H., A.A.E.-W., R.G., A.v.F., J.K. and C.V.; Visualization, B.C., V.W. and C.V.; Supervision, J.K. and C.V.; Project administration, C.B.H. and C.V.; Funding acquisition, J.K. and C.V. All authors have read and agreed to the published version of the manuscript.

Acknowledgments: We would like to thank the colleagues and animal keepers from the Institute for Animal Nutrition, University of Veterinary Medicine Hannover, Foundation for their support. In addition, we would like to thank Frances Sherwood-Brock for proof-reading the manuscript to ensure correct English.

References

1. WHO. Salmonella (non-typhoidal): Fact Sheets. Available online: https://www.who.int/en/news-room/fact-sheets/detail/salmonella-(non-typhoidal) (accessed on 11 March 2020).
2. Rosner, B.M.; Meinen, A.; Schmich, P.; Zeisler, M.-L.; Stark, K. Population-based food consumption survey as an additional tool for foodborne outbreak investigations, Germany, 2017. *Epidemiol. Infect.* **2020**, *148*. [CrossRef] [PubMed]
3. Rettenbacher-Riefler, S.; Ziehm, D.; Kreienbrock, L.; Campe, A.; Pulz, M.; Dreesman, J. Sporadic salmonellosis in Lower Saxony, Germany, 2011–2013: Raw ground pork consumption is associated with Salmonella

Typhimurium infections and foreign travel with Salmonella Enteritidis infections. *Epidemiol. Infect.* **2015**, *143*, 2777–2785. [CrossRef] [PubMed]
4. RKI. *Infektionsepidemiologisches Jahrbuch Meldepflichtiger Krankheiten für 2018*; Robert Koch Institute: Berlin, Germany, 2018; pp. 210–213.
5. WHO. *Global Antimicrobial Resistance Surveillance System (GLASS) Report: Early Implementation 2017–2018*; World Health Organization: Geneva, Switzerland, 2018.
6. Callegari, M.; Dalto, D.; Da Silva, C. A review of prevention and control methods of Salmonella species in swine production the role of dietary non-nutritional additives. *Asian J. Anim. Vet. Adv.* **2015**, *10*, 803–829. [CrossRef]
7. Visscher, C.; Winter, P.; Verspohl, J.; Stratmann-Selke, J.; Upmann, M.; Beyerbach, M.; Kamphues, J. Effects of feed particle size at dietary presence of added organic acids on caecal parameters and the prevalence of Salmonella in fattening pigs on farm and at slaughter. *J. Anim. Physiol. Anim. Nutr.* **2009**, *93*, 423–430. [CrossRef] [PubMed]
8. Boyen, F.; Haesebrouck, F.; Vanparys, A.; Volf, J.; Mahu, M.; Van Immerseel, F.; Rychlik, I.; Dewulf, J.; Ducatelle, R.; Pasmans, F. Coated fatty acids alter virulence properties of Salmonella Typhimurium and decrease intestinal colonization of pigs. *Vet. Microbiol.* **2008**, *132*, 319–327. [CrossRef]
9. Van Immerseel, F.; Russell, J.; Flythe, M.; Gantois, I.; Timbermont, L.; Pasmans, F.; Haesebrouck, F.; Ducatelle, R. The use of organic acids to combat Salmonella in poultry: A mechanistic explanation of the efficacy. *Avian Pathol.* **2006**, *35*, 182–188. [CrossRef]
10. Bederska-Łojewska, D.; Świątkiewicz, S.; Arczewska-Włosek, A.; Schwarz, T. Rye non-starch polysaccharides: Their impact on poultry intestinal physiology, nutrients digestibility and performance indices–a review. *Ann. Anim. Sci.* **2017**, *17*, 351–369. [CrossRef]
11. Schwarz, T.; Kuleta, W.; Turek, A.; Tuz, R.; Nowicki, J.; Rudzki, B.; Bartlewski, P.M. Assessing the efficiency of using a modern hybrid rye cultivar for pig fattening, with emphasis on production costs and carcass quality. *Anim.Prod. Sci.* **2015**, *55*, 467–473. [CrossRef]
12. Miedaner, T.; Geiger, H.H. Biology, genetics, and management of ergot (Claviceps spp.) in rye, sorghum, and pearl millet. *Toxins* **2015**, *7*, 659–678. [CrossRef]
13. Bach Knudsen, K.E. Fiber and nonstarch polysaccharide content and variation in common crops used in broiler diets. *Poult. Sci.* **2014**, *93*, 2380–2393. [CrossRef]
14. Wilke, V. Effects of increasing rye or rye and rapeseed meal (extracted) levels in diets for young pigs regarding digestibility and performance as well as diverse properties (milieu/substrate) of the digesta in the alimentary tract. Ph.D. Thesis, University of Veterinary Medicine Hannover, Hanover, Germany, 2020.
15. Grone, R. Zur Bedeutung physiko-chemischer Eigenschaften von Futtergetreide (Weizen, Roggen, Gerste) für die Herstellung und Verwendung in Mischfuttermitteln für Schweine. Ph.D. Thesis, University of Veterinary Medicine Hannover, Hanover, Germany, 2018.
16. Bach Knudsen, K.E. Nutritional modulation to improve health and welfare. In *Poultry and Pig Nutrition: Challenges of the 21st Century*; Hendriks, W.H., Verstegen, M.V.A., Babinszky, L., Eds.; Wageningen Academic Publishers: Wageningen, The Netherlands, 2019; pp. 87–96.
17. Rodehutscord, M.; Rückert, C.; Maurer, H.P.; Schenkel, H.; Schipprack, W.; Bach Knudsen, K.E.; Schollenberger, M.; Laux, M.; Eklund, M.; Siegert, W. Variation in chemical composition and physical characteristics of cereal grains from different genotypes. *Arch. Anim. Nutr.* **2016**, *70*, 87–107. [CrossRef] [PubMed]
18. Glitsø, L.; Brunsgaard, G.; Højsgaard, S.; Sandström, B.; Knudsen, K.B. Intestinal degradation in pigs of rye dietary fibre with different structural characteristics. *Br. J. Nutr.* **1998**, *80*, 457–468. [CrossRef]
19. Gantois, I.; Ducatelle, R.; Pasmans, F.; Haesebrouck, F.; Hautefort, I.; Thompson, A.; Hinton, J.; Van Immerseel, F. Butyrate specifically down-regulates Salmonella pathogenicity island 1 gene expression. *Appl. Environ. Microbiol.* **2006**, *72*, 946–949. [CrossRef] [PubMed]
20. Lawhon, S.D.; Maurer, R.; Suyemoto, M.; Altier, C. Intestinal short-chain fatty acids alter Salmonella typhimurium invasion gene expression and virulence through BarA/SirA. *Mol. Microbiol.* **2002**, *46*, 1451–1464. [CrossRef] [PubMed]
21. Mahu, M.; Boyen, F.; Ducatelle, R.; Decostere, A.; Van Immerseel, F.; Haesebrouck, F.; Pasmans, F. Short-and medium-chain fatty acids influence Salmonella Typhimurium virulence gene expression. In Proceedings of The International Symposium Salmonella and Salmonellosis, Saint-Malo, France, 10–12 May 2016; p. 297.

22. Carter, P.B.; Collins, F.M. The route of enteric infection in normal mice. *J. Exp. Med.* **1974**, *139*, 1189–1203. [CrossRef]
23. Naumann, C.; Bassler, R. *Methoden der landwirtschaftlichen Forschungs-und Untersuchungsanstalt, Biochemische Untersuchung von Futtermitteln. Methodenbuch III (einschließlich der achten Ergänzungen)*; VDLUFA: Darmstadt, Germany, 2012.
24. Wolf, P.; Arlinghaus, M.; Kamphues, J.; Sauer, N.; Mosenthin, R. Einfluss der Partikelgröße im Futter auf die Nährstoffverdaulichkeit und Leistung beim Schwein. *Übersichten zur Tierernährung* **2012**, *40*, 21–64.
25. Visscher, C.; Klein, G.; Verspohl, J.; Beyerbach, M.; Stratmann-Selke, J.; Kamphues, J. Serodiversity and serological as well as cultural distribution of Salmonella on farms and in abattoirs in Lower Saxony, Germany. *Int. J. Food Microbiol.* **2011**, *146*, 44–51. [CrossRef]
26. Buch, J.-M. Studies regarding the effects of the addition of a combination of different monoglycerides to compound feed on the success of experimental infection with Salmonella Typhimurium and on translocation in weaned piglets. Ph.D. Thesis, University of Veterinary Medicine Hannover, Hanover, Germany, 2019.
27. DIN ISO 6579-1:2017—Mikrobiologie der Lebensmittelkette-Horizontales Verfahren zum Nachweis, zur Zählung und zur Serotypisierung von Salmonellen. Teil 1: Horizontales Verfahren zum Nachweis von Salmonella spp. 2017. Available online: https://dx.doi.org/10.31030/2359254 (accessed on 20 December 2019).
28. DIN ISO 6579-2:2012—Mikrobiologie von Lebensmitteln und Futtermitteln-Horizontales Verfahren zum Nachweis, zur Zählung und zur Serotypisierung von Salmonellen. Teil 2: Zählung unter Anwendung eines miniaturisierten Verfahrens der wahrscheinlichsten Keimzahl. 2012. Available online: https://dx.doi.org/10.31030/1856259 (accessed on 20 December 2019).
29. Jarvis, B.; Wilrich, C.; Wilrich, P.T. Reconsideration of the derivation of Most Probable Numbers, their standard deviations, confidence bounds and rarity values. *J. Appl. Microbiol.* **2010**, *109*, 1660–1667. [CrossRef]
30. MPN Software Programme. Available online: http://standards.iso.org/iso/ts/6579/-2/ (accessed on 20 December 2019).
31. Abd El-Wahab, A.; Lingens, J.B.; Chuppava, B.; Ahmed, M.F.E.; Osman, A.; Langeheine, M.; Brehm, R.; Taube, V.; Grone, R.; von Felde, A.; et al. Impact of Rye Inclusion in Diets for Broilers on Performance, Litter Quality, Foot Pad Health, Digesta Viscosity, Organ Traits and Intestinal Morphology. *Sustainability* **2020**, *12*, 7753. [CrossRef]
32. Friend, D.; MacIntyre, T. Effect of rye ergot on growth and N-retention in growing pigs. *Can. J. Comp. Med.* **1970**, *34*, 198.
33. Bach Knudsen, K.E. Carbohydrate and lignin contents of plant materials used in animal feeding. *Anim. Feed Sci. Tech.* **1997**, *67*, 319–338. [CrossRef]
34. Fabà, L.; Litjens, R.; Allaart, J.; van den Hil, P.R. Feed additive blends fed to nursery pigs challenged with Salmonella. *J. Anim. Sci.* **2020**, *98*, skz382. [CrossRef]
35. Michiels, J.; Missotten, J.; Rasschaert, G.; Dierick, N.; Heyndrickx, M.; De Smet, S. Effect of organic acids on Salmonella colonization and shedding in weaned piglets in a seeder model. *J. Food Prot.* **2012**, *75*, 1974–1983. [CrossRef] [PubMed]
36. Boyen, F.; Pasmans, F.; Van Immerseel, F.; Donne, E.; Morgan, E.; Ducatelle, R.; Haesebrouck, F. Porcine in vitro and in vivo models to assess the virulence of Salmonella enterica serovar Typhimurium for pigs. *Lab. Anim.* **2009**, *43*, 46–52. [CrossRef] [PubMed]
37. Verspreet, J.; Dornez, E.; Van den Ende, W.; Delcour, J.A.; Courtin, C.M. Cereal grain fructans: Structure, variability and potential health effects. *Trends Food Sci. Tech.* **2015**, *43*, 32–42. [CrossRef]
38. Jürgens, H.-U.; Jansen, G.; Wegener, C.B. Characterisation of several rye cultivars with respect to arabinoxylans and extract viscosity. *J. Agric. Sci.* **2012**, *4*, 1–12. [CrossRef]
39. Hansen, H.B.; Rasmussen, C.V.; Bach Knudsen, K.E.; Hansen, Å. Effects of genotype and harvest year on content and composition of dietary fibre in rye (Secale cereale L) grain. *J. Sci. Food Agric.* **2003**, *83*, 76–85. [CrossRef]
40. De Ridder, L.; Maes, D.; Dewulf, J.; Pasmans, F.; Boyen, F.; Haesebrouck, F.; Méroc, E.; Butaye, P.; Van der Stede, Y. Evaluation of three intervention strategies to reduce the transmission of Salmonella Typhimurium in pigs. *Vet. J.* **2013**, *197*, 613–618. [CrossRef]
41. Walia, K.; Argüello, H.; Lynch, H.; Leonard, F.C.; Grant, J.; Yearsley, D.; Kelly, S.; Duffy, G.; Gardiner, G.E.; Lawlor, P.G. Effect of feeding sodium butyrate in the late finishing period on Salmonella carriage, seroprevalence, and growth of finishing pigs. *Prev. Vet. Med.* **2016**, *131*, 79–86. [CrossRef]

42. Knetter, S.M.; Bearson, S.M.; Huang, T.-H.; Kurkiewicz, D.; Schroyen, M.; Nettleton, D.; Berman, D.; Cohen, V.; Lunney, J.K.; Ramer-Tait, A.E. Salmonella enterica serovar Typhimurium-infected pigs with different shedding levels exhibit distinct clinical, peripheral cytokine and transcriptomic immune response phenotypes. *Innate Immun.* **2015**, *21*, 227–241. [CrossRef]
43. Casanova-Higes, A.; Andrés-Barranco, S.; Mainar-Jaime, R. Influence of on-farm pig salmonella status on salmonella shedding at slaughter. *Zoonoses Public Health* **2017**, *64*, 328–336. [CrossRef] [PubMed]
44. Latorre, J.; Hernandez-Velasco, X.; Bielke, L.; Vicente, J.; Wolfenden, R.; Menconi, A.; Hargis, B.; Tellez, G. Evaluation of a Bacillus direct-fed microbial candidate on digesta viscosity, bacterial translocation, microbiota composition and bone mineralisation in broiler chickens fed on a rye-based diet. *Br. Poult. Sci.* **2015**, *56*, 723–732. [CrossRef] [PubMed]
45. Tellez, G.; Latorre, J.D.; Kuttappan, V.A.; Kogut, M.H.; Wolfenden, A.; Hernandez-Velasco, X.; Hargis, B.M.; Bottje, W.G.; Bielke, L.R.; Faulkner, O.B. Utilization of rye as energy source affects bacterial translocation, intestinal viscosity, microbiota composition, and bone mineralization in broiler chickens. *Front. Genet.* **2014**, *5*. [CrossRef] [PubMed]
46. Thacker, P.A.; McLeod, J.G.; Campbell, G.L. Performance of Growing-Finishing Pigs Fed Diets Based on Normal or Low Viscosity Rye Fed With and Without Enzyme Supplementation. *Arch. Anim. Nutr.* **2002**, *56*, 361–370. [CrossRef]
47. Smit, M.N.; Zhou, X.; Landero, J.L.; Young, M.G.; Beltranena, E. Increasing hybrid rye level substituting wheat grain with or without enzyme on growth performance and carcass traits of growing-finishing barrows and gilts. *Trans. Anim. Sci.* **2019**, *3*, 1561–1574. [CrossRef]
48. McGhee, M.L.; Stein, H.H. Apparent and standardized ileal digestibility of AA and starch in hybrid rye, barley, wheat, and corn fed to growing pigs. *J. Anim. Sci.* **2018**, *96*, 3319–3329. [CrossRef]
49. Thacker, P.; Campbell, G.; Scoles, G. Performance of young growing pigs (17-34 kg) fed rye-based diets selected for reduced viscosity. *J. Anim. Feed Sci.* **1999**, *8*, 549–556. [CrossRef]
50. Friend, D.; MacIntyre, T. Digestibility of rye and its value in pelleted rations for pigs. *Can. J. Anim. Sci.* **1969**, *49*, 375–381. [CrossRef]
51. Kamphues, J.; Hartung, C.; Wilke, V.; Grone, R. Roggen: Renaissance einer altbekannten Getreideart in der Tierernährung? *Übers. Tierernährg.* **2019**, *44*, 107–163.
52. KWS. Rye-Rich Feed Mixes Can Reduce CO2 Emissions in Pork Production by More than 20%. Available online: https://www.kws.com/corp/en/media-innovation/press/rye-rich-feed-mixes-can-reduce-co2-emissions-in-pork-production-by-more-than-20/ (accessed on 30 August 2020).

4

A Role for the Microbiota in the Immune Phenotype Alteration Associated with the Induction of Disease Tolerance and Persistent Asymptomatic Infection of *Salmonella* in the Chicken

Annah Lee [1], Cristiano Bortoluzzi [1], Rachel Pilla [2] and Michael H. Kogut [3,*]

1 Department of Poultry Science, Texas A&M University, College Station, TX 77843, USA; annahlee89@gmail.com (A.L.); bortoluzzi.c@gmail.com (C.B.)

2 Department of Small Animal Clinical Sciences, Texas A&M University, College Station, TX 77843, USA; rpilla@cvm.tamu.edu

3 Food and Feed Safety Research Unit, United States Department of Agriculture/Agriculture Research Service, College Station, TX 77845, USA

* Correspondence: mike.kogut@usda.gov

Abstract: Previous studies have shown a tissue immune phenotype-altering event occurring on days 2 and 4 in the ceca post-*Salmonella* challenge. To evaluate the involvement of the cecal microbiota in the phenotype reprogramming, we hypothesized that the addition of subtherapeutic bacitracin (BMD) will affect the cecal microbiota. Therefore, the objective of this study was to determine if the antibiotic-mediated changes in the microbiota composition influenced the immune phenotype induced by *Salmonella enteritidis* infection of the chicken cecum. A total of 112 fertile eggs were obtained for each experiment, repeated for a total of three separate times. The ceca and cecal contents were collected on days 2 and 4 post-infection for mRNA expression TaqMan assay and 16S rRNA gene microbiota sequencing. The results demonstrate the effects of bacitracin on cecal composition and its interaction with *Salmonella enteritidis* in young chicks. There is a preliminary indication of phenotype change in the *Salmonella*-challenged group provided subtherapeutic BMD due to the shifting cecal microbiota and cecal immune response, indicating the addition of bacitracin during infection altered the cecal phenotype. These data demonstrate the potential involvement of the microbiota in reprogramming immune phenotype (disease resistance to disease tolerance) induced by *Salmonella* in the chicken cecum.

Keywords: *Salmonella enteritidis*; gut microbiota; antibiotics; immune phenotype

---

1. Introduction

Foodborne illnesses cause health and economic burden in the United States annually, affecting 48 million people every year. One of the major causes of human gastroenteritis is *Salmonella enterica* Enteritidis (*S.* Enteritidis) due to infected poultry products, accounting for 40–60% of all reported cases [1]. Although improved control measures have been implemented, *S. enterica* still continues to present an issue every year in US livestock [2]. One of the many reasons is due to the chickens' ability to co-exist with *Salmonella* without showing any outward clinical signs of distress, also referred to as disease tolerance, and increased antimicrobial resistance due to overuse of antibiotic growth promoters (AGPs) [3]. Although the mechanism of how AGPs improve animal performance is still unclear, Diaz Carrasco et al. [4] speculate it is through intestinal microbiota modulation, specifically in the ceca for the chicken, whether it is dietary related or pathogen related. Studies need to focus on identifying the mechanism of how broad-spectrum antibiotics work in the host gut towards improving the overall health of food production animals.

In the poultry industry, bacitracin methylene disalicylate (BMD) is used as an AGP to improve poultry health and growth development by reducing inflammatory markers [5]. The mechanism of action for BMD is targeting Gram-positive bacteria, which are usually associated with poorer animal performance and growth [6]. Furthermore, BMD promotes growth, proliferation, or intactness of beneficial and resident bacterial gut communities to confer protection against pathogens, such as *Salmonella enterica* [7]. What is important to note is that to promote an optimal immune system, the host needs a balanced pro-inflammatory and anti-inflammatory response. The suppression of pro-inflammatory responses does not always reap benefits to the host immunity. In fact, the initial immune response may be less effective while allowing pathogens to proliferate on the opportunity of imbalance [8]. However, most of these studies have been performed in vitro, which concluded in variable results of AGP and its effects on phagocyte or immune cell functions [8]. Therefore, focusing on the gut microbiota with subtherapeutic BMD inclusion may provide insights on improved mechanisms and health management strategies. Increasing studies are showing the importance of the gut microbiota and its role in digestion, host immunity, immune protection, and protection against pathogen colonization [9]. However, antibiotic usage in US poultry is facing scrutiny due to antibiotic resistance and increased consumer awareness [10]. Currently, many European countries have banned the usage of AGP in animal feed, even at subtherapeutic levels; in the US, subtherapeutic levels of AGP must now be provided under veterinary authorization [11].

Even before hatch, the chick can be infected with *S.* Enteritidis via vertical transmission [12]. Commercial broiler chicks are placed on used litter at hatch, which raises the risk of the naïve gut microbiota of neonatal chicks to be colonized by pathogenic *Salmonella* and take advantage of this susceptible environment [2,13–15]. The ceca contain the most diverse bacterial populations in the gastrointestinal tract (GIT): phyla *Bacteroides*, *Proteobacteria* and *Firmicutes* are the most dominantly observed [4,9,16]. Many of the taxa present in the chicken GIT are of human relevance, including *Salmonella* and certain *Campylobacter* species [16]. Recent findings have speculated a phenomenon occurring in the chicken ceca with *S.* Enteritidis infection, resulting in three distinct immune-metabolic phases: disease resistance (4–48 h post-infection), disease tolerance (3–4 days post-infection), and homeostasis (5–28 days post-infection) [17,18]. The study of the symbiosis between the metabolic and immunological (immunometabolic) changes occurring in the gut microbiota during *Salmonella* infection is a growing field, especially in the chicken. Once *Salmonella* enters the intestine, the interaction with the mucosal surface is crucial for successful attachment. Inflammatory responses can occur in as little as few hours after oral ingestion; however, the damage to the host does not occur in the chicken. Instead, a state of persistence occurs, allowing for minimized host defense action. While this is not harmful for the health of the chicken, it is not ideal downstream for human consumption. This phenotypic alteration event has been theorized as a survival mechanism of *Salmonella* in poultry to minimize host defenses [3].

Therefore, the objective of this study was to evaluate the effects of the broiler cecal microbiota and immunity induced by *Salmonella* infection with the addition of subtherapeutic level of BMD. The hypothesis is that tissue (cecal) phenotype will be altered due to the addition of subtherapeutic BMD during *Salmonella* infection. The results from this study will provide crucial perspectives on how broad range antibiotics act on the ceca, especially during a *Salmonella* infection, and potentially lead to better improvements on poultry intestinal health.

2. Materials and Methods

2.1. Experimental Animals, Housing, and Treatments

All experiments conducted were in accordance with the guidelines set by the United States Department of Agriculture Animal Care and Use Committee (IACUC #2019-003). By-product Cobb

500 broiler eggs were obtained from a commercial hatchery. Before incubation, the randomly selected eggs were swabbed for *Salmonella* detection on the shell surface. *Salmonella* were not detected on any of the tested surfaces. The fertile eggs were incubated (GQF Manufacturing Company, Savannah, GA, USA; Jamesway Incubator Company, Inc., Cambridge, ON, Canada; or Petersime Incubator Co., Gettysburg, PA, USA) and maintained at wet and dry bulb temperatures of 32 and 37 °C, presented as relative humidity. After 10 days of incubation, the eggs were candled and non-fertile or non-viable eggs were discarded. The viable eggs were returned to the incubator until day 18 when they were transferred to hatchers (Humidaire Incubator Company, New Madison, OH, USA) and maintained under the same temperature and humidity conditions until hatch. At hatch (n = 112), the chicks were randomly distributed into one of four groups (28 chicks/group): (T1) non-infected birds fed a broiler starter diet alone; (T2) *S.* Enteritidis-challenged birds fed a broiler starter diet alone; (T3) non-infected birds fed a broiler starter diet containing BMD (Zoetis Inc., Parsippany, NJ, USA) at the inclusion rate of 50 g/ton; (T4) *S.* Enteritidis-challenged birds fed a broiler starter diet containing BMD at the inclusion rate of 50 g/ton.

At day of hatch, the chicks were randomly distributed into each treatment group in pens with fresh pine shavings, water, and starter diet ad libitum. The chicks were maintained in biosafety level-2 (BSL-2) isolation units under 96 h light and then switched over to an 18 h light:6 h dark cycle until the end of the study. The temperature in the room was held between 90 to 95 °F (temperature decreasing to 90 °F by day 10). Birds were monitored daily for the entire experimental period. This study was repeated three times under identical parameters.

2.2. Bacteria Preparation

Upon hatching, all chicks were orally challenged with 10^{6-8} CFU/0.5 mL *S.* Enteritidis or mock challenge with 0.5 mL sterile 1xPBS. The *Salmonella enterica* serovar Enteritidis isolate was obtained from the National Veterinary Services Laboratory (Ames, IA, USA), selected for resistance to novobiocin (25 ug/mL) and nalidixic acid (20 ug/mL) in tryptic soy broth (Difco Laboratories, Sparks, MD, USA). Viable cell concentration of challenge were determined on XLT4 agar plates with XLT4 supplement (Difco Laboratories, Sparks, MD, USA), nalidixic acid and novobiocin (XLT-NN).

2.3. Bacterial Detection

The cecal contents (0.25 g/bird) were collected, serially diluted to 1:100, 1:1000, 1:10,000, 1:100,000, and spread onto XLT4 for *Salmonella* detection. These plates were incubated at 37 °C for 24 h. For the enrichment, 100 uL of the cecal contents were pre-enriched in Rappaport–Vassiliadis broth for 24 h at 37 °C.

2.4. Sample Collection and Processing

On each necropsy day (day 2 and 4 post-infection), 14 birds/group were selected by random and euthanized via cervical dislocation. The cecal contents were collected for bacterial detection and microbiota analysis. The ceca were stored in RNALater for gene expression studies. This trial was repeated two more times for three total separate experiments.

2.5. Microbiota Sequencing

For the microbiota studies, the remaining contents from each ceca (ranging from 300–500 mg per cecal sample) were submitted to a core sequencing facility at the University of Arkansas, Fayetteville (n = 14/treatment/day/experiment; 336 cecal contents submitted total). DNA was extracted from the ceca samples taken at the indicated time points (day 2 and 4) using the Qiagen Qiamp Fast DNA Stool Mini Kit (Qiagen, Hilden, Germany). The DNA purity was assessed, and all of the DNA samples were diluted to 10 ng/mL. The paired-end sequencing libraries were prepped by targeting the hypervariable region 4 of the 16S ribosomal RNA with PCR primers containing the linker and adapter sequence. The sequencing libraries were assessed for qualitative and quantitative homogeneity, and then sequenced using the Illumina MiSeq platform as previously described [19].

2.6. Microbiota Bioinformatic Analysis

Data sequences were uploaded onto BaseSpace (www.basespace.illumina.com) (Illumina, San Diego, CA, USA) to determine sequence run quality and run completion. De-multiplexed data were downloaded locally and uploaded onto QIIME2-2018.8. The sequences were demultiplexed and the amplicon variant sequence (ASV) table was created using DADA2 [20]. The representative sequences were then classified using VSEARCH, and ASVs were defined as sequences with at least 97% similarity with Greengenes v.13.8 database [21]. Sequences that were unassigned or identified as cyanobacteria, chloroplast, or mitochondria were removed. The ASV table was then rarefied at 6400 reads for even depth of analysis. Alpha diversity metrics calculated were Shannon's diversity index, observed OTUs (operational taxonomic units), and Chao1. Beta diversity metrics that were estimated with unweighted and weighted UniFrac distance and visualized using principle coordinate analysis (PCoA). Nonparametric test ANOSIM (analysis of similarities) was used to compare the similarity between the bacterial composition of each treatment to the baseline control (T1) using UniFrac.

2.7. Real-Time Quantitative RT-PCR

The immune genotyping portion was quantitated by mRNA expression, specifically through a TaqMan based assay adapted from Eldaghayes et al. [22]. The ceca that were previously stored in RNALater were cut longitudinally to expose the lumen, and any remaining fecal matter was gently removed with forceps. The total RNA was extracted using Qiagen RNeasy® Plus kits (Germantown, MD, USA), and RNA quality was evaluated with a NanoDrop™ 2000 Spectrophotometer (Thermo Fisher Scientific, Waltham, MA, USA).

Cytokine mRNA expression levels were determined using RT-PCR with 28S as the reference gene. The RNAs were stored in −80 °C until RT-PCR plate setup. The cytokines IL-1β, IL-6, IL-10, IFN-γ, and TNF-α were quantified utilizing the Eldaghayes et al. method [22]. Primer and probe sequences (Table 1) for amplification have been described previously by Kogut et al. [23] and Kaiser et al. [24]. The plates were run in the Applied Biosystems ABI StepOne Plus PCR system (ThermoFisher Scientific, Waltham, MA, USA) with the previously stated TaqMan Assay under the following conditions: one cycle of 48 °C for 30 min, 95 °C for 20 s, and 40 cycles of 95 °C for 3 s and 60 °C for 30 s. Normalization was carried out against 28S rRNA, which was used as a housekeeping gene. To correct for differences in RNA levels between samples within the experiment, the correction factor for each sample was calculated by dividing the mean threshold cycle (Ct) value for the 28S rRNA-specific product for each sample by the overall mean Ct value for the 28S rRNA-specific product from all samples. The corrected cytokine mean was calculated as follows: (average of each replicate × cytokine slope)/(28S slope × 28S correction factor). Fold changes in mRNA levels were calculated from mean 40 Ct values [22,25]. Each sample was run in triplicates for technical replication.

Table 1. Primer and probe sequences.

RNA Target		Probe/Primer Sequences	Accession No.
28S	Probe	5′-(FAM)-AGGACCGCTACGGACCTCCACCA-(TAMRA)-3′	X59733
	F	5′-GGCGAAGCCAGAGGAAACT-3′	
	R	5′-GACGACCGATTGCACGTC-3′	
IL-1β	Probe	5′-(FAM)-CCACACTGCAGCTGGAGGAAGCC-(TAMRA)-3′	AJ245728
	F	5′-GCTCTACATGTCGTGTGTGATGAG-3′	
	R	5′-TGTCGATGTCCCGCATGA-3′	
IL-6	Probe	5′-(FAM)-AGGAGAAATGCCTGACGAAGCTCTCCA-(TAMRA)-3′	AJ250838
	F	5′-GCTCGCCGGCTTCGA-3′	
	R	5′-GGTAGGTCTGAAAGGCGAACAG-3′	

Table 1. *Cont.*

RNA Target		Probe/Primer Sequences	Accession No.
TNF-α	Probe	5′-(FAM)-TGCTGAGAAGGAACAAACTGGTGGT-(TAMRA)-3′	MF000729
	F	5′-CCCATCCCTGGTCCGTAA-3′	
	R	5′- GGCGGCGTATACGAAGTAAAG-3′	
IL-10	Probe	5′-(FAM)-CGACGATGCGGCGCTGTCA-(TAMRA)-3′	AJ621614
	F	5′-CATGCTGCTGGGCCTGAA-3′	
	R	5′-CGTCTCCTTGATCTGCTTGATG-3′	
IFN-γ	Probe	5′-(FAM)-TGGCCAAGCTCCCGATGAACGA-(TAMRA)-3′	Y07922
	F	5′-GTGAAGAAGGTGAAAGATATATCATGGA-3′	
	R	5′-GCTTTGCGCTGGATTCTCA-3′	

2.8. Statistical Analysis for qRT-PCR and Microbiota Analysis

Cytokine mRNA expressions for control and treated ceca from days 2 and 4 were quantitated using a method described by Kaiser et al. [24] and Moody et al. [26]. Statistical analysis was performed with SAS (version 9.4, Cary, NC, USA) of the data collected from each trial for the qRT-PCR data. The Shapiro–Wilk's test for normality was used to determine if the fold change within each group was parametric or non-parametric, with an alpha of 0.05. For all analyses, statistical significance was considered if $p \leq 0.05$. All data were found to be non-parametric and were summarized as median values. An ad hoc analysis using the Kruskal–Wallis test was conducted to determine where the statistical differences lie between treatments. The ceca samples for the IL-1β, IL-6, IL-10, TNF-α, and IFN-γ were calculated with the 40-C_t method, as outlined by Eldaghayes et al. [22]. The results were reported in fold change values.

The frequencies of bacterial families were submitted to the Kruskal–Wallis test under non-parametric one-way ANOVA, and if there were significant differences seen ($p \leq 0.05$), a post hoc analysis using Dunn's multiple comparison test to separate the means using GraphPad Prism (version 8.0, La Jolla, CA, USA). For the microbiota correlation analysis, Pearson correlation analysis between the mean percentage of bacterial families and the fold change of cytokines was performed using SAS (version 9.4, Cary, NC, USA) with $\alpha \leq 0.05$. The Pearson correlation was carried out within each treatment on day 2 and day 4.

3. Results

3.1. Real-Time Quantitative RT-PCR Results

All results are reported as averaged triplicate experiments and compared to the control (T1). There was a significant upregulation of pro-inflammatory cytokines, specifically IL-1β and IL-6, in challenged birds fed with normal starter formula (T2), at day 2 post-infection (Figure 1A,B). This upregulation was much less marked in challenged birds fed with the subtherapeutic addition of BMD (T4 vs. T2). Furthermore, on day 2, both IL-10 and TNF-α were expressed in response to *Salmonella* challenge (T2 and T4), regardless of BMD addition in the feed (Figure 1C,D). The expression of IFN-γ in infected birds fed with the addition of BMD (T4) was significantly upregulated, in relation to the other treatments (Figure 1E).

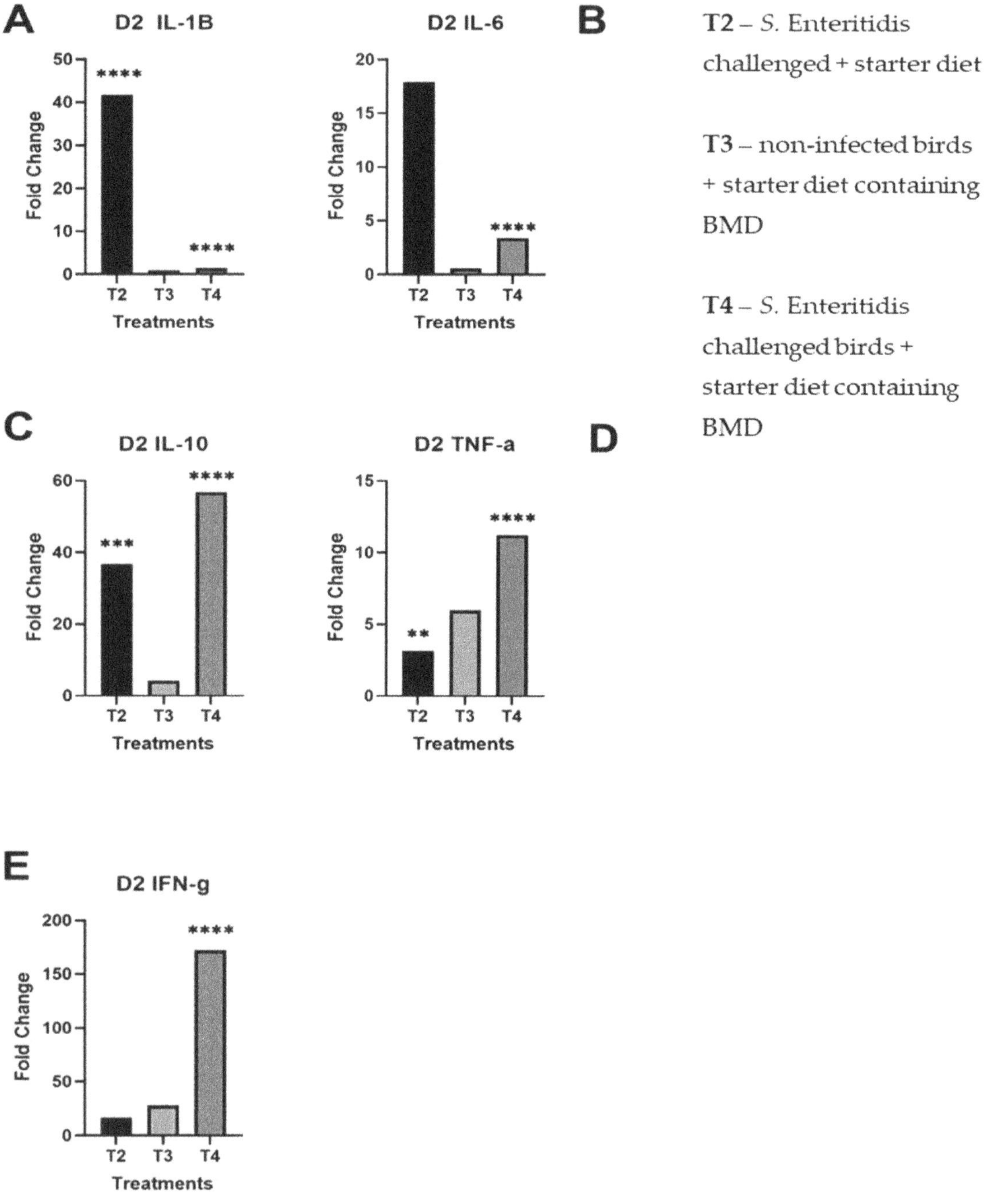

Figure 1. Fold changes of day 2 cecal samples by treatment per panel. These results for each treatment are compared against the control group (T1): (**A**) day 2 fold changes by treatment for IL-1β; (**B**) day 2 fold changes by treatment for IL-6; (**C**) day 2 fold changes by treatment for IL-10; (**D**) day 2 fold changes by treatment for TNF-α; (**E**) day 2 fold changes by treatment for IFN-γ. The starred bars indicate differing levels of significant *p*-values.

By day 4 post-infection, the expression of IL-10, TNF-α, and IFN-γ remained unchanged (Figure 2C–E) in comparison to day 2 post-infection. In contrast to day 2, the profile of pro-inflammatory cytokines IL-1β and IL-6 did not change much in upregulation at day 4 in challenged birds fed with normal starter formula (T2) (Figure 2A,B). However, the same pro-inflammatory cytokines were strongly upregulated at that time in challenged birds fed with subtherapeutic BMD (T4). For birds provided only subtherapeutic BMD (T3), the profile of pro-inflammatory cytokines IL-1β and IL-6 were slightly elevated; the other tested cytokines, IFN-γ, TNF-α, and IL-10, did not yield significant changes in fold change. Finally, the treatment with BMD appeared to invert the inflammatory profile of birds following infection with *S.* Enteritidis at days 2 and 4 post-infection.

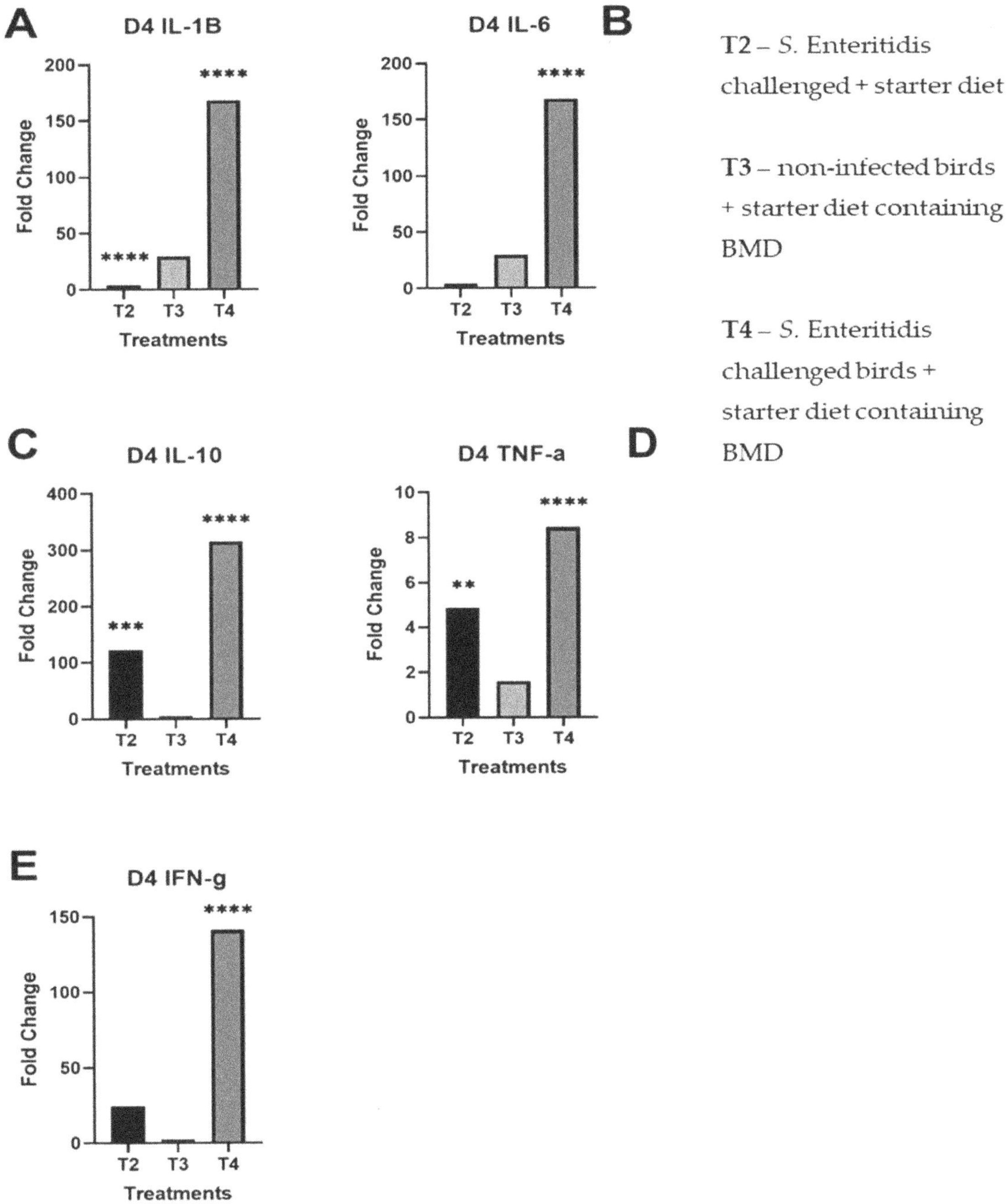

Figure 2. Fold changes of day 4 cecal samples by treatment per panel. These results for each treatment are compared against the control group (T1): (**A**) day 4 fold changes by treatment for IL-1β; (**B**) day 4 fold changes by treatment for IL-6; (**C**) day 4 fold changes by treatment for IL-10; (**D**) day 4 fold changes by treatment for TNF-α; (**E**) day 4 fold changes by treatment for IFN-γ. The starred bars indicate differing levels of significant *p*-values.

Overall, there was significant upregulation of pro-inflammatory and regulatory cytokines in *S.* Enteritidis-challenged birds given subtherapeutic BMD on day 4 than non-infected birds given BMD, indicating a stimulation of the immune system. Notably, there were statistically significant fold changes on day 2 of IL-1β in T2, IL-6 in T4, IL-10 in T2 and T4, TNF-α in T2 and T4, and IFN-γ in T4 (Figure 1). In day 4, there were statistically significant fold changes of IL-1β in T2 and T4,

IL-6 in T4, IL-10 in T2 and T4, TNF-α in T2 and T4, and IFN-γ in T4. As previously shown, *Salmonella* induces pro-inflammatory response within 2 days of infection and reprogrammed to anti-inflammatory response by day 4. However, the treatment of birds with bacitracin inhibited the immune alteration in the *Salmonella*-challenged birds (T4) (Figure 2).

3.2. Microbiota Composition

To understand whether bacitracin treatment alteration of the cecal microbiota composition could account for the inhibition of immune phenotype in *Salmonella*-challenged birds, the cecal microbiota was evaluated for both days 2 and 4 for all treatment groups. Relative abundances are reported as median values (Table 2), and only the high-frequency bacterial families are reported. The most abundant bacterial families observed in the ceca were *Enterobacteriaceae* and *Clostridiaceae* at day 2 (Figure 3A). There was noticeable increase in bacterial diversity according to age.

Table 2. The top listed median relative abundance (by %) of observed families in the ceca of day 2 and day 4 birds.

Group	*Paenibacillaceae*		*Lachnospiraceae*		*Clostridiaceae*		*Enterobacteriaceae*		*Bacillaceae*	
	Day 2	Day 4	Day 2	Day 4	Day 2	Day 4	Day 2	Day 4	Day 2	Day 4
T1	0.11 ^{a,b}	8.23 ^{a}	0	1.32 ^{b}	95.9 ^{a}	69.1 ^{a}	0.55 ^{a}	0.94 ^{a,c}	0.14 ^{a,c}	1.70 ^{a}
T2	0 ^{b,d}	3.02 ^{a,b}	0	0.14 ^{b}	23.5 ^{b}	23.8 ^{b}	73.6 ^{b}	58.9 ^{b}	0 ^{b}	0.02 ^{b}
T3	0.18 ^{a,c}	7.25 ^{a,b}	0.04	12.33 ^{a}	86.5 ^{c}	40.3 ^{b}	4.45 ^{c}	0.19 ^{c}	0.20 ^{c}	0.07 ^{b}
T4	0 ^{d}	1.98 ^{b}	0	1.25 ^{b}	25.0 ^{b}	34.3 ^{b}	68.1 ^{b}	48.5 ^{b}	0 ^{b}	0 ^{b}

^{a,b,c,d} The differing superscripts indicate varying significant values ($p \leq 0.001$).

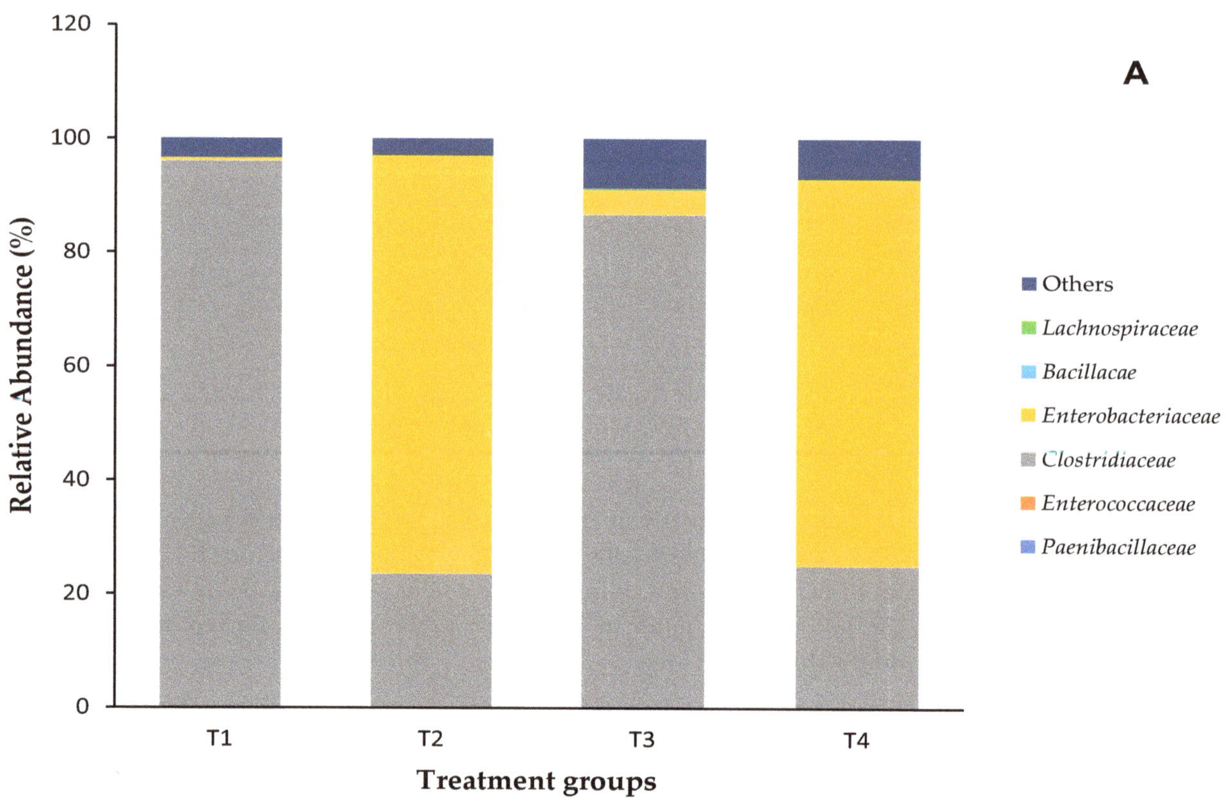

Figure 3. *Cont.*

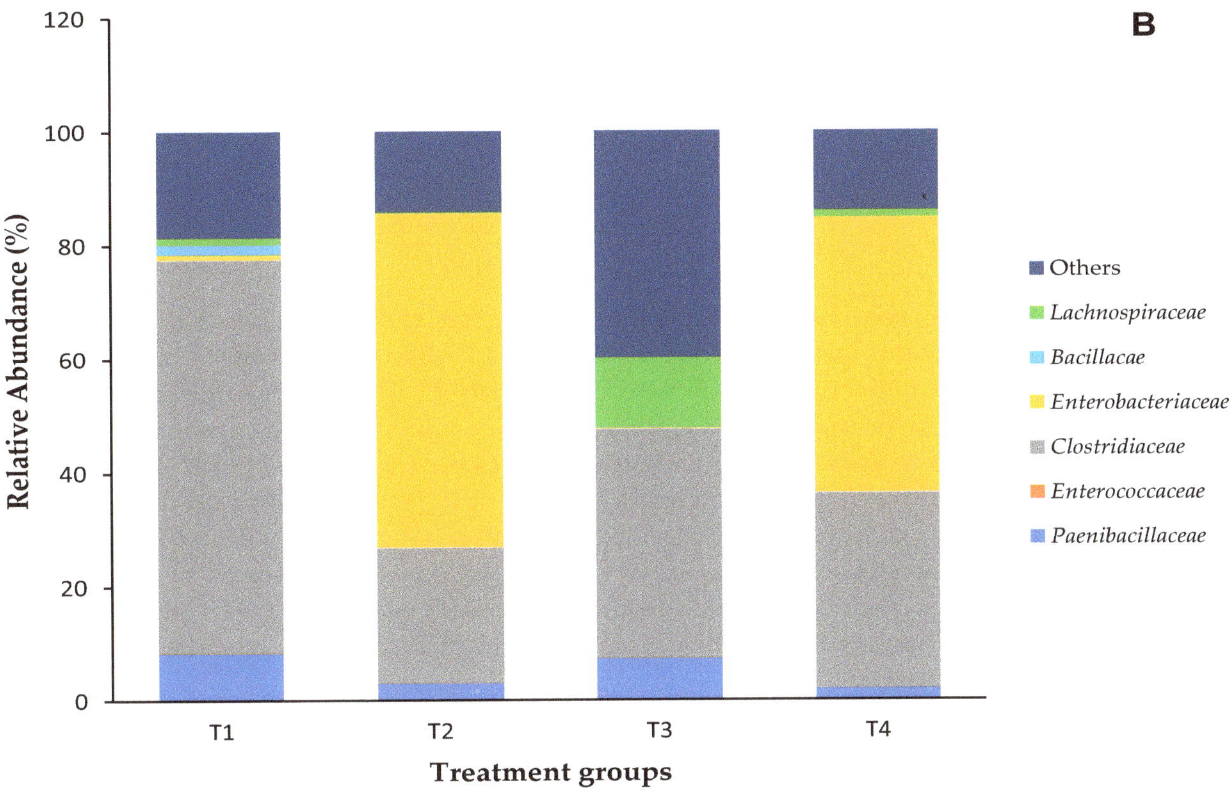

Figure 3. (**A**) Microbiota composition of day 2 chicken ceca; (**B**) microbiota composition of day 4 chicken ceca.

On day 2, the 16S rRNA sequence analysis of the cecal microbiota of control birds fed normal starter feed (T1) revealed a microbiota composition dominated by the family *Clostridiaceae*. Birds infected with *Salmonella* and fed normal starter feed (T2) were dominated by *Enterobacteriaceae* (73.6%) followed by lesser presence of *Clostridiaceae* (23.5%). Birds fed bacitracin (T3) had mostly the presence of *Clostridiaceae* (86.5%) followed by a much lesser presence of *Enterobacteriaceae* (4.45%). In the final group with birds challenged with *S.* Enteritidis and provided subtherapeutic BMD in the starter feed (T4), there was mostly the presence of *Enterobacteriaceae* (68.1%) followed by *Clostridiaceae* (25%) in day 2 ceca.

By day 4, there were still mostly *Enterobacteriaceae* and *Clostridiaceae* but with increased presence of *Paenibacillaceae* across all treatment groups. The control group (T1) was still mostly dominated by *Clostridiaceae* (69.1%) but with a marked increase in *Paenibacillaceae* (8.23%) and starting presence of *Bacillaceae* (1.7%). In the treatment group with *S.* Enteritidis challenge fed the control feed (T2), there were mostly *Enterobacteriaceae* (58.9%) followed by *Clostridiaceae* (23.8%). In the non-infected group fed with bacitracin (T3), the cecal composition had varying changes: large *Clostridiaceae* frequency (40.3%) but with an increased frequency of *Lachnospiraceae* (12.3%) and *Paenibacillaceae* (7.25%). The final group of birds challenged with *S.* Enteritidis with subtherapeutic BMD addition (T4) also had increased frequency of *Lachnospiraceae* (1.25%) and *Paenibacillaceae* (1.98%) but was still dominated by *Enterobacteriaceae* (48.5%) and *Clostridiaceae* (34.3%).

The infection by *Salmonella* seemed to provoke an increase in *Enterobacteriaceae* at the detriment of *Clostridiaceae*, regardless of the age of the birds. When comparing the *Salmonella*-challenged group (T2) with the *Salmonella*-challenged with bacitracin in feed group (T4), there is not much difference in diversity and frequency of families on day 2, but there is a notable decrease in *Enterobacteriaceae* and increase in *Lachnospiraceae*, and to a lesser degree, increased frequency of *Clostridiaceae* and decreased frequency of *Paenibacillaceae*. Birds infected with *Salmonella* and fed control feed (T2) were observed to have decreased frequency of *Enterobacteriaceae* (58.9%) as compared to day 2, and a starting presence of *Paenibacillaceae* (3.02%) with not much change in the *Clostridiaceae* frequency (23.8%). The addition of subtherapeutic BMD feed had no major effect on the bacterial composition at day 2 (T3 vs. T1); however, in non-infected birds at day 4, it provoked an increase in *Lachnospiraceae* and other species at the detriment of *Clostridiaceae* (T3 vs. T1). In contrast, *S.* Enteritidis-challenged birds at day 4 with added BMD provoked a significant 10% increase in *Clostridiaceae* compared to a 10% decrease in *Enterobacteriaceae* (T4 vs. T2).

3.3. Beta Diversity Index of Cecal Composition

Unifrac was utilized to compare similarities between bacterial communities in the cecal samples across independent time points (day 2 and day 4). Weighted UniFrac plots showed better separation on day 2 than day 4 where more clustering occurred (Figure 4A–F). There were large differences in the weighted UniFrac, but not in the unweighted UniFrac (data not shown) between groups. The ANOSIM of the weighted Unifrac across different ages within each treatment group (Table 3) displays large quantitative differences between T2 and control on day 2 and T4 and control on day 2. However, the differences in microbiota composition between T2 and control ($R = 0.62$, $p \leq 0.001$) and T4 ($R = 0.59$, $p \leq 0.001$) and control, while still significant, are not as large by day 4, as indicated by lower R values. Overall, while the effect of bacitracin feed was significant both at days 2 and 4, the difference in microbiota composition compared to controls was small, as shown by the small R value between T1 vs. T3 in the ANOSIM analysis.

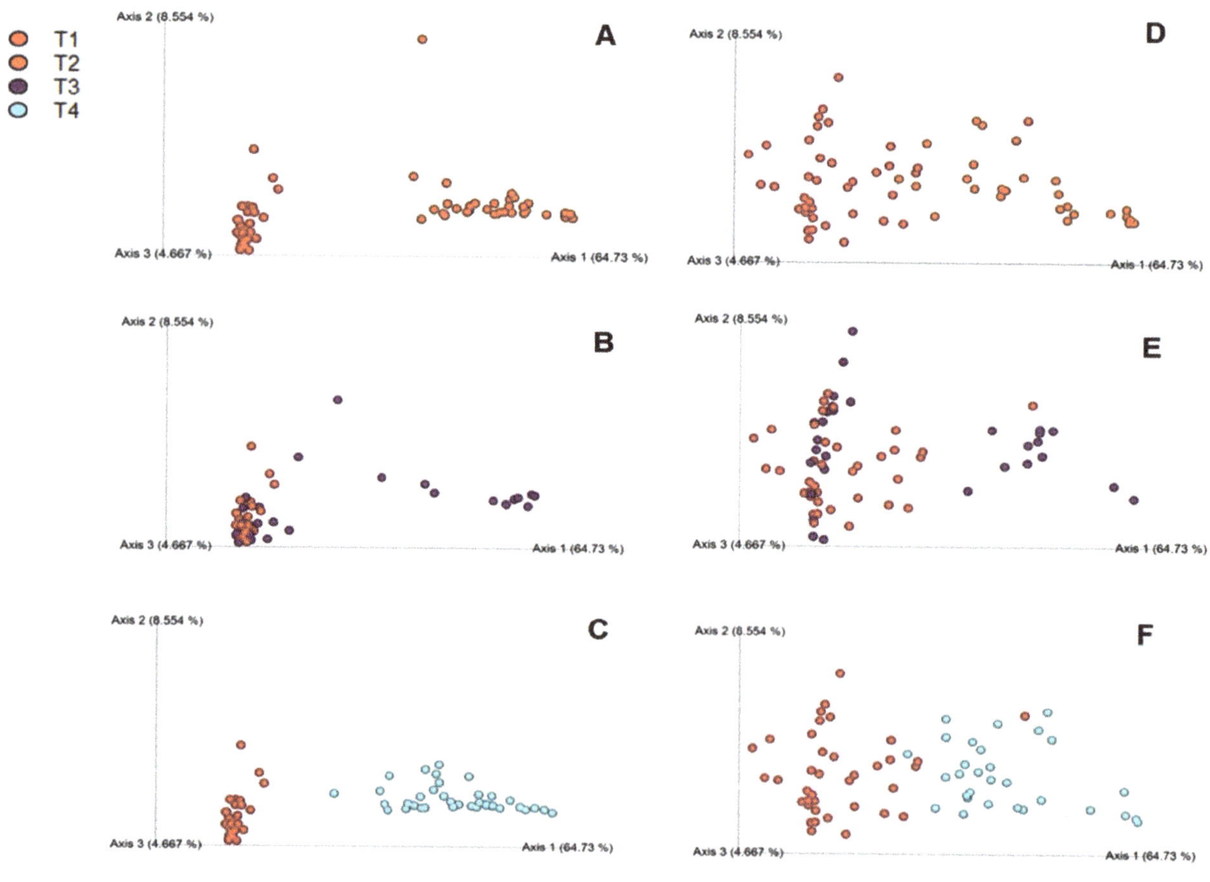

Figure 4. (**A–C**) Principle coordinate analysis (PCoA) charts using Unifrac for day 2 comparison of treatments: (**A**) T1 vs. T2, (**B**) T1 vs. T3, (**C**) T1 vs. T4; (**D–F**) PCoA charts using Unifrac for day 4 comparison of treatments: (**D**) T1 vs. T2, (**E**) T1 vs. T3, (**F**) T1 vs. T4. The legend is located at the top left of the figure.

Table 3. ANOSIM analysis of weighted Unifrac on different day comparisons within each of the treatment groups.

Age	Comparison	R [1]	Probability [2]
Day 2	T1 vs. T2	0.96	**0.001**
	T1 vs. T3	0.1	0.002
	T1 vs. T4	0.98	**0.001**
Day 4	T1 vs. T2	0.62	**0.001**
	T1 vs. T3	0.15	0.002
	T1 vs. T4	0.59	**0.001**

[1] R is the similarity of comparison: 0 means equally similar, 1 means completely dissimilar. [2] Significant differences are set at $p \leq 0.001$. Significant differences between treatments are bolded.

4. Discussion

As sites of persistent colonization of bacteria, the avian ceca are important sites to study and better understand how the poultry GIT microbiota interact with pathogens. Generally, taxonomic diversity increases as the bird ages, enriched mainly with bacteria in the phylum Firmicutes [6]. Immediately after hatch, the chicks are exposed to numerous environmental factors that activate their immune system, leading to low-grade inflammation by increased cytokine and chemokine expression [2]. Previous studies have already observed bacterial families in the ceca, including *Clostridiaceae*, *Lachnospiraceae*, and *Streptococcaceae* as shown in the present results [27]. These results highlight some key bacterial alterations between the gut bacterial communities and a potential link to changes in the intestinal immune function in the crucial first days post-hatch. Therefore, the goal was met to observe the effects of how introducing subtherapeutic BMD during *Salmonella* challenge would affect the phenotype alteration of the ceca.

The addition of subtherapeutic BMD group (T3) affected the pro-inflammatory cytokines IL-1β and IL-6 by the upregulated expression between day 2 and 4, compared to the control (T1). The other cytokine profiles, namely, TNF-α, IL-10, and IFN-γ, were also affected but with a downregulated expression. Meanwhile, the cecal composition comparing day 2 and day 4 showed increasing bacterial diversity, with a marked increase in *Lachnospiraceae* and other species at the detriment of *Clostridiaceae* (T3 vs. T1). This may be due to the subtherapeutic levels provided, in which previous studies [28,29] also did not see significant changes in the cecal community structure but did see changes in the community structure overall. In fact, the addition of pro-inflammatory mediators increases the resistance of the animal to pathogen challenge, specifically a rapid and efficient inflammatory response during pathogen invasion [18].

When an opportunistic pathogen such as *S.* Enteritidis is involved, the results are distinctly different when compared to the control. The pro-inflammatory cytokines IL-1β and IL-6 were significantly upregulated on day 2 and even more upregulated by day 4 for T4, indicating a strong inflammatory response during these two days in the chicks. However, the other cytokines, IL-10, TNF-α, and IFN-γ, were also significantly upregulated on day 2 but then observed to be downregulated overall by day 4. Infections with *S.* Enteritidis and treatment with BMD affected the overall bacterial composition in the ceca, which has also been shown in previous studies with mammalian models as well [30]. Generally, AGPs like BMD improve growth performance through an anti-inflammatory effect in the GI tract [31]. In fact, it is speculated that AGPs may eliminate some members of *Enterobacteriaceae*, but this allows for opportunistic bacteria to proliferate as a result [14]. In this study, the addition of subtherapeutic BMD in the *S.* Enteritidis challenge model (T4) altered the immune system by the induced inflammatory response, compared to the treatment group with just the challenge on starter feed (T2) which was downregulated by day 4. The addition of subtherapeutic BMD in the *S.* Enteritidis-challenged group (T4) also reduced the *Enterobacteriaceae* population by almost 20% from day 2 to day 4. In previous studies from our group [3,32], the phenomenon of phenotypic switch occurred between days 2 and 4 from a pro-inflammatory response to an anti-inflammatory,

Salmonella disease tolerance response. The inflammatory response, defined by the IL-1β and the IL-6 response, was inhibited on day 2 compared to the *Salmonella*-challenged chicks without BMD treatment. Infected hosts undergo phenotypic shifts in tissue metabolism, metabolic sensors such as mTOR and AMPK, and immune cell functions [33]. The *Salmonella*-challenged treatment (T2) follows the previously documented studies: IL-6 and IL-1β are highly upregulated on day 2 and dramatically reduced by day 4 post-infection [33]. Therefore, it can be speculated that bacitracin is preventing an overstimulation in the earlier stage of *Salmonella* infection. This disruption of the microbiota increases the pathogen's drive to survive by changing the state of inflammatory response.

According to the UniFrac results, the overall data demonstrated species disappearing or showing up, but with strong differences in abundances of those that were already present. As seen in Figure 4A–F and Table 3, there were large quantitative differences between *S.* Enteritidis-challenged group (T2) and control (T1) on day 2 and *S.* Enteritidis-challenged group with the addition of the subtherapeutic BMD group (T4) and control (T1) on day 2. However, the differences between T2 and control and T4 and control are not as similar by day 4. Juricova et al. [13] concluded that infection with *Salmonella enteritidis* caused delays in the microbiota development of young chicks, which could explain the phenomenon occurring in the present study. This interaction could also affect the immune system of the host, adding another layer of variability that has not been well classified in broilers. Interesting, there were bacterial community differences seen in T2 and T4 compared to the control, but not much between T3 and control. Oakley and Kogut [6] concluded that Proteobacteria, which includes *Salmonella* spp., had strong correlations to IL-6 pro-inflammatory response. We also observed increased IL-10 expression which can be attributed to the gut modulation via bacitracin and young age of the birds [34]. While the presence of these pro-inflammatory cytokines could be attributed to the fluctuations of an unstable gut microbiota environment of young chicks, antibody-mediated immune response has been confirmed due to modulated gut microbiota via antibiotics [6,34].

While increased inflammation may affect the animal's performance level, appetite and muscle catabolism, the shifting gut microbiota of young broilers would eventually adjust for the imbalance and lead to less inflammation and energy expenditure for the animal as it ages [5,35]. The presence of *Enterobacteriaceae* has been shown to influence the amount of metabolites expressed in the GIT, especially with short-chain fatty acids (SCFAs) [36]. SCFAs are important for energy production for epithelial cells and immune cells including T cells and macrophages [37]. We also observed high frequency of *Enterobacteriaceae*, which *Salmonella enterica* is a part of, on both days in *Salmonella* infected birds treated with subtherapeutic bacitracin (T4). This could be due to bacitracin's inhibitory action primarily against Gram-positive bacteria even though it is a broad-spectrum antibiotic. Similarly seen in a study by Kumar et al. [38], this may be occurring due to *Salmonella* outcompeting the resident microflora for nutrients, which allows *Enterobacteriaceae* to flourish in the ceca.

The family *Clostridiaceae*, including *Clostridium perfringens*, is of interest in both humans and chickens. On both days tested, the family *Clostridiaceae* persisted, although in varying percentages, since it is generally part of the resident microbiota of the gut [16]. In chickens, pathogenic *C. perfringens* causes necrotic enteritis and is usually prevented by AGPs such as bacitracin [16]. A previous study by Ballou et al. [39] reports increased cecal diversity of bacterial communities, mainly within the order Clostridiales, which our present study confirms. The high frequency of members of the order Clostridiales in the ceca has also been linked to improved growth performance in chickens, which is an important factor for the broiler industry to consider [4,40].

Another minorly present bacterial family was *Lachnospiraceae*, identified as poultry probiotic bacteria, which appears to remain low in abundance until the chickens are much older in age, but this family of bacteria was one of the most modulated members of the cecal community when bacitracin was provided (Figure 3A,B) [4,40]. Depending on the genera, this family has been widely associated for the ability to produce beneficial metabolites, specifically SCFAs, influence dietary digestion, and influence metabolic disease regulation for mammalian hosts as well [41]. This family has been found in mucosal folds of the GI tract, suggesting that their interaction with the lamina propria immune cells makes

Lachnospiraceae, immune regulators that prevent pathogen colonization [42]. Furthermore, studies have documented an overall reduction of probiotic-related bacteria in the intestinal tract of chickens with the usage of AGPs [4,43,44]. The addition of an SCFA like butyrate has demonstrated to reduce invasion abilities and colonization abilities of *Salmonella* in the host [14,45]. Interestingly, the effects of SCFAs tend to produce anti-inflammatory effects on host immunity [46]. This study has observed the continual upregulation of pro-inflammatory cytokines with chicks provided subtherapeutic BMD (T3) and chicks provided subtherapeutic BMD with *S.* Enteritidis challenge (T4). However, this could be attributed to the unstable microbiota of young chicks or metabolic interactions causing pro-inflammatory effects. The presence of certain SCFAs could explain how bacitracin prevents infection of the cecal epithelium by *Salmonella,* thereby reducing the inflammatory response overall by day 2. Then, by day 4, a response against *Salmonella* is induced at a higher level, as indicated by the large upregulation of pro-inflammatory cytokines in the mRNA expression data. Further studies will need to be conducted to identify what SCFAs are present and how they affect the tissues histologically (lesion scoring or inflammatory evaluation) and immunologically during this crucial time point of chick development.

Overall, our results demonstrate the effects of bacitracin on cecal composition and its interaction with *S.* Enteritidis in young chicks. There is preliminary evidence of a phenotype change in the ceca due to the shifting microbiota with the addition of BMD; the phenotype has been altered by adding subtherapeutic BMD. This is supported by the decrease in *Enterobacteriaceae* and the increase in *Lachnospiraceae* and *Clostridiaceae* from day 2 to day 4. This is further supported by the upregulated inflammatory response of IL-6 and IL-1β on day 2 and day 4 in the *S.* Enteritidis-challenged group provided subtherapeutic BMD. Our group has previously reported the initial occurrence of an immunometabolic reprogramming in the cecal tissue during infection with *S. enterica* [3,32]. The current study validates this phenotype switch event while also providing initial evidence of a phenotype switch in birds provided subtherapeutic BMD and challenged with *S.* Enteritidis. While the study looked at a short time frame, the study demonstrated that the shift in microbiota can affect the immune reaction. These results provide initial insight of the phenotype changes occurring with the cecal bacterial population and the influence on the immune system. Future studies should look at a longer duration period and other segments of the GIT for a wider overview of bacterial communities.

Author Contributions: Conceptualization, A.L. and M.H.K.; methodology, A.L.; SAS software, C.B.; formal analysis, C.B., A.L., R.P.; investigation, A.L., C.B., M.H.K.; resources, M.H.K.; data curation, A.L.; writing—original draft preparation, A.L.; writing—review and editing, A.L., C.B., M.H.K.; visualization, A.L. and C.B.; supervision, M.H.K.; project administration, M.H.K.; funding acquisition, M.H.K. All authors have read and agreed to the published version of the manuscript.

Acknowledgments: We thank the USDA ARS Animal Care Staff and lab colleagues Gabriela Cardoso Dal Pont and Cinthia Eyng for all their help during the animal experiments.

References

1. Boore, A.L.; Hoekstra, R.M.; Iwamoto, M.; Fields, P.I.; Bishop, R.D.; Swerdlow, D.L.; Chaturvedi, V. Salmonella enterica infections in the United States and assessment of coefficients of variation: A novel approach to identify epidemiologic characteristics of individual serotypes, 1996–2011. *PLoS ONE* **2015**, *10*, e0145416. [CrossRef]
2. Crhanova, M.; Hradecka, H.; Faldynova, M.; Matulova, M.; Havlickova, H.; Sisak, F.; Rychlik, I. Immune response of chicken gut to natural colonization by gut microflora and to Salmonella enterica serovar Enteritidis infection. *Infect. Immun.* **2011**, *79*, 2755–2763. [CrossRef]
3. Kogut, M.H.; Arsenault, R.J. Immunometabolic phenotype alterations associated with the induction of disease tolerance and persistent asymptomatic infection of Salmonella in the chicken intestine. *Front. Immunol.* **2017**, *8*, 372. [CrossRef]
4. Carrasco, J.M.D.; Redondo, E.A.; Viso, N.D.P.; Redondo, L.M.; Farber, M.D.; Miyakawa, M.E.F. Tannins and bacitracin differentially modulate gut microbiota of broiler chickens. *BioMed Res. Int.* **2018**, *2018*, 1–11. [CrossRef]

5. Niewold, T.A. The nonantibiotic anti-inflammatory effect of antimicrobial growth promoters, the real mode of action? A hypothesis. *Poult. Sci.* **2007**, *86*, 605–609. [CrossRef] [PubMed]
6. Oakley, B.B.; Kogut, M.H. Spatial and temporal changes in the broiler chicken cecal and fecal microbiomes and correlations of bacterial taxa with cytokine gene expression. *Front. Vet. Sci.* **2016**, *3*. [CrossRef]
7. Wan, M.L.Y.; Ling, K.H.; El-Nezami, H.; Wang, M.F. Influence of functional food components on gut health. *Crit. Rev. Food Sci. Nutr.* **2019**, *59*, 1927–1936. [CrossRef]
8. Broom, L.J. The sub-inhibitory theory for antibiotic growth promoters. *Poult. Sci.* **2017**, *96*, 3104–3108. [CrossRef]
9. Azcarate-Peril, M.A.; Butz, N.; Cadenas, M.B.; Koci, M.; Ballou, A.; Mendoza, M.; Ali, R.; Hassan, H. An attenuated *Salmonella enterica* serovar Typhimurium strain and galacto-oligosaccharides accelerate clearance of *Salmonella* infections in poultry through modifications to the gut microbiome. *Appl. Environ. Microbiol.* **2017**, *84*, e02526-17. [CrossRef]
10. Lillehoj, H.; Liu, Y.; Calsamiglia, S.; Fernandez-Miyakawa, M.E.; Chi, F.; Cravens, R.L.; Oh, S.; Gay, C.G. Phytochemicals as antibiotic alternatives to promote growth and enhance host health. *Vet. Res.* **2018**, *49*. [CrossRef]
11. Center for Veterinary Medicine. Veterinary Feed Directive (VFD) [Online]. *FDA* 2020. Available online: https://www.fda.gov/animal-veterinary/development-approval-process/veterinary-feed-directive-vfd (accessed on 18 October 2020).
12. Barrow, P.A.; Methner, U. *Salmonella in Domestic Animals*, 2nd ed.; CABI: Wallingford, UK, 2013.
13. Juricova, H.; Videnska, P.; Lukac, M.; Faldynova, M.; Babak, V.; Havlickova, H.; Sisak, F.; Rychlik, I. Influence of Salmonella enterica serovar Enteritidis infection on the development of the cecum microbiota in newly hatched chicks. *Appl. Environ. Microbiol.* **2013**, *79*, 745–747. [CrossRef] [PubMed]
14. Mon, K.K.Z.; Saelao, P.; Halstead, M.M.; Chanthavixay, G.; Chang, H.; Garas, L.; Maga, E.A.; Zhou, H. Salmonella enterica serovars Enteritidis infection alters the indigenous microbiota diversity in young layer chicks. *Front. Vet. Sci.* **2015**, *2*. [CrossRef] [PubMed]
15. Kogut, M.H. The effect of microbiome modulation on the intestinal health of poultry. *Anim. Feed Sci. Technol.* **2019**, *250*, 32–40. [CrossRef]
16. Oakley, B.B.; Lillehoj, H.S.; Kogut, M.H.; Kim, W.K.; Maurer, J.J.; Pedroso, A.; Lee, M.D.; Collett, S.R.; Johnson, T.J.; Cox, N.A. The chicken gastrointestinal microbiome. *FEMS Microbiol. Lett.* **2014**, *360*, 100–112. [CrossRef] [PubMed]
17. Kogut, M.H.; Arsenault, R.J. Gut health: The new paradigm in food animal production. *Front. Vet. Sci.* **2016**, *3*. [CrossRef]
18. Kogut, M.H.; Yin, X.; Yuan, J.; Broom, L. Gut health in poultry. *CAB Rev.* **2017**, *12*, 1–7. [CrossRef]
19. Kozich, J.J.; Westcott, S.L.; Baxter, N.T.; Highlander, S.K.; Schloss, P.D. Development of a dual-index sequencing strategy and curation pipeline for analyzing amplicon sequence data on the MiSeq Illumina sequencing platform. *Appl. Environ. Microbiol.* **2013**, *79*, 5112–5120. [CrossRef]
20. Callahan, B.; McMurdie, P.; Han, A.; Johnson, A.J.A.; Holmes, S. DADA2: High-resolution sample inference from Illumina amplicon data. *Nat. Methods* **2020**, *13*, 581–583. [CrossRef]
21. Callahan, B. The RDP and GreenGenes taxonomic training sets formatted for DADA2 [software]. *Zenodo* **2016**. [CrossRef]
22. Eldaghayes, I.; Rothwell, L.; Williams, A.; Withers, D.; Balu, S.; Davison, F.; Kaiser, P. Infectious bursal disease virus: Strains that differ in virulence differentially modulate the innate immune response to infection in the chicken bursa. *Viral Immunol.* **2003**, *19*, 83–91. [CrossRef]
23. Kogut, M.H.; Rothwell, L.; Kaiser, P. Differential regulation of cytokine gene expression by avian heterophils during receptor-mediated phagocytosis of opsonized and nonopsonized *Salmonella enteritidis*. *J. Interferon Cytokine Res.* **2003**, *23*, 319–327. [CrossRef] [PubMed]
24. Kaiser, P.; Wigley, P.; Burnside, J.; Barrow, P.A.; Galyov, E.E.; Rothwell, L. Differential 498 cytokine expression in avian cells in response to invasion by Salmonella typhimurium, Salmonella enteritidis and Salmonella gallinarum. *Microbiology* **2000**, *146*, 3217–3226. [CrossRef] [PubMed]
25. Swaggerty, C.L.; Kogut, M.H.; He, H.; Genovese, K.J.; Johnson, C.; Arsenault, R.J. Differential levels of cecal colonization by Salmonella Enteritidis in chickens triggers distinct immune kinome profiles. *Front. Vet. Sci.* **2017**, *4*. [CrossRef]
26. Moody, A.; Sellers, S.; Bumstead, N. Measuring infectious bursal disease virus RNA in blood by multiplex real-time quantitative RT-PCR. *J. Virol. Methods* **2000**, *85*, 55–64. [CrossRef]
27. Shang, Y.; Kumar, S.; Oakley, B.; Kim, W.K. Chicken gut microbiota: Importance and detection technology. *Front. Vet. Sci.* **2018**, *5*. [CrossRef] [PubMed]

28. Costa, M.C.; Bessegatto, J.A.; Alfieri, A.A.; Weese, J.S.; Filho, J.A.B.; Oba, A. Different antibiotic growth promoters induce specific changes in the cecal microbiota membership of broiler chicken. *PLoS ONE* **2017**, *12*, e0171642. [CrossRef]
29. Gong, J.; Yu, H.; Liu, T.; Gill, J.J.; Chambers, J.R.; Wheatcroft, R.; Sabour, P.M. Effects of zinc bacitracin, bird age and access to range on bacterial microbiota in the ileum and caeca of broiler chickens. *J. Appl. Microbiol.* **2008**, *104*, 1372–1382. [CrossRef]
30. Bratburd, J.R.; Keller, C.; Vivas, E.; Gemperline, E.; Li, L.; Rey, F.E.; Currie, C.R.; Blaser, M.J. Gut microbial and metabolic responses to *Salmonella enterica* serovar Typhimurium and *Candida albicans*. *mBio* **2018**, *9*. [CrossRef]
31. Gadde, U.D.; Oh, S.; Lillehoj, H.S.; Lillehoj, E.P. Antibiotic growth promoters virginiamycin and bacitracin methylene disalicylate alter the chicken intestinal metabolome. *Sci. Rep.* **2018**, *8*. [CrossRef]
32. Arsenault, R.J.; Napper, S.; Kogut, M.H. *Salmonella enterica* Typhimurium infection causes metabolic changes in chicken muscle involving AMPK, fatty acid and insulin/mTOR signaling. *Vet. Res.* **2013**, *44*, 35. [CrossRef]
33. Kogut, M.H.; Genovese, K.J.; He, H.; Arsenault, R.J. AMPK and mTOR: Sensors and regulators of immunometabolic changes during *Salmonella* infection in the chicken. *Poult. Sci.* **2016**, *95*, 345–353. [CrossRef] [PubMed]
34. Mwangi, W.N.; Beal, R.K.; Powers, C.; Wu, X.; Humphrey, T.; Watson, M.; Bailey, M.; Friedman, A.; Smith, A.L. Regional and global changes in TCRαβ T cell repertoires in the gut are dependent upon the complexity of the enteric microflora. *Dev. Comp. Immunol.* **2010**, *34*, 406–417. [CrossRef] [PubMed]
35. Huyghebaert, G.; Ducatelle, R.; Immerseel, F.V. An update on alternatives to antimicrobial growth promoters for broilers. *Vet. J.* **2011**, *187*, 182–188. [CrossRef] [PubMed]
36. Sorbara, M.T.; Pamer, E.G. Interbacterial mechanisms of colonization resistance and the strategies pathogens use to overcome them. *Mucosal. Immunol.* **2019**, *12*, 1–9. [CrossRef] [PubMed]
37. Rychlik, I.; Elsheimer-Matulova, M.; Kyrova, K. Gene expression in the chicken caecum in response to infections with non-typhoid Salmonella. *Vet. Res.* **2014**, *45*, 119. [CrossRef] [PubMed]
38. Blacher, E.; Levy, M.; Tatirovsky, E.; Elinav, E. Microbiome-modulated metabolites at the interface of host immunity. *J. Immunol.* **2017**, *198*, 572–580. [CrossRef]
39. Buck, M.D.; O'Sullivan, D.; Pearce, E.L. T cell metabolism drives immunity. *J. Exp. Med.* **2015**, *212*, 1345–1360. [CrossRef]
40. Kumar, S.; Chen, C.; Indugu, N.; Werlang, G.O.; Singh, M.; Kim, W.K.; Thippareddi, H. Effect of antibiotic withdrawal in feed on chicken gut microbial dynamics, immunity, growth performance and prevalence of foodborne pathogens. *PLoS ONE* **2018**, *13*, e0192450. [CrossRef]
41. Ballou, A.L.; Ali, R.A.; Mendoza, M.A.; Ellis, J.C.; Hassan, H.M.; Croom, W.J.; Koci, M.D. Development of the chick microbiome: How early exposure influences future microbial diversity. *Front. Vet. Sci.* **2016**, *3*. [CrossRef]
42. Stanley, D.; Hughes, R.J.; Geier, M.S.; Moore, R.J. Bacteria within the gastrointestinal tract microbiota correlated with improved growth and feed conversion: Challenges presented for the identification of performance enhancing probiotic bacteria. *Front. Microbiol.* **2016**, *7*. [CrossRef]
43. Vacca, M.; Celano, G.; Calabrese, F.M.; Portincasa, P.; Gobbetti, M.; de Angelis, M. The controversial role of human gut Lachnospiraceae. *Microorganisms* **2020**, *8*, 573. [CrossRef] [PubMed]
44. Chen, L.; Wilson, J.; Koenigsknecht, M.; Chou, W. The intracellular innate immune sensor NLRP12 attenuates colon inflammation by maintaining colonic microbial diversity and promoting protective commensal bacterial growth. *Nat. Immunol.* **2017**, *18*, 541–551. [CrossRef] [PubMed]
45. Danzeisen, J.L.; Kim, H.B.; Isaacson, R.E.; Tu, Z.J.; Johnson, T.J. Modulations of the chicken cecal microbiome and metagenome in response to anticoccidial and growth promoter treatment. *PLoS ONE* **2011**, *6*, e27949. [CrossRef] [PubMed]
46. Lin, J.; Hunkapiller, A.A.; Layton, A.C.; Chang, Y.J.; Robbins, K.R. Response of intestinal microbiota to antibiotic growth promoters in chickens. *Foodborne Pathog. Dis.* **2013**, *10*, 331–337. [CrossRef] [PubMed]

5

Salmonella Pathogenicity Island 1 (SPI-1): The Evolution and Stabilization of a Core Genomic type Three Secretion System

Nicole A. Lerminiaux [1,2], Keith D. MacKenzie [1,2] and Andrew D. S. Cameron [1,2,*]

1 Department of Biology, Faculty of Science, University of Regina, Regina, SK S4S 0A2, Canada; lerminin@uregina.ca (N.A.L.); keith.mackenzie@uregina.ca (K.D.M.)

2 Institute for Microbial Systems and Society, Faculty of Science, University of Regina, Regina, SK S4S 0A2, Canada

* Correspondence: Andrew.Cameron@uregina.ca

Abstract: *Salmonella* Pathogenicity Island 1 (SPI-1) encodes a type three secretion system (T3SS), effector proteins, and associated transcription factors that together enable invasion of epithelial cells in animal intestines. The horizontal acquisition of SPI-1 by the common ancestor of all *Salmonella* is considered a prime example of how gene islands potentiate the emergence of new pathogens with expanded niche ranges. However, the evolutionary history of SPI-1 has attracted little attention. Here, we apply phylogenetic comparisons across the family Enterobacteriaceae to examine the history of SPI-1, improving the resolution of its boundaries and unique architecture by identifying its composite gene modules. SPI-1 is located between the core genes *flhA* and *mutS*, a hotspot for the gain and loss of horizontally acquired genes. Despite the plasticity of this locus, SPI-1 demonstrates stable residency of many tens of millions of years in a host genome, unlike short-lived homologous T3SS and effector islands including *Escherichia* ETT2, *Yersinia* YSA, *Pantoea* PSI-2, *Sodalis* SSR2, and *Chromobacterium* CPI-1. SPI-1 employs a unique series of regulatory switches, starting with the dedicated transcription factors HilC and HilD, and flowing through the central SPI-1 regulator HilA. HilA is shared with other T3SS, but HilC and HilD may have their evolutionary origins in *Salmonella*. The *hilA*, *hilC*, and *hilD* gene promoters are the most AT-rich DNA in SPI-1, placing them under tight control by the transcriptional repressor H-NS. In all *Salmonella* lineages, these three promoters resist amelioration towards the genomic average, ensuring strong repression by H-NS. Hence, early development of a robust and well-integrated regulatory network may explain the evolutionary stability of SPI-1 compared to T3SS gene islands in other species.

Keywords: genomic island; SPI-1; *Salmonella*; pathogenicity island; comparative genomics; type III secretion system

---

1. Introduction

Bacterial genomes are highly dynamic, able to gain and lose genes over short evolutionary times. Comparative genomics enables the differentiation of genes that are shared by all members of a species (core genes) from the genes with variable distributions across a species (accessory genes). *Escherichia coli* is a prime example of genomic variability. Although gene content ranges from 3744 to 6844 open reading frames in individual *E. coli* isolates, only 1000 genes are shared by the over 21,000 whole genome sequences that represent this species and are currently available in GenBank [1]. As accessory genes constitute the bulk of an average bacterial genome, understanding their evolutionary histories and genetic dynamics is central to understanding bacterial functions, and capabilities.

Accessory genes often become physically linked on contiguous segments of DNA, and these islands can range from two to dozens of genes. Horizontal gene transfer (HGT) is a driver of this coalescence because a physical connection between functionally linked genes increases the frequency of successful transfer [2–4]. HGT disconnects the phylogenetic history of a genomic island from that of its host genome [5], which can be reflected in islands having nucleotide and codon frequencies that differ from a genomic average [6–8]. Further signatures of HGT are that islands often insert adjacent to genetic elements that facilitate recombination, such as tRNA genes and mobile genetic elements [8–11].

Acquisition of genomic islands can provide new ecological functions and facilitate the invasion of new niches, enabling evolutionary leaps and even speciation [12]. Examples of biological functions that mobilize as genomic islands include sugar catabolism [13], plant symbioses [14], antibiotic resistance [15], virulence factors [6], and other pathogenicity determinants [8]. The contributions of "pathogenicity islands" to bacterial evolution and niche adaptation is best understood in the model pathogen *Salmonella*. A total of 24 pathogenicity islands have been identified in this genus, though not all of these islands have been experimentally validated to contribute to virulence phenotypes [16–18]. The largest is *Salmonella* Pathogenicity Island 1 (SPI-1) [19], which encodes a type three secretion system (T3SS) and type three secretion effectors (T3SEs) that mediate intracellular invasion of intestinal cells in animal hosts [20–23].

Acquisition of SPI-1 is a defining event in the evolution of *Salmonella*, occurring after divergence from the common ancestor with *Escherichia* over 100 million years ago [24–26]. The boundaries of SPI-1 were initially determined through DNA hybridization, then later through alignment with *E. coli* DNA sequence [21–23] (Figure 1A). Homologous T3SS and T3SE genes have been acquired by lineages of *E. coli*, but these are rare and a prominent example in *E. coli* O157:H7 is losing functionality [27]. Broader phylogenetic comparisons have identified homologous T3SS in facultative human pathogens such as *Yersinia*, *Chromobacterium*, and *Shigella*, and plant pathogens such as *Pantoea* (Table 1) [28–34]. These T3SSs are found only in select members of each genus. For example, PSI-2 appears to be undergoing frequent HGT and loss in the genus *Pantoea* [32]. Similarly, *Yersinia* YSA is present in *Yersinia enterocolitica* but is absent from *Yersinia pestis* [35]. The Mxi-Spa T3SS has entered the *Shigella* clade multiple times on several types of pINV plasmids [36–38].

Despite its prominence as the archetypal pathogenicity island and intensive research attention for several decades, little is known about why SPI-1 is uniquely stable among T3SS genomic islands in Enterobacteriaceae. Previous studies of T3SS genetic architecture have included cursory analyses of the evolutionary transitions that differentiate T3SS-containing gene islands in bacteria [27,28,31,32,39–42]. Pathogenicity islands can have mosaic structures arising from the merger of smaller islands that were acquired at different points in evolutionary history [8]. While several studies have suggested that SPI-1 has a mosaic structure [43,44], an in-depth evolutionary analysis of the island's history has not yet been conducted.

The most robust approach to find genomic islands and their boundaries is through comparative genomics. xenoGI is a recently released comparative genomics program that identifies genomic islands that are shared by a clade of bacteria as well as islands that are unique to certain strains by grouping genes by origin on a phylogenetic tree [45]. Using this locus-based approach, the objectives of our study were to: (1) identify the genomic islands of SPI-1, (2) examine the evolutionary history of the SPI-1 locus, and (3) evaluate the evolutionary history of SPI-1-encoded transcriptional regulators *hilA*, *hilC*, and *hilD*. Tracking how genomic islands originate, spread, and decay is key to determining how islands enable genomic diversification and adaptation. Connecting the evolutionary history of an infection-relevant pathogenicity island, SPI-1, to extensive experimental characterization of its molecular components helps develop and improve our understanding of pathogen emergence.

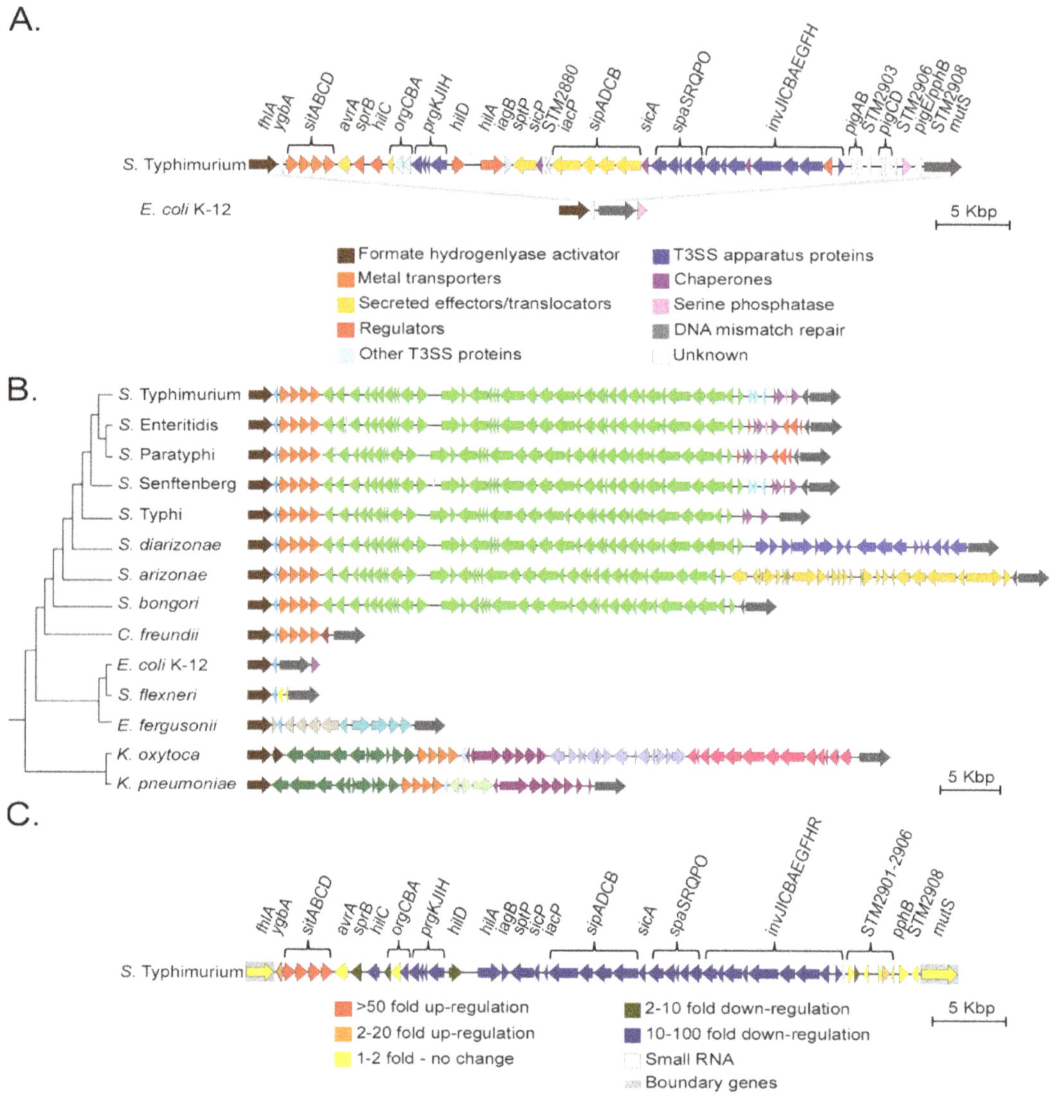

Figure 1. Comparative genomic analysis of *Salmonella* Pathogenicity Island 1 (SPI-1). (**A**) Alignment of *Salmonella enterica* serovar Typhimurium LT2 SPI-1 to the same locus in *Escherichia coli* K12. Genes are coloured by function based on annotations in Genbank and SalCom [46,47]. Grey bars represent sequence homology determined by blastx (minimum length 100 bp, e-value < 0.00001). (**B**) Alignment of the SPI-1 locus in *Salmonella, Escherichia, Citrobacter,* and *Klebsiella*. Whole-genome phylogeny was constructed with PATRIC. Gene colouring corresponds to different gene clusters identified by xenoGI [45]: *fhlA* (dark brown), *ygbA* (blue), *sitABCD* (orange), *avrA – invH* (green), *pig* genes and *pphB* (light blue/purple) and *mutS* (grey). *S. enterica* Senftenberg strain ATCC 43845 is included in this figure. Small open reading frames (white) between *sitD* and *hilA* in *S. enterica* Enteriditis, *S. enterica* Paratyphi, *S. enterica* Senftenberg may be due to different annotation pipelines and will not be examined here. (**C**) The transcriptional response to the intra-macrophage environment by *S.* Typhimurium 4/74 reflects that SPI-1 is an island composed of transcriptionally-cohesive modules. Genes are coloured according to the fold differences quantified by RNA-seq in the macrophage vacuole compared to early stationary phase in Lennox broth; data from [48].

2. Materials and Methods

2.1. Bacterial Strains

Table 2 has a complete list of 29 bacterial strains and accession numbers included in xenoGI analysis. These strains were chosen to capture phylogenetic and GC content diversity. Unless otherwise specified, all gene and ortholog names will be as annotated as in *Salmonella enterica* serovar Typhimurium LT2 to avoid confusion over different annotations for the same genes. All genome sequence files and corresponding annotations were downloaded from NCBI Genbank. Several other strains that were used for genomic comparison but not included in xenoGI analysis are *S.* Senftenberg strain N17-509 (accession: CP026379.1), *E. coli* ISCII (accession: CBWP010000030.1), and *E. coli* O104:H11 strain RM14721 plasmid RM14721 (accession: NZ_CP027106.1). Strains with genomes at the NCBI assembly level of "complete" (gapless chromosome) were selected over draft genomes due to the higher quality and ability to distinguish independent units such as plasmids.

2.2. Whole-Genome Phylogenetic Tree Building for xenoGI Input

The phylogenetic tree was built using PATRIC 3.4.2 [49], which constructs trees based on coding sequence similarity. All bacteria strains listed in Table 1 were the focal group, except for *Pseudomonas aeruginosa* which was used as the outgroup (Supplementary Figure S1).

2.3. xenoGI Parameters

Analysis was run using default parameters in xenoGI v2.2.0 [45] with the following exceptions: rootFocalClade was set to i26 (Figure S1) and evalueThresh was set to 1e-8. Computing time took approximately 3 h with 29 strains. Bed files were generated from xenoGI scripts and were used to visualize islands in Integrated Genome Browser version 9.1.0 [50] and Easyfig version 2.2.3 [51]. Analysis of islands was done with the interactiveAnalysis.py script. Annotations used to determine gene function were obtained from the Genbank flat files (.gbff) and SalCom (Table 1) [46,47,52]. Raw analysis output from xenoGI is found in Supplementary Table S1.

2.4. AT Content Analysis

AT content was calculated from the Genbank flat files (.gbff) for select strains in Table 1 using Geneious R11 (https://www.geneious.com) [53] and plotted as a heatmap. The average GC content for each nucleotide position was determined using a 100 base sliding window.

2.5. Hil Phylogenies

We used blastx 2.10.0+ [54] to search for *hil* gene homologs in other bacteria excluding the *Salmonella* clade (taxid:590) and filtering for hits that covered > 80% of the query sequence. *Salmonella enterica* serotype Typhimurium LT2 HilA (AAL21756.1), HilC (NP_461788.1), and HilD (NP_461796.1) were used as the query sequences. Because *S. enterica* Typhimurium LT2 HilC and HilD have high sequence similarity (36.4 % identity over 88 % query coverage, e-value < 3e-51, bit score = 168), we chose a 80% query cut-off filter when searching for HilC and HilD homologs to capture both regulators of interest and sufficient diversity. In other words, when searching in the *Salmonella* clade using HilC as a query with these settings, HilD would return as a hit and vice versa. The accession numbers included in the phylogenetic analysis for HilA are listed in Supplementary Table S2 and accession numbers for HilC/D are listed in Supplementary Table S3. *Salmonella bongori* NCTC 12419 HilA (CCC31553.1), HilC (WP_000243993.1) and HilD (WP_000432692.1) and *Salmonella enterica* serotype Typhi CT18 HilA (CAD05983.1) were included as representatives in the phylogenetic trees. Multiple protein alignments were done using MUSCLE [55] in MEGA 7 [56]. Maximum likelihood trees were constructed using the LG+G amino acid substitution model for HilA in Figure 6, the LG+G+I amino acid substitution model for HilA in Supplementary Figure S2 and the JTT+G amino acid substitution model for HilC/D in MEGA X [57]. The maximum-likelihood phylogenies were supported with 1000 bootstrap replicates. Tree visualization was done with iTOL [58].

Table 1. Nomenclature of genes in T3SSs related to SPI-1 [1].

Salmonella SPI-1	*Pantoea* PSI-2	*Shigella* Mxi-Spa	*Escherichia* ETT2	*Escherichia* LEE	*Yersinia* YSA	*Yersinia* YSC	*Sodalis* SSR1	*Sodalis* SSR2	*Pseudomonas* Psc/Pcr/Pop/Exs	*Chromobacterium* CPI-1	Universal [2]	Function [3]
avrA						*yopP*						Effector
sprB												Regulator
hilC		*S0103*										Regulator
orgC										*corC*		Effector
orgB		*mxiL/mxiN*	*orgB*	*escL*	YE3555	*yscL*		*orgAb*	*pscL*	*corB*	*sctL*	Needle assembly
orgA		*mxiK*	*orgA*		YE3554	*yscK*		*orgA*	*pscK*	*corA*	*sctK*	Needle assembly
prgK	*psaJ*	*mxiJ/yscJ*	*eprK*	*escJ*	*ysaJ*	*yscJ*	*ysaJ*	*prgK*	*pscJ*	*cprK*	*sctJ*	Inner mb ring
prgJ	*psaI*	*mxiI*	*eprJ*	*escI*	*ysaI*	*yscI*	*ysaI*	*prgJ*	*pscI*	*cprJ*	*sctI*	Needle subunit
prgI	*psaG*	*mxiH*	*eprI*	*escF*	YE3551	*yscF*	*ysaG*	*prgI*	*pscF*	*cprI*	*sctF*	Needle subunit
prgH	*psaF*	*mxiG*	*eprH*	*escD*	YE3550	*yscD*	*ysaF*	*prgH*	*pscD*	*cprH*	*sctD*	Inner mb ring
hilD												Regulator
hilA			*ygeH*					*hilA*		*cilA*		Regulator
iagB	*psaH*	*ipgF*	*ipgF*	*etgA*	*ysaH*		*ysaH*			*iagB*		Transglosylase
sptP					*yspP*	*yopH*				CV0974		Effector
sicP	*psa7*											Chaperone
iacP	*psaC/acpM*	*ipgG*			*acpY*		*ysaC*			*iacP*		Acyl carrier
STM2880												Unknown
sipA		*ipaA*			*yspA*		*yspA*			*cipA*		Effector
sipD	*pspD*	*ipaD*		*espA*	*yspD*	*lcrV*	*yspD*		*pcrV*	*cipD*		Tip complex
sipC	*pspC*	*ipaC*		*espB*	*yspC*	*yopD*	*yspC*		*popD*	*cipC*		Effector
sipB	*pspB*	*ipaB*		*espD*	*yspB*	*yopB*	*yspB*		*popB*	*cipB*		Effector
sicA	*pchA*	*ipgC*	*ygeG*	*cesD*	*sycB*	*sycD*	*sycB*	*sicA*	*pcrH*	*cicA*		Chaperone
spaS	*psaU*	*spa40*	*epaS*	*escU*	*ysaU*	*yscU*	*ysaU*	*spaS*	*pscU*	*cpaS*	*sctU*	Export apparatus
spaR	*psaT*	*spa29*	*epaR*	*escT*	*ysaT*	*yscT*	*ysaT*	*spaR*	*pscT*	*cpaR*	*sctT*	Export apparatus
spaQ	*psaS*	*spa9*	*epaQ*	*escS*	*ysaS*	*yscS*	*ysaS*	*spaQ*	*pscS*	*cpaQ*	*sctS*	Export apparatus
spaP	*psaR*	*spa24*	*epaP*	*escR*	*ysaR*	*yscR*	*ysaR*	*spaP*	*pscR*	*cpaP*	*sctR*	Export apparatus
spaO	*psaQ*	*spa33*	*epaO*	*escQ/sepQ*	*ysaQ*	*yscQ*	*ysaQ*	*spaO*	*pscQ/hrcQ*	*cpaO*	*sctQ*	Cytoplasmic ring
invJ	*psaP*	*spa32/spaN*	*eivJ*	*escP/orf16*	*yspN*	*yscP*	*ysaP*	*spaN*	*pscP*	*cpaN*	*sctP*	Needle assembly
invI	*psaO*	*spa13/spaM*	*eivI*	*escO/escA/orf15*	YE3543A	*yscO*	*ysaO*	*spaM*	*pscO*	*cpaM*	*sctO*	Needle assembly
invC/spaL	*psaN*	*spa47/spaL*	*eivC*	*escN*	*ysaN*	*yscN*	*ysaN*	*invC*	*pscN*	*civC*	*sctN*	ATPase
invB	*psaK*	*spa15/spaK*			*ysaK*		*ysaK*	*invB*		*civB*		Chaperone
invA	*psaV*	*mxiA*	*eivA*	*escV*	*ysaV*	*yscV/lcrD*	*ysaV*	*invA*	*pcrD*	*civA*	*sctV*	Export apparatus
invE	*psaW*	*mxiC*	*eivE*	*sepL/sepD*	*ysaW*	*yopN/tyeA*	*ysaW*	*invE*	*popN*	*civE*	*sctW*	Export regulator

Table 1. *Cont.*

Salmonella SPI-1	*Pantoea* PSI-2	*Shigella* Mxi-Spa	*Escherichia* ETT2	*Escherichia* LEE	*Yersinia* YSA	*Yersinia* YSC	*Sodalis* SSR1	*Sodalis* SSR2	*Pseudomonas* Psc/Pcr/Pop/Exs	*Chromobacterium* CPI-1	Universal [2]	Function [3]
invG	*psaC*	*mxiD*	*eivG*	*escC*	*ysaC*	*yscC*	*ysaC*	*invG*	*pscC*	*civG*	*sctC*	Outer mb ring
invF	*mxiE/ysaE*	*mxiE*	*eivF*		*ysaE*	*virF*	*ysaE*	*invF*	*exsA*	*civF*		Regulator
invH		*mxiM*				*yscW*			*exsB*			Export apparatus
pigA												Unknown
pigB												Unknown
STM2903												Insertion element
pigC												Unknown
pigD												Unknown
STM2906												Transposase
pphB												Phosphatase
STM2908												Unknown

[1] Gene names curated for Pantoea PSI-2 [32,40], Shigella Mxi-Spa [39,41,59], Escherichia ETT2 Sakai [27], Escherichia EPEC LEE [39], Yersinia YSA [30,40,41,60,61], Yersinia YSC [39,42], Sodalis SSR1 [29,40], Sodalis SSR2 [29], Pseudomonas aeruginosa Psc/Pcr/Pop/Exs [39,42], Chromobacterium CPI-1 [28]. [2] Universal gene names from [31,52]. [3] Functions from [46,47,52]. Mb = membrane.

Table 2. List of bacterial strains and genome assembly versions used in xenoGI analysis.

Genus	Species	Strain	% GC	Mbp	Genbank Accession	Genbank Assembly Version
Citrobacter	*freundii*	CFNIH1	52.2	5.09	NZ_CP007557.1	GCA_000648515.1_ASM64851v1
Citrobacter	*koseri*	ATCC BAA-895	53.8	4.72	NC_009792.1	GCA_000018045.1_ASM1804v1
Enterobacter	*cloacae* subsp. *cloacae*	ATCC 13047	52.47	5.32	NC_014121.1	GCA_000025565.1_ASM2556v1
Enterobacter	*lignolyticus*	SCF1	57.2	4.81	NC_014618.1	GCA_000164865.1_ASM16486v1
Escherichia	*albertii*	KF1	49.7	4.7	NZ_CP007025.1	GCA_000512125.1_ASM51212v1
Escherichia	*coli*	O157:H7 Sakai	50.45	5.59	NC_002695.1	GCA_000008865.1_ASM886v1
Escherichia	*coli*	K12 MG1655	50.8	4.64	NC_000913.3	GCA_000005845.2_ASM584v2
Escherichia	*coli*	IAI39	50.6	5.13	NC_011750.1	GCA_000026345.1_ASM2634v1
Escherichia	*coli*	O104:H4 str 2011C-3493	50.63	5.44	NC_018658.1	GCA_000299455.1_ASM29945v1
Escherichia	*fergusonii*	ATCC 35469	49.88	4.64	NC_011740.1	GCA_000026225.1_ASM2622v1
Klebsiella	*pneumoniae* subsp. *pneumoniae*	HS11286	57.14	5.68	NC_016845.1	GCA_000240185.2_ASM24018v2
Klebsiella	*oxytoca*	CAV1374	55.26	7.23	NZ_CP011636.1	GCA_001022195.1_ASM102219v1
Pantoea	*agglomerans*	IG1	55.02	5.12	NZ_CP016889.1	GCA_001709315.1_ASM170931v1
Pantoea	*ananatis*	LMG 5342	53.4	4.14	NC_016816.1	GCA_000283875.1_ASM28387v1
Pantoea	*stewartii*	DC283	54.2	4.53	NZ_CP017581.1	GCA_002082215.1_ASM208221v1
Pseudomonas	*aeruginosa*	PAO1	66.6	6.26	NC_002516.2	GCA_000006765.1_ASM676v1
Salmonella	*bongori*	NCTC 12419	51.3	4.46	NC_015761.1	GCA_000252995.1_ASM25299v1
Salmonella	*enterica* subsp. *enterica* Enteritidis	P125109	52.2	4.69	NC_011294.1	GCA_000009505.1_ASM950v1
Salmonella	*enterica* subsp. *enterica* Typhi	CT18	51.88	5.13	NC_003198.1	GCA_000195995.1_ASM19599v1
Salmonella	*enterica* subsp. *enterica* Typhimurium	LT2	52.22	4.95	NC_003197.2	GCA_000006945.2_ASM694v2
Salmonella	*enterica* subsp. *enterica* Paratyphi C	RKS4594	52.21	4.89	NC_012125.1	GCA_000018385.1_ASM1838v1
Salmonella	*enterica* subsp. *enterica* Senftenberg	ATCC 43845	51.93	5.26	CP019194.1	GCA_000486525.2_ASM48652v2
Salmonella	*enterica* subsp. *arizonae*	62z23 RSK2980	51.4	4.6	NZ_CP006693.1	GCA_000018625.1_ASM1862v1
Salmonella	*enterica* subsp. *diarizonae*	HZS154	51.4	5.09	CP023345.1	GCA_002794415.1_ASM279441v1
Shigella	*flexneri*	2a 301	50.67	4.83	NC_004337.2	GCA_000006925.2_ASM692v2
Sodalis	*glossinidius*	mortisans	54.51	4.29	NC_007712.1	GCA_000010085.1_ASM1008v1
Sodalis	*praecaptivus*	HS1	57.13	4.29	NZ_CP006569.1	GCA_000517425.1_ASM51742v1
Yersinia	*enterocolitica* subsp. *enterocolitica*	8081	47.25	4.68	NC_008800.1	GCA_000009345.1_ASM934v1
Yersinia	*pestis*	CO92	47.61	4.83	NC_003143	GCA_000009065.1_ASM906v1

3. Results

3.1. *SPI-1 is a Mosaic of Gene Islands*

We conducted a fine scale analysis of gene content and architecture at the *fhlA/-/mutS* locus using xenoGI, a program based explicitly on phylogenetic comparisons to identify islands. Briefly, xenoGI sorts genes into families, then sorts families into islands based on synteny or location within a genome, while also accounting for amino acid similarity. Many genomic island-finding programs exist [reviewed in [62,63]], but unlike other methodologies, xenoGI requires a phylogenetic tree for input. The phylogeny is used to determine which islands are shared by a clade and to identify at which branch they were acquired [45].

The core chromosomal genes that have been previously defined as the boundaries of the SPI-1 locus are *fhlA*, encoding the formate hydrogenlyase transcriptional activator, and *mutS*, encoding a DNA mismatch repair protein, as noted previously from direct comparison of *E. coli* K-12 to *S.* Typhimurium [23,64] (Figure 1A). Comparing this locus in *Salmonella* to homologs in closely related genera *Citrobacter*, *Escherichia*, *Shigella*, *Enterobacter* and *Klebsiella* confirmed that *fhlA* and *mutS* define the boundaries of a plastic locus across these Enterobacteriaceae. In the reference *Salmonella* Typhimurium genome, xenoGI divided SPI-1 into three gene islands, which are coloured in Figure 1B: *sitABCD* (orange), *avrA-invH* (green), and *pigA*-STM2908 (purple & blue). The distinct nature of these three islands is reflected in their independent transcriptional output in infection-relevant conditions [46,48] (Figure 1C). Each of these islands is examined separately below.

3.2. *A Cohesive SPI-1 Gene Set is Highly Conserved in* Salmonella

To evaluate SPI-1 conservation across the genus *Salmonella*, we selected representative strains from both species (*S. enterica* and *S. bongori*), three *S. enterica* subspecies (*arizonae*, *diarizonae*, and *enterica*), and four serotypes of model pathogens (Typhimurium, Typhi, Paratyphi, and Enteritidis). This selection includes the deepest branches within the genus [65] and a range of genome sizes (4.46-5.26 Mbp). Figure 1B shows that the *avrA-invH* island (green), which encodes the T3SS and associated effectors (T3SE), is conserved across all eight *Salmonella* genomes but is absent from this locus in other Enterobacteriaceae.

A single gene in the *avrA-invH* island is not conserved across the eight representative *Salmonella* genomes. The effector gene *avrA* is absent in *S. enterica* Typhi, *S. enterica* Paratyphi and *S. enterica arizonae* (Figure 1B). The frequent loss of *avrA* in independent lineages of *Salmonella* is illustrated more comprehensively in the analysis 445 *Salmonella* strains by Worley and colleagues [66]. We note that *avrA* expression is unchanged during macrophage infection (Figure 1C), suggesting its dispensability is reflected in low integration into the SPI-1 regulatory network.

3.3. *The* ygbA *and* sitABCD *Islands Predate Core SPI-1*

The *sitABCD* island identified by xenoGI is conserved across *Salmonella*, *Citrobacter*, and *Klebsiella* (orange genes in Figure 1B). Hypothetical protein *ygbA* at this locus was classified into two islands: one in *Salmonella*, *Citrobacter*, *Escherichia* and *Enterobacter lignolyticus* and one in *Klebsiella* where is has a reverse orientation at the other side of the *sitABCD* operon (Figure 1B, blue). The simplest interpretation of this phylogeny is that the common ancestor of these Enterobacteriaceae had *ygbA* and *sitABCD* at this locus, but the *sitABCD* operon was subsequently lost from the *Escherichia/Shigella* clade and some minor reorganization has placed *ygbA* in two alternate positions either adjacent to *sitD* or *sitA*. Furthermore, the *ygbA* and *sitABCD* islands predate the insertion of the *avrA-invH* (T3SS) island in the *Salmonella* ancestor.

To test whether *E. coli* strains might encode the *sitABCD* operon at other genomic locations, we used blastx to search for orthologs in whole genome sequences. *Shigella flexneri* strain 2a 301 and *E. coli* IAI39 have *ygbA* at the *fhlA/-/mutS* locus and *sitABCD* at another location in their genome. We also examined a small number of species from sister families in the order Enterobacterales. The *sitABCD* operon is present in these bacterial families located either at chromosomal locations separate from *mutS* in *Sodalis glossinidius* and *Sodalis praecaptivus* (Pectobacteriaceae) and *Yersinia pestis* (Yersiniaceae), or on a plasmid in *Pantoea ananatis* (Erwiniaceae) (Figure 2). These species all lack *ygbA* homologs.

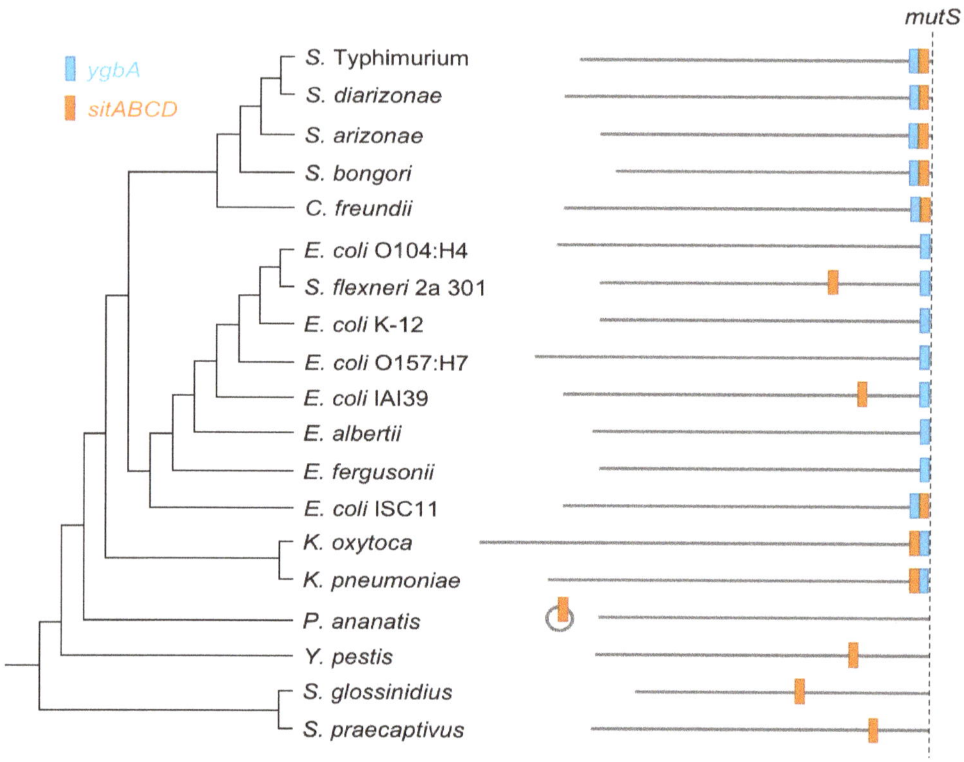

Figure 2. Genomic positions of *ygbA* and *sitABCD* relative to *mutS* in select Enterobacterales. The whole-genome phylogeny was constructed by PATRIC [49]. Variations of the *ygbA* and *sitABCD* gene clusters are coloured for *ygbA* (blue) and *sitABCD* (orange). Chromosome lengths are drawn to scale.

In *E. coli* K12, *ygbA* is the only gene located between the core genes *fhlA* and *mutS* (Figure 1A). However, the broader phylogenetic comparison in Figure 2 shows the presence of *ygbA* and *sitABCD* at this locus in the deepest-branching *E. coli* considered here (strain ISC11). This evidence further supports the supposition that many lineages of *E. coli* have lost *sitABCD* while in others the operon has relocated.

3.4. *The Highly Variable* mutS*-Proximal Region*

The region adjacent to the *mutS* gene promoter is highly variable in gene content, demonstrating gene gain and loss in all Enterobacteriaceae lineages examined here (Figure 1B). In the reference *Salmonella* genome, *S. enterica* Typhimurium, this region encodes several pathogenicity island genes (*pig* genes) and mobile elements (Figure 3). Several of the *pig* genes are regulated by SPI-1-encoded HilC, but they do not seem to contribute to *Salmonella*'s virulence phenotype and their specific functions remain unknown [43]. Reconstructing the temporal events in gene gain and loss in the representative *Salmonella* suggests an initial gain of *pigC, pigD, pphB* (purple) and a transposase (pink). This was followed by gain of *pigA, pigB* and an insertion element (blue) then loss of these elements by *S.* Enteritidis and *S.* Paratyphi. The *S.* Enteritidis and *S.* Paratyphi lineage acquired four hypothetical proteins (red) (Figure 3). No *pig* genes are found at the *fhlA*/-/*mutS* locus in other Enterobacteriaceae. *pphB* encodes a serine phosphatase that is ancestral at this locus but is located on the opposing side of *mutS* in *E. coli* (Figure 1A).

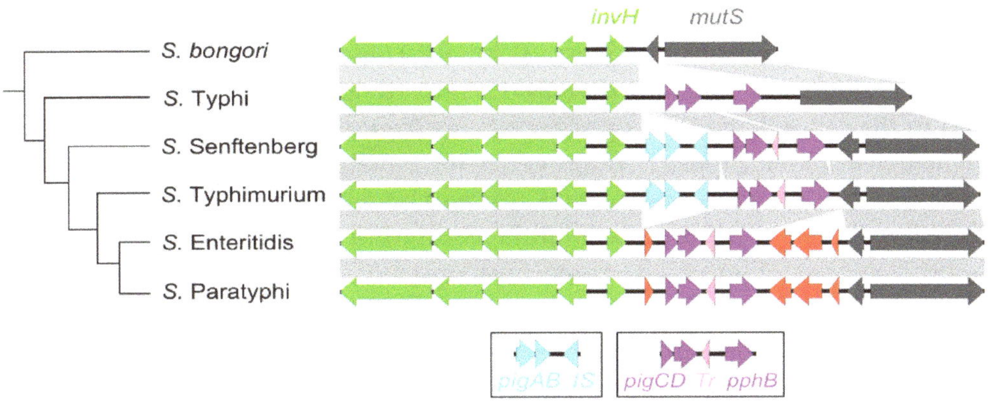

Figure 3. Alignment of the SPI-1 downstream boundary across the *Salmonella* clade. Whole-genome phylogeny was constructed with PATRIC [49]. Gene colouring corresponds to different gene clusters identified by xenoGI [45]: *invAEGFH* (green), *pigAB* and insertion element (blue), *pigCD* (purple), transposase (pink), *pphB* (purple), hypothetical coding sequences (red, grey). *S. enterica* Senftenberg strain ATCC 43845 is included in this figure. Grey bars represent sequence homology determined by blastx (min length 100 bp, e-value < 0.00001). IS, insertion element; Tr, transposase.

3.5. Decay and Loss of SPI-1

The core SPI-1 island is exceptional among related T3SS-T3SE systems in its long-term residency and stability in a bacterial clade. Nevertheless, SPI-1 can be lost, as observed in *S. enterica* serotype Senftenberg [67–72]. *S.* Senftenberg ATCC 43845 was included in the analysis presented in Figure 1B. However, the presence of pseudogenes in the *avrA-invH* island, including the SPI-1 regulator *hilD*, indicates genetic decay that is expected to cause loss of invasion functions.

To understand the genetic changes associated with the loss of SPI-1, we aligned *S.* Senftenberg ATCC 43845 to *S.* Senftenberg strain N17-509, a strain that has lost SPI-1 [72]. *S.* Senftenberg N17-509 has lost the entire SPI-1 core region (*avrA-invH*) but retains homologs to the *ygbA*, *sitABCD* and *pig* genes (Figure 4). Another gene island containing mobile elements, a toxin-antitoxin system, and a restriction endonuclease has inserted between the *pig* genes and *mutS* (Figure 4).

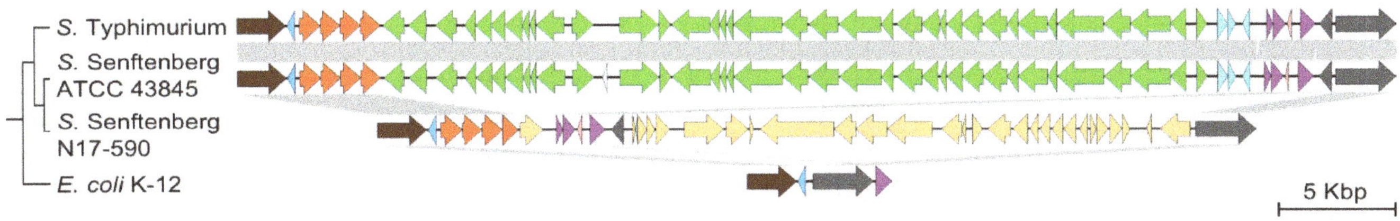

Figure 4. Alignment of the SPI-1 locus in *S. enterica* Typhimurium LT2, *S. enterica* Senftenberg strains ATCC 43845 and N17-590 and *Escherichia coli* K12. Gene colouring corresponds to different gene clusters identified by xenoGI [45]: *fhlA* (dark brown), *ygbA* (blue), *sitABCD* (orange), *avrA – invH* (green), *pig* genes and *pphB* (light blue/purple) and *mutS* (grey). Genomic island in *S.* Senftenberg N17-509 with no homology to SPI-1 is coloured beige. Grey bars represent sequence homology determined by blastx (min length 100 bp, e-value < 0.00001).

3.6. The fhlA/-/mutS Locus is a Hotspot for Island Acquisition

Our analysis shows that SPI-1 inserted at a highly plastic locus that is a hotspot for the acquisition of small and large gene islands. In *S. enterica* subsp. *diarizonae* and subsp. *arizonae*, a second island exists in each strain between *invH* and *mutS* (blue and gold, respectively, in Figure 1B). These islands consist largely of hypothetical proteins and encode mobile elements such as integrases (*S. enterica* subsp. *arizonae*) and transposases (*S. enterica* subsp. *diarizonae*).

Various *Escherichia* species and strains were included in the xenoGI analysis to capture lineage diversity (Table 2). *S. flexneri* has two integrases encoded between *ygbA* and *mutS*, but no other genes. Several *Escherichia* strains (*E. albertii, E. fergusonii* and *E. coli* IAI39) have a single transcriptional regulator *modE* located between *fhlA* and *ygbA*. *E. coli* O104:H4 2011C-3493 has a hypothetical protein between *ygbA* and *mutS*. *E. coli* K12 and *E. coli* O157:H7 are identical at this locus. Of the *Escherichia* species included in the xenoGI analysis, only *Escherichia fergusonii* had islands larger than single genes inserted at the *fhlA/-/mutS* locus; these contain genes for metabolism functions and sugar transport.

Representatives of two *Klebsiella* species, *K. oxytoca* and *K. pneumoniae*, were included in xenoGI analysis. Both strains have multiple gene islands inserted between *fhlA* and *mutS*, and two islands are shared by both species (Figure 1B, green and purple). The shared islands encode genes for an iron transport system and homologs of the sugar translocation proteins EIIB and EIIC in the phosphotransferase system, suggesting that these islands enable nutrient acquisition in *Klebsiella*.

3.7. AT Nucleotide Content and the Evolution of Transcriptional Control

A paradigm in bacterial genomics is that AT-rich DNA is a signature of horizontally acquired genes [73]. SPI-1 has been resident in *Salmonella* for many tens of million years, yet the island has a high AT content that has resisted amelioration to match the nucleotide composition of the core genome [65]. AT-richness of SPI-1 is maintained by a higher GC-to-AT substitution rate compared to a higher AT-to-GC substitution rate in core genes [65]. Protein-DNA interactions in gene regulatory networks may explain nucleotide frequencies that resist amelioration to genomic averages [65]. In bacteria, several global transcription factors favour the nucleotide composition and physical properties of AT-rich DNA [73,74]. One such protein is the nucleoid-associated protein H-NS, a global repressor of gene expression [75,76]. The strong repression of SPI-1 gene expression by H-NS suggest that SPI-1 resists amelioration to remain within the H-NS regulon.

We compared AT content at SPI-1 in the eight representative *Salmonella* genomes, which confirmed the expectation that all eight lineages have maintained an amazingly consistent pattern of high AT content (Supplementary Figure S3). This heatmap of nucleotide composition shows the level of conservation and resilience of the high AT content of SPI-1. Moreover, it illustrates how gene islands can be internally consistent in nucleotide composition and can differ dramatically from neighbouring islands, which is especially apparent in the cases of the GC-rich islands in *Klebsiella* (Supplementary Figure S3).

Two regions in SPI-1 are very AT-rich: the *hilD-hilA* and *hilC* loci (Figure 5A). This pattern fits particularly well with the model that AT content is selected to maintain membership in the H-NS regulon. Transcriptional activation of SPI-1 begins with antagonism of H-NS repression by the transcriptional activators HilC and HilD [77–79] (Figure 5B). When active in DNA binding, HilC and HilD activate their own promoters to create a feed-forward signal that counteracts H-NS silencing of the *hilA* promoter [80]. HilA, in turn, activates transcription of the regulator *invF* and acts directly at the T3SS and T3SE gene promoters.

3.8. Evolution of Transcriptional Control: Acquisition of hilA

HilA, a DNA binding protein in the OmpR/ToxR family of transcription factors, is the master activator of SPI-1 transcription. HilA binds to the *invF* and *prgH* promoters, triggering the activation of T3SS and T3SE genes [81–83]. A recent survey of T3SS in ~20,000 bacterial genomes classified SPI-1 according to gene conservation and synteny into what the authors termed category II [31]. Category II T3SS are scattered among Gammaproteobacteria and Betaproteobacteria, but *hilA* is missing from most genomes with a category II T3SS [31], suggesting this regulatory module is a relatively recent addition within this family of homologous T3SSs. We examined the evolutionary connection between *hilA*, T3SS, and T3SE genes in Proteobacteria (Figure 6, Supplementary Figure S2). The HilA phylogeny does not recapitulate organismal phylogeny, consistent with the role of HGT in distributing T3SS across diverse strains and species. The dynamic architecture of SPI-1 homologs is further illustrated by aligning genes according to the largest conserved island, *spaS-invF*. This alignment helps illustrate how the T3SS and T3SE components are genetically divisible into distinct islands, *orgCBA-prgKJIH*, *hilA-iagB*, *iacP-sipADCB-sicA*, and *spaSRQPO-invJICBAEGF* (Figure 6). These constituent islands are illustrated at the bottom of Figure 6, and correspond approximately to the microsynteny blocks described by Hu and colleagues [31]: MSB1+*orgC*, MSB5+*iacP/sipA*, and MSB3+MSB4+MSB2 is island *spaSRQPO/invJICBAEGF*. The shuffled orientation and composition of these blocks means that no two genera possess the same island architecture.

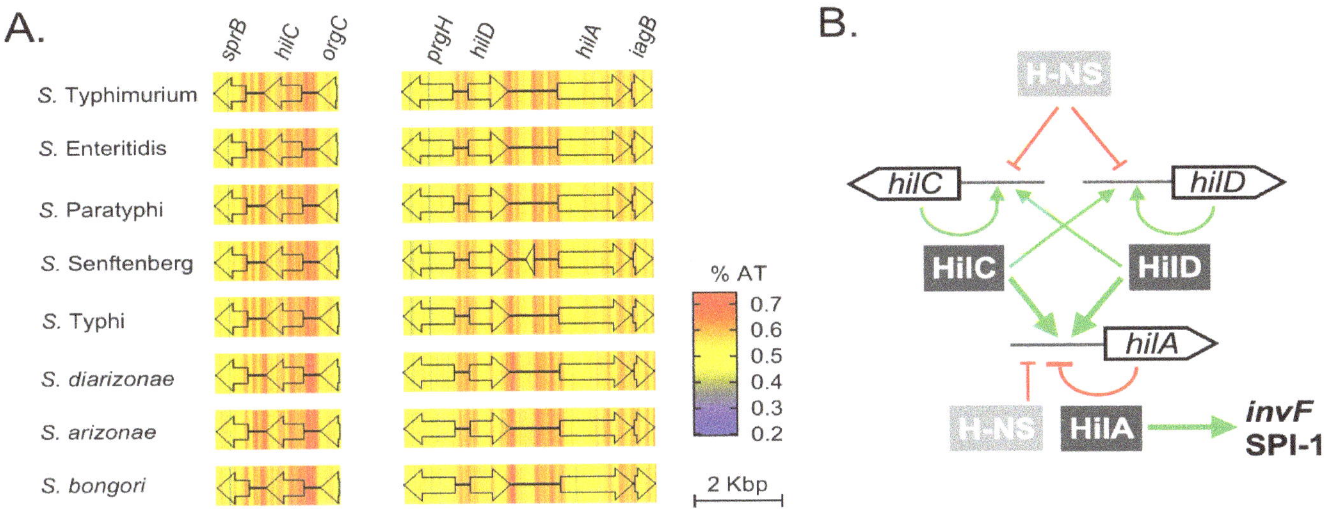

Figure 5. Nucleotide composition and gene regulation in SPI-1. (**A**) AT content schematic of *hil* gene promoters across eight *Salmonella* strains. AT content was overlaid as a heatmap on the regions surrounding *hilC*, *hilD* and *hilA*. Heatmap values were generated with a 100 base sliding window using Geneious R11 [53]. (**B**) Core elements of the SPI-1 transcriptional regulatory network.

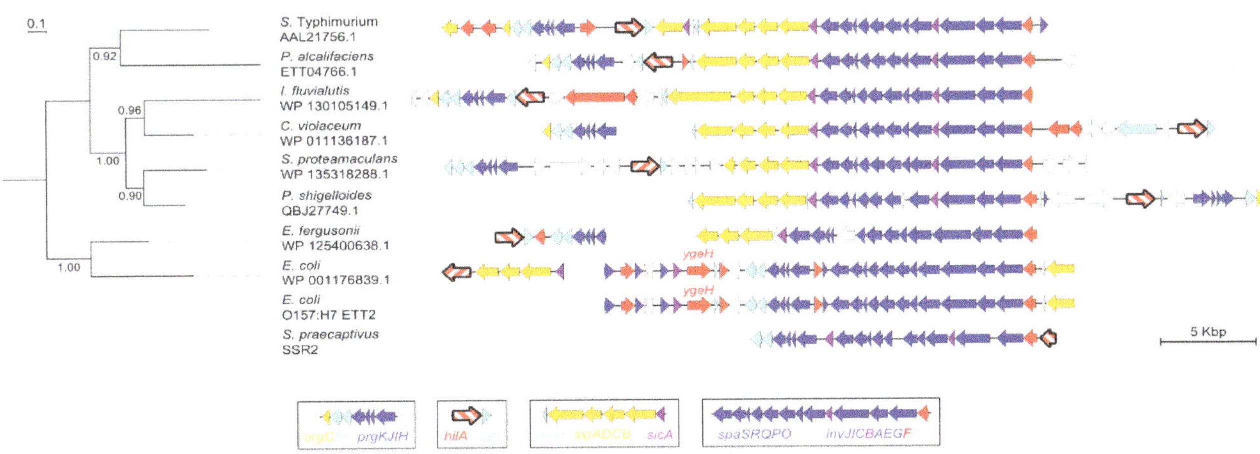

Figure 6. HilA phylogeny and genetic context for *hilA* in T3SS islands. Best blastx hits covering at least 80% of the query (*S. enterica* Typhimurium LT2 HilA) were identified and one representative protein sequence was selected from each species to capture phylogenetic diversity. Protein sequences were aligned using MUSCLE [55] and phylogeny was built using a maximum-likelihood model LG+G with 1000 bootstrap replicates [57]. *hilA* is illustrated in bold with white and red hashes and genes are coloured according to function (see Figure 1 legend). Conserved gene modules in T3SSs with *hilA* are identified at the bottom of the figure. Two strains (bottom) were included in xenoGI analysis but not the phylogenetic tree. Both have a T3SS but are either missing *hilA* (*E. coli* O157:H7 Sakai) or have a truncated *hilA* (*S. praecaptivus*). For a more detailed reconstruction of *hilA* evolution, see Supplementary Figure S2.

hilA is contiguous with T3SS genes in 26 of 30 representative genomes we examined. In the other four genomes, (three strains of *Escherichia* and one strain of *Chromobacterium vaccinii*), *hilA* is either located alone on the chromosome or is absent from the genome (Figure 6). In *E. coli* O42 and *E. coli* O157:H7, an alternate transcription factor, *ygeH*, occupies the approximate location of *hilA*, adjacent to the T3SS genes (Figure 6). YgeH has low (29%) similarity to HilA, yet the *E. coli* O42 YgeH can functionally replace HilA in *Salmonella* and like HilA, its expression is regulated by H-NS [84,85].

The *E. coli* O157:H7 ETT2 is undergoing mutational attrition and becoming a cryptic gene island [27,84]. The accumulation of pseudogenes is accompanied by a loss of *hilA*, and the *ygeH* ortholog is non-functional as a transcription factor [84]. *Sodalis* presents another genus where the evolutionary stages in the decline of T3SS can be observed through comparative genomics. Members of this genus encode two T3SS homologs of SPI-1: SSR1 and SSR2. In *Sodalis praecaptivus*, SSR1 lacks *hilA* and SSR2 encodes a truncated *hilA* (Figure 6). In the endosymbiont *Sodalis glossinidius*, no *hilA* is present in the genome, and SSR1 and SSR2 are accumulating pseudogenes, consistent with a loss of island function due to the host occupying a highly specialized and obligate niche in tsetse flies.

3.9. Evolution of Transcriptional Control: Addition of the HilC/D Paralogs

Regulation of SPI-1 by the AraC-family proteins HilC and HilD appears to be unique because related T3SS and T3SE islands in Enterobacteriaceae do not include *hilC* or *hilD* homologs (Figure 6, Table 1). We reconstructed the evolutionary history of *hilC* and *hilD* by searching for all homologs in GenBank that are similar across 80% or more of the length of each query protein. With this search parameter, using HilC as a query recovers HilD, and vice versa, because the two proteins are closely related (36.4 % identity over 88 % query coverage, e-value < 3e-51). *hilC* and *hilD* are core elements of SPI-1 (Figure 1B), and so a GenBank search for homologs was conducted after excluding all *Salmonella* genomes from the search. Seventy-two non-redundant proteins were identified when either HilC or HilD served as a query sequence, whereas each individual query identified four unique proteins. Although HilC and HilD are ubiquitous in *Salmonella* (except for the case of *S*. Senftenberg that has lost SPI-1), searching all non-*Salmonella* genome sequences in GenBank revealed that HilC and HilD homologs are rare and sporadically distributed, occurring in only five genera outside *Salmonella* (Figure 7, Supplementary Figure S4). Moreover, each genome outside of *Salmonella* has a single HilC/D homolog, highlighting another unique feature of the SPI-1 regulatory network.

A HilC/D phylogeny has low bootstrap support that prevents ordering the deepest branches (illustrated as a polytomy in Figure 7). Nevertheless, the ubiquity of HilC and HilD in *Salmonella* compared to the sporadic distribution of homologs is consistent with the two genes arising from gene duplication in *Salmonella*. The phylogeny is consistent with a series of horizontal gene transfer events that spread HilD to *Edwardsiella*, *Enterobacter*, and *Escherichia*. The largest number of homologs were detected in incomplete *Escherichia* genomes in GenBank.

In most *Escherichia*, HilC/D homologs are located adjacent to type IV pilus genes and plasmid-specific genes. For example, the complete genome of *E. coli* O104:H11 strain RM14721 includes a 106 kb plasmid, and a HilC/D homolog labeled as CofS is found on the plasmid [86] (Figure 7). This protein is part of the *cof* operon, which encodes a type 4b pilus colonization factor antigen in enterotoxigenic *E. coli* and is used to attach to host cells [87]. A homolog of HilC/D in *Enterobacter lignolyticus* was also found located near type IV pilus genes, albeit on a chromosome. A small number of HilC/D homologs were found in *Citrobacter*, *Edwardsiella*, and *Hafnia* (Figure 7). Most of these strains have complete genome sequence available, and the HilC/D homolog appears to be in the same chromosomal location across these genera. Of these genomes, only one *C. freundii* strain has a T3SS, which is located at a different position in the chromosome from the HilC/D homolog. Based on GenBank annotations, the T3SS genes are converting to pseudogenes as mutations accumulate, suggesting that this is most likely a non-functional gene island.

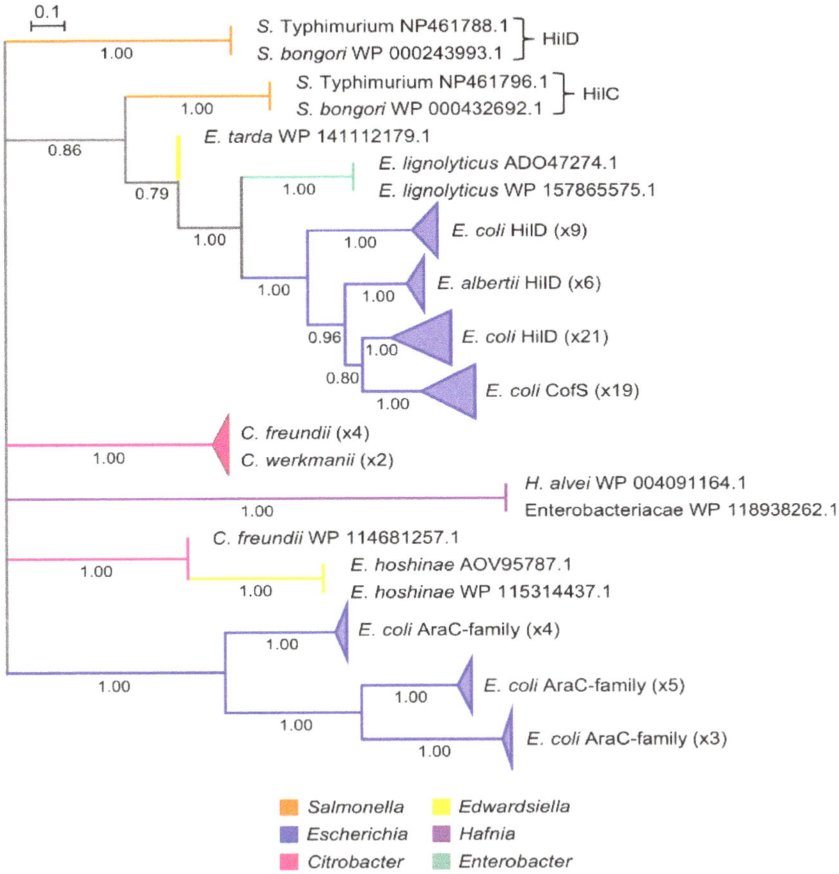

Figure 7. HilCD phylogeny. Nodes with bootstrap support below 0.70 are condensed to polytomies, and branches are coloured by genus. The number of strains in each collapsed node is indicated on the figure. *S. bongori* and *S. enterica* Typhimurium HilC and HilD sequences were included as representatives from the *Salmonella* clade. The top 100 best blastx hits covering at least 80% of the query for *S. enterica* Typhimurium LT2 HilC and HilD sequences were aligned using MUSCLE [55] and the phylogeny was inferred using a maximum-likelihood model JTT+G with 1000 bootstrap replicates [57]. For the full unrooted phylogeny, see Supplementary Figure S4.

4. Discussion

In bacteria, the forces of horizontal gene transfer and recombination have significant impacts on genome content and organization, accelerating evolution and community diversity. The consequences are etched across bacterial genomes in the form of vast numbers of accessory genes and gene islands, each with distinct phylogenetic histories. Genomic islands are born from HGT: physical linkage between cooperative genes is beneficial for the simultaneous transfer of the genetic information required to assemble a cellular machine or perform a metabolic process. For example, contiguity increases the odds of successful transfer of large islands, like the genomic island replacement and serogroup conversion that drove the emergence of pathogenic *Vibrio cholerae* O139 [88].

Specific genomic regions can be hotspots for the gain and loss of islands. The plasticity of a genomic region is often attributed to the presence of DNA sequences that facilitate the integration or excision of mobile genetic elements. Prominent examples include sequences that facilitate intramolecular and intermolecular recombination such as direct repeat sequences, inverted repeat sequences, bacteriophage attachment sites, and the 3′ end of tRNA genes [9,42,89]. SPI-1 is located in a hotspot for island insertion, as revealed in our comparative analysis across multiple genera of Enterobacteriaceae (Figure 1B). However, the genetic features such as tRNA sites, phage integration sites and repeat sequence elements associated with high recombination rates are not apparent at the SPI-1 locus [23].

Even in the absence of recognizable DNA elements that facilitate recombination, *mutS* and the surrounding region are known to have high rates of horizontal exchange relative to other regions in *Salmonella* and *E. coli* genomes [43,90–97]. A defective *mutS* results in higher recombination rates, which can be beneficial in times of stress but can also have long-term negative consequences on the cell [93,94,98]. As a result of higher recombination rates, there is a more frequent changing of *mutS* alleles, which increases the likelihood that a defective *mutS* allele will be rescued by a new, functioning allele [90,93]. As the *mutS* region favours horizontal gene transfer, *Salmonella* may have concurrently acquired a *mutS* allele and a T3SS that rose to dominance in the population.

The sporadic distribution of gene islands related to SPI-1 outside the genus *Salmonella* suggests that many independent gain and loss events have scattered variant SPI-1-like islands across Proteobacteria (Figure 6). In *Shigella, Pantoea,* and *Yersinia,* T3SSs are located on plasmids, which helps explain their sporadic distribution [32,35–38,59,99]. SPI-1 has different GC content, genetic organization and phylogenetic histories than the plasmid-borne islands in *Yersinia* and *Shigella,* indicating that these plasmids were not the original source of SPI-1 in *Salmonella* [64]. Alternatively, it is unlikely that SPI-1 represents a progenitor that has been subdivided after transfer from a *Salmonella* donor to other Proteobacteria (Figure 6). *Salmonella* HilA form a distinct, highly-supported clade, providing further evidence that *Salmonella* is not the ancestral source of HilA and linked T3SS islands in other Proteobacteria.

Even archetypal islands like SPI-1 are themselves mosaics composed of smaller islands. For example, as part of the validation of xenoGI, Bush and colleagues evaluated the SPI-2 locus in *Salmonella* and found that it is composed of several smaller gene islands. SPI-2 is composed of a T3SS gene island and a tetrathionate reductase operon island [45]. These findings are consistent with a previous analysis of genetic flux in *Salmonella* that identified the *ttr* gene island as a more ancient acquisition than the SPI-2 T3SS gene island [100]. Similarly, three phylogenetically distinct T3SS islands –including homologs of SPI-1 and SPI-2– are distributed sporadically across the *Pantoea* genus, and each island is a composite of reassorting subcomponents [31,32].

During macrophage infection, the distinct transcriptional profiles of gene modules in and around SPI-1 confirms the phylogenetic evidence for the locus being an archipelago of smaller islands with distinct evolutionary histories and regulatory programs (Figure 1C). In the macrophage vacuole, transcription of *ygbA* and *sitABCD* is very high, whereas transcription of genes in the *avrA-invH* island is repressed. In contrast, transcription of genes STM2901-STM2908 is largely unchanged between laboratory and intracellular environments [48] (Figure 1C). Thus, the genes that contribute to shared cellular functions, such as the T3SS or metal ion import, are co-regulated. Additional examples of island-specific transcriptional responses in and around SPI-1 can be visualized in the *Salmonella* compendium of transcriptomic data [46], further confirming that the boundaries between differentially regulated transcriptional units align well with the xenoGI assignment of gene islands based on evolutionary histories.

Another aspect of the mosaicism within a genomic island is the gain and loss of transcription factors. This is pertinent in the study of SPI-1 because it encodes an unusually high number of transcription factors (five), at least four of which are required to activate transcription of SPI-1 genes. HilA is a central regulator of SPI-1 transcription, but most homologous T3SSs do not have HilA (Table 1) [31]. Some lineages in Figure 6 have lost HilA, but this is always correlated with mutational attrition of the T3SS and T3SE genes, suggesting HilA is dispensable only after its regulatory targets have lost their biological function. Although HilA is a diffusible trans-acting factor, it is almost always contiguous with the T3SS genes it regulates, further highlighting how selection for effective HGT builds and maintains the composition of genomic islands.

Xenogeneic silencing of transcription at genomic islands by H-NS and counter-silencing by transcriptional activators like HilC and HilD has been thoroughly reviewed elsewhere [73,79]. Scientists have observed that winged helix-turn-helix proteins like HilA are effective activators of horizontally-acquired AT-rich DNA because their low specificity for DNA binding sites enables competition and displacement of H-NS across broad regions of gene promoters [101]. Less well understood are the mechanisms and evolutionary steps through which local-acting dedicated transcription factors, like HilA, HilC, and HilD are gained and integrated into a functionally cohesive island. We posit that the unusually long-term stability of SPI-1 is *Salmonella* arises from the fine-tuning of transcriptional activation only when ecologically appropriate. Further, we suspect that integration is reinforced by coordination of SPI-1 expression with core housekeeping functions by regulators like H-NS, in addition to development of cross-talk between SPI-1 regulators and the transcriptional control of other genomic islands [102]

SPI-1 has many features consistent with the classical model of a genomic island: a history of insertion revealed by comparative genomics plus a high AT content exceeding the genomic average. Yet in other respects, SPI-1 is unusual as a genomic island. For example, unlike its related islands that demonstrate short residency times in bacterial strains, SPI-1 has been resident in its host for many tens of millions of years. The average residency time of a genomic island is difficult to estimate due to the absence of a calibrated evolutionary record in the vast majority of bacteria. In laboratory conditions, pathogenicity islands have natural deletion frequencies ranging from 10^{-4} to 10^{-7} [reviewed in [103]], including several pathogenicity islands (PAIs) in uropathogenic *E. coli* [104] and the High-Pathogenicity Island (HPI) in *Yersinia* [105]. Residency and lasting integration will depend on organismal biology, stochastic molecular genetic events, and broader ecological pressures acting on the host organism and the host's ability to use the genetic potential in the island.

The *sitABCD* genes are traditionally treated as members of the SPI-1 island. Yet they have been previously been suggested to have an alternate history than the other SPI-1 genes based on the similarity of their AT content to the genomic average, which contrasts with the AT-rich SPI-1 [44] (Supplementary Figure S3). Our analysis supports this hypothesis, as the *sitABCD* genes are found at the same locus in *Klebsiella* and at other locations in other Enterobacteriaceae (Figure 2). There are conflicting reports on whether *sitABCD* is essential for SPI-1 virulence, but the majority argue that is it required for infection [44,106–108]. Although *sitABCD* may be useful for iron and/or manganese acquisition during infection, this operon was present at the *fhlA/-/mutS* locus prior to acquisition of the structural T3SS genes. If *sitABCD* and SPI-1 do cooperate during infection, their physical proximity on the genome may be purely coincidence.

xenoGI is an easy-to-use program that was able to conduct our multi-genome analysis in under three hours. Basing comparative analysis on a phylogenetic tree makes xenoGI a powerful tool to analyze the history of genomic islands. When released, xenoGI was validated with several examples using similar clades of bacteria to our analysis (*Salmonella* and *Escherichia*, with *Klebsiella* and *Serratia* used as outgroups) [45]. Our analysis covers a larger phylogenetic breadth than previously tested, and xenoGI resolved *sitABCD*, *fhlA*, and *mutS* gene conservation consistent with the whole genome phylogenies. xenoGI is constrained to the analysis of coding sequences from complete genomes, meaning that it is unable to recognize small RNAs and promoter sequences. There is a small RNA, *invR*, adjacent to *invH* that is an important regulator of SPI-1 [109], but it was not considered in this analysis for this reason.

SPI-1 can almost be considered a core gene set in *Salmonella*, but it fails the bioinformatic definition of a "core" genetic element due to its loss from some members of the genus. Similar to the loss from strains of *S.* Senftenberg [67–72], isolates of *S.* Litchfield have also lost SPI-1 [68,71]. These strains were isolated from environmental samples, not from animals or human infections [68,71]. These strains remain able to invade animal cells, albeit at a reduced rate [69]. After many millions of years of integration and a near ubiquity in extant members of the diverse *Salmonella* genus, SPI-1 is expected to perform key ecological functions, including in the less-studied species *S. bongori*. The natural loss of SPI-1 presents a test case for predicting ecological functions based on gene content [110]. Specifically, a reduced ability to colonize animal hosts may be accompanied by a loss of metabolic pathways for host-derived nutrients. Loss of SPI-1 may not be strongly selected against in some niches, but the lineages lacking SPI-1 may be evolutionary dead ends [111].

Supplementary Materials:
Figure S1: Cladogram of bacterial strains used as input for xenoGI analysis, Figure S2: AT content values of the *flhA*/-/*mutS* locus overlaid as a heatmap on genomic islands in Enterobacteriaceae, Figure S3: HilA phylogeny alongside genomic context for *hilA* in various T3SSs, Figure S4: Unrooted HilCD phylogeny of homologs found outside the *Salmonella* clade, Table S1: Summary of xenoGI island classification for genes at the *flhA*/-/*mutS* locus, Table S2: HilA homolog accession list from representative species, Table S3: HilC/D homolog accession list from best blastx hits.

Author Contributions: Conceptualization, N.A.L. and A.D.S.C.; Formal analysis, N.A.L and A.D.S.C.; Funding acquisition, N.A.L., K.D.M. and A.D.S.C.; Investigation, N.A.L.; Methodology, N.A.L.; Visualization, N.A.L., K.D.M. and A.D.S.C.; Writing—original draft, N.A.L., K.D.M. and A.D.S.C.; Writing—review & editing, N.A.L., K.D.M. and A.D.S.C. All authors have read and agreed to the published version of the manuscript.

Acknowledgments: The authors thank Charles Dorman and three anonymous reviewers for their comments that helped improve the quality of this manuscript. We thank Eliot Bush, Chris Yost, Illona Monkman, and Emre Islam for helpful discussions.

References

1. Gonzalez-Alba, J.; Baquero, F.; Cantón, R.; Galán, J.E. Stratified reconstruction of ancestral *Escherichia coli* diversification. *BMC Genom.* **2019**, *20*, 936. [CrossRef]
2. Maddamsetti, R.; Lenski, R.E. Analysis of bacterial genomes from an evolution experiment with horizontal gene transfer shows that recombination can sometimes overwhelm selection. *PLoS Genet.* **2018**, *14*, e1007199. [CrossRef]
3. Ochman, H.; Lawrence, J.G.; Groisman, E.A. Lateral gene transfer and the nature of bacterial innovation. *Nature* **2000**, *405*, 299–304. [CrossRef]
4. Summers, A.O. Genetic linkage and horizontal gene transfer, the roots of the antibiotic multi-resistance problem. *Anim. Biotechnol.* **2006**, *17*, 125–135. [CrossRef] [PubMed]
5. Hacker, J.; Carniel, E. Ecological fitness, genomic islands and bacterial pathogenicity. *EMBO Rep.* **2001**, *21*, 376–381. [CrossRef] [PubMed]
6. Hacker, J.; Blum-Oehler, G.; Tschäpe, H.; Mühldorfer, I. Pathogenicity islands of virulent bacteria: Structure, function and impact on microbial evolution. *Mol. Microbiol.* **1996**, *23*, 1089–1097. [CrossRef] [PubMed]
7. Juhas, M.; van der Meer, J.R.; Gaillard, M.; Harding, R.M.; Hood, D.W.; Crook, D.W. Genomic islands: Tools of bacterial horizontal gene transfer and evolution. *FEMS Microbiol. Rev.* **2009**, *33*, 376–393. [CrossRef]
8. Schmidt, H.; Hensel, M. Pathogenicity islands in bacterial pathogenesis. *Clin. Microbiol. Rev.* **2004**, *17*, 14–56. [CrossRef]
9. Gal-Mor, O.; Finlay, B.B. Pathogenicity islands: A molecular toolbox for bacterial virulence. *Cell. Microbiol.* **2006**, *8*, 1707–1719. [CrossRef]
10. Hacker, J.; Kaper, J. Pathogenicity islands and the evolution of microbes. *Annu. Rev. Microbiol.* **2000**, *54*, 641–679. [CrossRef]
11. Ou, H.-Y.; Chen, L.-L.; Lonnen, J.; Chaudhuri, R.R.; Thani, A.; Smith, R.; Garton, N.J.; Hinton, J.; Pallen, M.; Barer, M.R.; et al. A novel strategy for the identification of genomic islands by comparative analysis of the contents and contexts of tRNA sites in closely related bacteria. *Nucleic Acids Res.* **2006**, *34*, 1–11. [CrossRef] [PubMed]
12. Groisman, E.A.; Ochman, H. Pathogenicity islands: Bacterial evolution in quantum leaps. *Cell* **1996**, *87*, 791–794. [CrossRef]
13. Hochhut, B.; Jahreis, K.; Lengeler, J.W.; Schmid, K. CTnsct94, a conjugative transposon found in Enterobacteria. *J. Bacteriol.* **1997**, *179*, 2097–2102. [CrossRef]
14. Sullivan, J.T.; Trzebiatowski, J.R.; Cruickshank, R.W.; Gouzy, J.; Brown, S.D.; Elliot, R.M.; Fleetwood, D.J.; McCallum, N.G.; Rossbach, U.; Stuart, G.S.; et al. Comparative sequence analysis of the symbiosis island of *Mesorhizobium loti* strain R7A. *J. Bacteriol.* **2002**, *184*, 3086–3095. [CrossRef] [PubMed]

15. Novick, R.P.; Schlievert, P.; Ruzin, A. Pathogenicity and resistance islands of staphylococci. *Microbes Infect.* **2001**, *3*, 585–594. [CrossRef]
16. Fookes, M.; Schroeder, G.N.; Langridge, G.C.; Blondel, C.J.; Mammina, C.; Connor, T.R.; Seth-Smith, H.; Vernikos, G.S.; Robinson, K.S.; Sanders, M.; et al. *Salmonella bongori* provides insights into the evolution of the Salmonellae. *PLoS Pathog.* **2011**, *7*, e1002191. [CrossRef]
17. Hayward, M.R.; AbuOun, M.; La Ragione, R.M.; Tchórzewska, M.A.; Cooley, W.A.; Everest, D.J.; Petrovska, L.; Jansen, V.; Woodward, M.J. SPI-23 of S. Derby: Role in adherence and invasion of porcine tissues. *PLoS ONE* **2014**, *9*, e107857. [CrossRef]
18. Urrutia, I.M.; Fuentes, J.A.; Valenzuela, L.M.; Ortega, A.P.; Hidalgo, A.A.; Mora, G.C. Salmonella Typhi shdA: Pseudogene or allelic variant? *Infect. Genet. Evol.* **2014**, *26*, 146–152. [CrossRef]
19. Wisner, A.; Desin, T.; White, A.; Köster, W. The *Salmonella* pathogenicity island-1 and -2 encoded type III secretion systems. In *Salmonella—A Diversified Superbug*; InTech: Rijeka, Croatia, 2012; pp. 469–494.
20. Fàbrega, A.; Vila, J. *Salmonella enterica* serovar Typhimurium skills to succeed in the host: Virulence and regulation. *Clin. Microbiol. Rev.* **2013**, *26*, 308–341. [CrossRef]
21. Galán, J.E. Molecular genetic bases of *Salmonella* entry into host cells. *Mol. Microbiol.* **1996**, *20*, 263–271. [CrossRef]
22. Hensel, M.; Shea, J.E.; Gleeson, C.; Jones, M.D.; Dalton, E.; Holden, D.W. Simultaneous identification of bacterial virulence genes by negative selection. *Science* **1995**, *269*, 400–403. [CrossRef] [PubMed]
23. Mills, D.M.; Bajaj, V.; Lee, C.A. A 40 kB chromosomal fragment encoding *Salmonella typhimurium* invasion genes is absent from the corresponding region on the *Escherichia coli* K-12 chromosome. *Mol. Microbiol.* **1995**, *15*, 749–759. [CrossRef] [PubMed]
24. Bäumler, A.J. The record of horizontal gene transfer in *Salmonella*. *Trends Microbiol.* **1997**, *5*, 318–322. [CrossRef]
25. Doolittle, R.; Feng, D.; Tsang, S.; Cho, G.; Little, E. Determining divergence times of the major kingdoms of living organisms with a protein clock. *Science* **1996**, *26*, 470–477. [CrossRef] [PubMed]
26. Ochman, H.; Wilson, A. Evolution in bacteria: Evidence for a universal substitution rate in cellular genomes. *J. Mol. Evol.* **1987**, *26*, 74–86. [CrossRef] [PubMed]
27. Ren, C.-P.; Chaudhuri, R.R.; Fivian, A.; Bailey, C.M.; Antonio, M.; Barnes, W.M.; Pallen, M.J. The ETT2 gene cluster, encoding a second type III secretion system from *Escherichia coli*, is present in the majority of strains but has undergone widespread mutational attrition. *J. Bacteriol.* **2004**, *186*, 3547–3560. [CrossRef]
28. Betts, H.J.; Chaudhuri, R.R.; Pallen, M.J. An analysis of type-III secretion gene clusters in *Chromobacterium violaceum*. *Trends Microbiol.* **2004**, *12*, 476–482. [CrossRef]
29. Dale, C.; Jones, T.; Pontes, M. Degenerative evolution and functional diversification of type-III secretion systems in the insect endosymbiont *Sodalis glossinidius*. *Mol. Biol. Evol.* **2005**, *22*, 758–765. [CrossRef]
30. Haller, J.C.; Carlson, S.; Pederson, K.J.; Pierson, D.E. A chromosomally encoded type III secretion pathway in *Yersinia enterocolitica* is important in virulence. *Mol. Microbiol.* **2000**, *36*, 1436–1446. [CrossRef]
31. Hu, Y.; Huang, H.; Cheng, X.; Shu, X.; White, A.; Stavrinides, J.; Köster, W.; Zhu, G.; Zhao, Z.; Wang, Y. A global survey of bacterial type III secretion systems and their effectors. *Environ. Microbiol.* **2017**, *19*, 3879–3895. [CrossRef]
32. Kirzinger, M.W.B.; Butz, C.J.; Stavrinides, J. Inheritance of *Pantoea* type III secretion systems through both vertical and horizontal transfer. *Mol. Genet. Genom.* **2015**, *290*, 2075–2088. [CrossRef] [PubMed]
33. Ménard, R.; Prévost, M.C.; Gounon, P.; Sansonetti, P.; Dehio, C. The secreted Ipa complex of *Shigella flexneri* promotes entry into mammalian cells. *Proc. Natl. Acad. Sci. USA* **1996**, *93*, 1254–1258. [CrossRef] [PubMed]
34. Batista, J.; da Silva Neto, J. *Chromobacterium violaceum* pathogenicity: Updates and insights from genome sequencing of novel *Chromobacterium* species. *Front. Microbiol.* **2017**, *8*. [CrossRef] [PubMed]
35. Parkhill, J.; Wren, B.W.; Thomson, N.R.; Titball, R.; Holden, M.; Prentice, M.B.; Sebaihia, M.; James, K.; Churcher, C.; Mungall, K.; et al. Genome sequence of *Yersinia pestis*, the causative agent of plague. *Nature* **2001**, *413*, 523–527. [CrossRef] [PubMed]
36. Lan, R.; Lumb, B.; Ryan, D.; Reeves, P.R. Molecular evolution of large virulence plasmid in *Shigella* and enteroinvasive *Escherichia coli*. *Infect. Immun.* **2001**, *69*, 6303–6309. [CrossRef] [PubMed]
37. The, H.C.; Thanh, D.P.; Holt, K.E.; Thomson, N.R.; Baker, S. The genomic signatures of *Shigella evolution*, adaptation and geographical spread. *Nat. Rev. Microbiol.* **2016**, *14*, 235–250. [CrossRef]

38. Yang, J.; Nie, H.; Chen, L.; Zhang, X.; Yang, F.; Xu, X.; Zhu, Y.; Yu, J.; Jin, Q. Revisiting the molecular evolutionary history of *Shigella* spp. *J. Mol. Evol.* **2007**, *64*, 71–79. [CrossRef]
39. Burkinshaw, B.J.; Strynadka, N.C.J. Assembly and structure of the T3SS. *Biochim. Biophys. Acta* **2014**, *1843*, 1649–1663. [CrossRef]
40. Correa, V.R.; Majerczak, D.R.; Ammar, E.-D.; Merighi, M.; Pratt, R.C.; Hogenhout, S.A.; Coplin, D.L.; Redinbaugh, M.G. The bacterium *Pantoea stewartii* uses two different type III secretion systems to colonize its plant host and insect vector. *Appl. Environ. Microbiol.* **2012**, *78*, 6327–6336. [CrossRef]
41. Foultier, B.; Troisfontaines, P.; Müller, S.; Opperdoes, F.R.; Cornelis, G.R. Characterization of the ysa pathogenicity locus in the chromosome of *Yersinia enterocolitica* and phylogeny analysis of type III secretion systems. *J. Mol. Evol.* **2002**, *55*, 37–51. [CrossRef]
42. Hueck, C.J. Type III protein secretion systems in bacterial pathogens of animals and plants. *Microbiol. Mol. Biol. Rev.* **1998**, *62*, 379–433. [CrossRef] [PubMed]
43. Pancetti, A.; Galán, J.E. Characterization of the *mutS*-proximal region of the *Salmonella typhimurium* SPI-1 identifies a group of pathogenicity island-associated genes. *FEMS Microbiol. Lett.* **2001**, *197*, 203–208. [CrossRef] [PubMed]
44. Zhou, D.; Hardt, W.D.; Galán, J.E. *Salmonella typhimurium* encodes a putative iron transport system within the centisome 63 pathogenicity island. *Infect. Immun.* **1999**, *67*, 1974–1981. [CrossRef] [PubMed]
45. Bush, E.C.; Clark, A.E.; DeRanek, C.A.; Eng, A.; Forman, J.; Heath, K.; Lee, A.B.; Stoebel, D.M.; Wang, Z.; Wilber, M.; et al. xenoGI: Reconstructing the history of genomic island insertions in clades of closely related bacteria. *BMC Bioinform.* **2018**, *19*, 32. [CrossRef] [PubMed]
46. Kröger, C.; Colgan, A.; Srikumar, S.; Händler, K.; Sivasankaran, S.K.; Hammarlöf, D.L.; Canals, R.; Grissom, J.E.; Conway, T.; Hokamp, K.; et al. An infection-relevant transcriptomic compendium for *Salmonella enterica* serovar Typhimurium. *Cell Host Microbe* **2013**, *14*, 683–695.
47. O'Leary, N.A.; Wright, M.W.; Brister, J.R.; Ciufo, S.; Haddad, D.; McVeigh, R.; Rajput, B.; Robbertse, B.; Smith-White, B.; Ako-Adjei, D.; et al. Reference sequence (RefSeq) database at NCBI: Current status, taxonomic expansion, and functional annotation. *Nucleic Acids Res.* **2016**, *44*, D733–D745. [CrossRef]
48. Srikumar, S.; Kröger, C.; Hébrard, M.; Colgan, A.; Owen, S.; Sivasankaran, S.K.; Cameron, A.; Hokamp, K.; Hinton, J. RNA-seq brings new insights to the intra-macrophage transcriptome of *Salmonella* Typhimurium. *PLoS Pathog.* **2015**, *11*, e1005262. [CrossRef]
49. Wattam, A.R.; Davis, J.J.; Assaf, R.; Boisvert, S.; Brettin, T.; Bun, C.; Conrad, N.; Dietrich, E.M.; Disz, T.; Gabbard, J.L.; et al. Improvements to PATRIC, the all-bacterial Bioinformatics Database and Analysis Resource Center. *Nucleic Acids Res.* **2017**, *45*, D535–D542. [CrossRef]
50. Freese, N.H.; Norris, D.C.; Loraine, A.E. Integrated genome browser: Visual analytics platform for genomics. *Bioinformatics* **2016**, *32*, 2089–2095. [CrossRef]
51. Sullivan, M.; Petty, N.K.; Beatson, S. Easyfig: A genome comparison visualizer. *Bioinformatics* **2011**, *27*, 1009–1010. [CrossRef]
52. Galán, J.E.; Lara-Tejero, M.; Marlovits, T.C.; Wagner, S. Bacterial type III secretion systems: Specialized nanomachines for protein delivery into target cells. *Nucleic Acids Res.* **2014**, *68*, 415–438. [CrossRef] [PubMed]
53. Kearse, M.; Moir, R.; Wilson, A.; Stones-Havas, S.; Cheung, M.; Sturrock, S.; Buxton, S.; Cooper, A.; Markowitz, S.; Duran, C.; et al. Geneious Basic: An integrated and extendable desktop software platform for the organization and analysis of sequence data. *Bioinformatics* **2012**, *15*, 1647–1649. [CrossRef] [PubMed]
54. Altschul, S.F.; Madden, T.L.; Schäffer, A.A.; Zhang, J.; Zhang, Z.; Miller, W.; Lipman, J.L. Gapped BLAST and PSI-BLAST: A new generation of protein database search programs. *Nucleic Acids Res.* **1997**, *25*, 3389–3402. [CrossRef] [PubMed]
55. Edgar, R. MUSCLE: Multiple sequence alignment with high accuracy and high throughput. *Nucleic Acids Res.* **2004**, *32*, 1792–1797. [CrossRef]
56. Kumar, S.; Stecher, G.; Tamura, K. MEGA7: Molecular Evolutionary Genetic Analysis Version 7.0 for bigger datasets. *Mol. Biol. Evol.* **2016**, *33*, 1870–1874. [CrossRef]
57. Kumar, S.; Stecher, G.; Li, M.; Knyaz, C.; Tamura, K. MEGA X: Molecular Evolutionary Genetics Analysis across computing platforms. *Mol. Biol. Evol.* **2018**, *35*, 1547–1549. [CrossRef]
58. Letunic, I.; Bork, P. Interactive Tree Of Life (iTOL) v4: Recent updates and new developments. *Nucleic Acids Res.* **2019**, *47*, W256–W259. [CrossRef]

59. Venkatesan, M.M.; Goldberg, M.B.; Rose, D.J.; Grotbeck, E.J.; Burland, V.; Blattner, F.R. Complete DNA sequence and analysis of the large virulence plasmid of *Shigella flexneri*. *Infect. Immun.* **2001**, *69*, 3271–3285. [CrossRef]
60. Matsumoto, H.; Young, G. Proteomic and functional analysis of the suite of Ysp proteins exported by the Ysa type III secretion system of *Yersinia enterocolitica* Biovar 1B. *Mol. Microbiol.* **2005**, *59*, 689–706. [CrossRef]
61. Walker, K.; Miller, V.L. Regulation of the Ysa Type III secretion system of *Yersinia enterocolitica* by YsaE/SycB and YrsS/YsrR. *J. Bacteriol.* **2004**, *186*, 4056–4066. [CrossRef]
62. Bertelli, C.; Tilley, K.; Brinkman, F. Microbial genomic island discovery, visualization and analysis. *Brief. Bioinform.* **2019**, *20*, 1685–1698. [CrossRef] [PubMed]
63. Lu, B.; Leong, H.W. Computational methods for predicting genomic islands in microbial genomes. *Comput. Struct. Biotechnol. J.* **2016**, *14*, 200–206. [CrossRef] [PubMed]
64. Groisman, E.A.; Ochman, H. Cognate gene clusters govern invasion of host epithelial cells by *Salmonella* typhimurium and *Shigella flexneri*. *EMBO J.* **1993**, *12*, 3779–3787. [CrossRef] [PubMed]
65. Desai, P.; Porwollik, S.; Long, F.; Cheng, P.; Wollam, A.; Clifton, S.W.; Weinstock, G.M.; McClelland, M. Evolutionary genomics of *Salmonella enterica* subspecies. *mBio* **2013**, *4*, e00579-12. [CrossRef]
66. Worley, J.; Meng, J.; Allard, M.; Brown, E.W.; Timme, R. *Salmonella enterica* phylogeny based on whole-genome sequencing reveals two new clades and novel patterns of horizontally acquired genetic elements. *mBio* **2018**, *9*, e02303-18. [CrossRef]
67. El Ghany, M.; Shi, X.; Li, Y.; Ansari, H.; Hill-Cawthorne, G.; Ho, Y.; Naeem, R.; Pickard, D.; Klena, J.; Xu, X.; et al. Genomic and phenotypic analyses reveal the emergence of an atypical *Salmonella enterica* serovar Senftenberg variant in China. *J. Clin. Microbiol.* **2016**, *54*, 2014–2022. [CrossRef]
68. Ginocchio, C.; Rahn, K.; Clarke, R.; Galán, J.E. Naturally occurring deletions in the centisome 63 pathogenicity island of environmental isolates of *Salmonella* spp. *Infect. Immun.* **1997**, *65*, 1267–1272. [CrossRef]
69. Hu, Q.; Coburn, B.; Deng, W.; Li, Y.; Shi, X.; Lan, Q.; Wang, B.; Coombes, B.K.; Finlay, B.B. *Salmonella enterica* serovar Senftenberg human clinical isolates lacking SPI-1. *J. Clin. Microbiol.* **2008**, *46*, 1330–1336. [CrossRef]
70. Morita, M.; Shimada, K.; Baba, H.; Morofuji, K.; Oda, S.; Izumiya, H.; Ohnishi, M. Genome sequence of a *Salmonella enterica* serotype Senftenberg strain lacking *Salmonella* Pathogenicity Island-1 and isolated in Japan. *Microbiol. Resour. Announc.* **2019**, *9*, e00653-19. [CrossRef]
71. Rahn, K.; De Grandis, S.; Clarke, R.; McEwen, S.A.; Galán, J.E.; Ginocchio, C.; Curtiss III, R.; Gyles, C. Amplification of an *invA* gene sequence of *Salmonella typhimurium* by polymerase chain reaction as a specific method of detecting *Salmonella*. *Mol. Cell. Probes* **1992**, *6*, 271–279. [CrossRef]
72. Stevens, M.; Zurfluh, K.; Althaus, D.; Corti, S.; Lehner, A.; Stephan, R. Complete and assembled genome sequence of *Salmonella enterica* subsp. *enterica* serotype Senftenberg N17-509, a strain lacking *Salmonella* Pathogen Island 1. *Genome Announc.* **2018**, *6*, e00156-18.
73. Singh, K.; Milstein, J.; Navarre, W. Xenogeneic silencing and its impact on bacterial genomes. *Nucleic Acids Res.* **2016**, *70*, 199–213. [CrossRef]
74. Dillon, S.C.; Cameron, A.; Hokamp, K.; Lucchini, S.; Hinton, J.; Dorman, C.J. Genome-wide analysis of the H-NS and Sfh regulatory networks in *Salmonella* Typhimurium identifies a plasmid-encoded transcription silencing mechanism. *Mol. Microbiol.* **2010**, *76*, 1250–1265. [CrossRef]
75. Lucchini, S.; Rowley, G.; Goldberg, M.B.; Hurd, D.; Harrison, M.; Hinton, J. H-NS mediates the silencing of laterally acquired genes in bacteria. *PLoS Pathog.* **2006**, *2*, e81. [CrossRef] [PubMed]
76. Navarre, W.; Porwollik, S.; Wang, Y.; McClelland, M.; Rosen, H.; Libby, S.J.; Fang, F.C. Selective silencing of foreign DNA with low GC content by the H-NS protein in *Salmonella*. *Science* **2006**, *313*, 236–238. [CrossRef]
77. Cameron, A.; Dorman, C.J. A fundamental regulatory mechanism operating through OmpR and DNA topology that controls expression of *Salmonella* pathogenicity islands SPI-1 and SPI-2. *PLoS Genet.* **2012**, *8*, e1002615. [CrossRef] [PubMed]
78. Schechter, L.M.; Lee, C.A. AraC/XylS family members, HilC and HilD, directly bind and derepress the *Salmonella typhimurium hilA* promoter. *Mol. Microbiol.* **2001**, *40*, 1289–1299. [CrossRef] [PubMed]
79. Will, W.; Navarre, W.; Fang, F.C. Integrated circuits: How transcriptional silencing and counter-silencing facilitate bacterial evolution. *Curr. Opin. Microbiol.* **2015**, *23*, 8–13. [CrossRef]
80. Olekhnovich, I.; Kadner, R. Crucial roles of both flanking sequences in silencing of the *hilA* promoter in *Salmonella enterica*. *J. Mol. Biol.* **2006**, *357*, 373–386. [CrossRef]

81. Bajaj, V.; Hwang, C.; Lee, C.A. *hilA* is a novel *ompR/toxR* family member that activates the expression of *Salmonella typhimurium* invasion genes. *Mol. Microbiol.* **1995**, *18*, 715–727. [CrossRef]
82. Daly, R.; Lostroh, C. Genetic analysis of the *Salmonella* transcription factor HilA. *Can. J. Microbiol.* **2008**, *54*, 854–860. [CrossRef] [PubMed]
83. Lostroh, C.; Bajaj, V.; Lee, C.A. The *cis* requirements for transcriptional activation by HilA, a virulence determinant encoded on SPI-1. *Mol. Microbiol.* **2000**, *37*, 300–315. [CrossRef] [PubMed]
84. Hüttener, M.; Dietrich, M.; Paytubi, S.; Juárez, A. HilA-like regulators in *Escherichia coli* pathotypes: The YgeH protein from the enteroaggregative strain 042. *BMC Microbiol.* **2014**, *14*, 268. [CrossRef] [PubMed]
85. Pallen, M.J.; Francis, M.; Fütterer, K. Tetratricopeptide-like repeats in type-III-secretion chaperones and regulators. *FEMS Microbiol. Lett.* **2003**, *223*, 53–60. [CrossRef]
86. Carter, M.; Pham, A. Complete genome sequence of a natural *Escherichia coli* O145:H11 isolate that belongs to phylogroup A. *Genome Announc.* **2018**, *6*, e00349-18.
87. Taniguchi, T.; Akeda, Y.; Haba, A.; Yasuda, Y.; Yamamoto, K.; Honda, T.; Tochikubo, K. Gene cluster for assembly of pilus colonization factor antigen III of enterotoxigenic *Escherichia coli*. *Infect. Immun.* **2001**, *69*, 5864–5873. [CrossRef]
88. Blokesch, M.; Schoolnik, G. Serogroup conversion of *Vibrio cholerae* in aquatic reservoirs. *PLoS Pathog.* **2007**, *3*, e81. [CrossRef]
89. Reiter, W.; Palm, P.; Yeats, S. Transfer RNA genes frequently serve as integration sites for prokaryotic genetic elements. *Nucleic Acids Res.* **1989**, *17*, 1907–1914. [CrossRef]
90. Brown, E.W.; LeClerc, E.; Li, B.; Payne, W.L.; Cebula, T.A. Phylogenetic evidence for horizontal transfer of mutS alleles among naturally occurring *Escherichia coli* strains. *J. Bacteriol.* **2001**, *183*, 1631–1644. [CrossRef]
91. Brown, E.W.; Mammel, M.K.; LeClerc, E.; Cebula, T.A. Limited boundaries for extensive horizontal gene transfer among Salmonella pathogens. *Proc. Natl. Acad. Sci. USA* **2003**, *100*, 15676–15681. [CrossRef]
92. Cao, G.; Meng, J.; Strain, E.; Stones, R.; Pettengill, J.; Zhao, S.; McDermott, P.; Brown, E.; Allard, M. Phylogenetics and differentiation of Salmonella Newport lineages by whole genome sequencing. *PLoS ONE* **2013**, *8*, e55687. [CrossRef] [PubMed]
93. Denamur, E.; Lecointre, G.; Darlu, P.; Tenaillon, O.; Acquaviva, C.; Sayada, C.; Sunjevaric, I.; Rothstein, R.; Elion, J.; Taddei, F.; et al. Evolutionary implications of the frequent horizontal transfer of mismatch repair genes. *Cell* **2000**, *103*, 711–721. [CrossRef]
94. Funchain, P.; Yeung, A.; Stewart, J.L.; Lin, R.; Slupska, M.M.; Miller, J.H. The consequences of growth of a mutator strain of *Escherichia coli* as measured by loss of function among multiple gene targets and loss of fitness. *Genetics* **2000**, *154*, 959–970. [PubMed]
95. Kotewicz, M.L.; Li, B.; Levy, D.D.; LeClerc, E.; Shifflet, A.W.; Cebula, T.A. Evolution of multi-gene segments in the mutS-rpoS intergenic region of Salmonella enterica serovar Typhimurium LT2. *Microbiology* **2002**, *148*, 2531–2540. [CrossRef]
96. Herbelin, C.; Chirillo, S.; Melnick, K.; Whittam, T.S. Gene conservation and loss in the *mutS-rpoS* genomic region of the pathogenic *Escherichia coli*. *J. Bacteriol.* **2000**, *182*, 5381–5390. [CrossRef]
97. Brown, E.W.; Kotewicz, M.L.; Cebula, T.A. Detection of recombination among *Salmonella enterica* strains using the incongruence length difference test. *Mol. Phylogenetics Evol.* **2002**, *24*, 102–120. [CrossRef]
98. LeClerc, J.; Li, B.; Payne, W.L.; Cebula, T.A. High mutation frequencies among *Escherichia coli* and *Salmonella* pathogens. *Science* **1996**, *274*, 1208–1211. [CrossRef]
99. Duong, D.A.; Stevens, A.M.; Jensen, R.V. Complete genome assembly of *Pantoea stewartii* subsp. *stewartii* DC283, a corn pathogen. *Genome Announc.* **2017**, *5*, e00435-17.
100. Vernikos, G.S.; Thomson, N.R.; Parkhill, J. Genetic flux over time in the *Salmonella* lineage. *Genome Biol.* **2007**, *8*, R100. [CrossRef]
101. Dorman, C.J.; Dorman, M. Control of virulence gene transcription by indirect readout in *Vibrio cholerae* and *Salmonella enterica* serovar Typhimurium. *Environ. Microbiol.* **2017**, *19*, 3834–3845. [CrossRef]
102. Bustamante, V.; Martínez, L.; Santana, F.; Knodler, L.; Steele-Mortimer, O.; Puente, J.L. HilD-mediated transcriptional cross-talk between SPI-1 and SPI-2. *Proc. Natl. Acad. Sci. USA* **2008**, *105*, 14591–14596. [CrossRef] [PubMed]
103. Hacker, J.; Blum-Oehler, G.; Mühldorfer, I.; Tschäpe, H. Pathogenicity islands of virulent bacteria: Structure, function and impact on microbial evolution. *Mol. Microbiol.* **1997**, *23*, 1089–1097. [CrossRef] [PubMed]

104. Blum, G.; Ott, M.; Lischewski, A.; Ritter, A.; Imrich, H.; Tschäpe, H.; Hacker, J. Excision of large DNA regions termed pathogenicity islands from tRNA-specific loci in the chromosome of an *Escherichia coli* wild-type pathogen. *Infect. Immun.* **1994**, *62*, 606–614. [CrossRef] [PubMed]
105. Bach, S.; Buchrieser, C.; Prentice, M.; Guiyoule, A.; Msadek, T.; Carniel, E. The High-Pathogenicity Island of *Yersinia enterocolitica* Ye8081 undergoes low-frequency deletion but not precise excision, suggesting recent stabilization in the genome. *Infect. Immun.* **1999**, *67*, 5091–5099. [CrossRef]
106. Fisher, C.R.; Davies, N.; Wyckoff, E.E.; Feng, Z.; Oaks, E.V.; Payne, S.M. Genetics and virulence association of the *Shigella flexneri* Sit iron transport system. *Infect. Immun.* **2009**, *77*, 1992–1999. [CrossRef]
107. Janakiraman, A.; Slauch, J.M. The putative iron transport system SitABCD encoded on SPI1 is required for full virulence of *Salmonella typhimurium*. *Mol. Microbiol.* **2000**, *35*, 1146–1155. [CrossRef]
108. Sun, W.-S.W.; Syu, W.-J.; Ho, W.-L.; Lin, C.-N.; Tsai, S.-F.; Wang, S.-H. SitA contributes to the virulence of *Klebsiella pneumoniae* in a mouse infection model. *Microbes Infect.* **2014**, *16*, 161–170. [CrossRef]
109. Pfeiffer, V.; Sittka, A.; Tomer, R.; Tedin, K.; Brinkmann, V.; Vogel, J. A small non-coding RNA of the invasion gene island (SPI-1) represses outer membrane protein synthesis from the Salmonella core genome. *Mol. Microbiol.* **2007**, *66*, 1174–1191. [CrossRef]
110. Shapiro, B.; Polz, M.F. Ordering microbial diversity into ecologically and genetically cohesive units. *Trends Microbiol.* **2014**, *22*, 235–247. [CrossRef]
111. Redfield, R.J.; Findlay, W.; Bossé, J.; Kroll, J.; Cameron, A.; Nash, J. Evolution of competence and DNA uptake specificity in the Pastuerellaceae. *BMC Evol. Biol.* **2006**, *6*, 82. [CrossRef] [PubMed]

6

The not so Good, the Bad and the Ugly: Differential Bacterial Adhesion and Invasion Mediated by *Salmonella* PagN Allelic Variants

Yanping Wu [1,2,†], Qiaoyun Hu [1,†,‡], Ruchika Dehinwal [1], Alexey V. Rakov [1,§], Nicholas Grams [1], Erin C. Clemens [3,||], Jennifer Hofmann [3], Iruka N. Okeke [3,4] and Dieter M. Schifferli [1,*]

1 Department of Pathobiology, University of Pennsylvania, School of Veterinary Medicine, Philadelphia, PA 19104, USA; ypwu0902@163.com (Y.W.); huqiaoyun2020@163.com (Q.H.); druchika@vet.upenn.edu (R.D.); rakovalexey@gmail.com (A.V.R.); gramsn@pennmedicine.upenn.edu (N.G.)

2 College of Animal Science and Technology, College of Veterinary Medicine, Zhejiang Agriculture and Forestry University, Hangzhou 311300, China

3 Department of Biology, Haverford College, Haverford, PA 19041, USA; eclemen1@swarthmore.edu (E.C.C.); hofmann.jen@gmail.com (J.H.); iruka.n.okeke@gmail.com (I.N.O.)

4 Department of Pharmaceutical Microbiology, Faculty of Pharmacy, University of Ibadan, Ibadan 200284, Oyo State, Nigeria

* Correspondence: dmschiff@vet.upenn.edu

† These authors contributed equally to this work.

‡ Current address: Hunan Center for Animal Disease Control and Prevention, Changsha, Hunan, China.

§ Current address: Somov Institute of Epidemiology and Microbiology, Vladivostok, Russia.

|| Current address: Swarthmore College, Swarthmore, PA, USA.

Abstract: While advances in genomic sequencing have highlighted significant strain variability between and within *Salmonella* serovars, only a few protein variants have been directly related to evolutionary adaptation for survival, such as host specificity or differential virulence. The current study investigated whether allelic variation of the *Salmonella* adhesin/invasin PagN influences bacterial interaction with their receptors. The *Salmonella enterica, subspecies enterica* serovar Typhi (*S.* Typhi) allelic variant of PagN was found to bind significantly better to different enterocytes as well as to the extracellular matrix protein laminin than did the major *Salmonella enterica, subspecies enterica* serovar Typhimurium (*S.* Typhimurium) allele. The two alleles differed at amino acid residues 49 and 109 in two of the four predicted PagN surface loops, and residue substitution analysis revealed that a glutamic acid at residue 49 increased the adhesive and invasive properties of *S.* Typhi PagN. PagN sequence comparisons from 542 *Salmonella* strains for six representative *S. enterica* serovars and *S. diarizonae* further supported the role of glutamic acid at residues 49 and 109 in optimizing adhesion to cells and laminin, as well as for cell invasion. In summary, this study characterized unique residues in allelic variants of a virulence factor that participates in the colonization and invasive properties of different *Salmonella* stains, subspecies and serovars.

Keywords: *Salmonella*; *S.* Typhi; *S.* Typhimurium; S. diarizonae; PagN; adhesin; invasin; alleles; allelic variants

---

1. Introduction

Salmonella enterica subsp. *enterica* (*S. enterica*) is an entero-invasive bacterial pathogen that utilizes a type three secretion system (T3SS) encoded on the *Salmonella* pathogenicity island 1 (SPI-1) to invade intestinal epithelial cells. T3SS-driven uptake is particularly critical for intestinal *S. enterica* infections in mammals, as demonstrated with several experimental animal models [1]. *S. enterica* strains are differentiated by their flagella and O-antigens, which are highly variable and provide the basis for identification of over 2500 different serovars [2,3]. There is a direct correlation between the range of host adaptation of different *S. enterica* serovars with their levels of virulence and types of pathogenesis [4]. Serovars that are better adapted to a specific host species, such as the human-restricted *S. enterica* serovar Typhi (*S.* Typhi), are extremely pathogenic due to their ability to leave the intestines and spread hematogenously, resulting in sepsis. In contrast, serovars such as *S. enterica* serovar Typhimurium (*S.* Typhimurium) that have a broad host range are restricted to local invasion, and their containment by host inflammatory responses narrows their pathogenesis to gastrointestinal symptoms in humans. Finally, some *Salmonella* such as *S. enterica* subsp. *diarizonae* (*S. diarizonae*) are primarily associated with cold-blooded animals, and only rarely result in invasive diseases in sheep or humans [5,6].

Even though all *Salmonella* have and express SPI-1 genes [7], variations in the sequence of specific SPI-1 proteins and the unique repertoire of translocated SPI-1 effector proteins by different species, serovars and even strains within the same serovar has a direct impact on the invasion efficiency of different cell types [8–10]. Moreover, the diversity of *S. enterica* invasion levels for various cell types and host species can be partially attributed to variations in the regulation and export efficiencies of effector proteins through the SPI-1 T3SS [11]. In addition to the SPI-1 T3SS, cell invasion by *S. enterica* involves two outer membrane proteins (OMP), Rck and PagN, that have been designated adhesins–invasins due to their ability to promote both bacterial binding to host receptors and cellular uptake [12–14]. Rck has several adhesive properties: it binds to factor H to mediate bacterial resistance to complement and adheres to laminin and interacts with the epidermal growth factor receptor for a zipper mechanism of cell invasion [13,15–17]. Rck also contains a self-association motif that has the potential to mediate interbacterial attachment, as described for Hra1/Hek, an integral outer membrane protein of enteroaggregative *Escherichia coli* (*E. coli*) [18,19]. The adhesins/invasins Hra1/Hek, Hra2 and Tia of enteroaggregative or enterotoxigenic *E. coli* share homologies with membrane spanning domains of PagN, but their surface-exposed loops are less similar, alluding to variable binding affinities for different host receptors [18,20–22].

Unlike *rck*, which is plasmid-encoded and absent in many virulent *S. enterica* serovars and strains, *pagN* is encoded on the bacterial chromosome and present in most, if not all, *S. enterica*. One study indicated that deletion of *pagN* in *S.* Typhimurium SL1344 grown under PhoPQ-activating conditions to inhibit SPI-1 gene transcription decreased bacterial adhesion and invasion of HT-29 cells [12]. In contrast, deletion of *pagN* in the *S.* Typhimurium strain LT2 did not impact adhesion to HT-29 or other cells [23], potentially due to the expression of other adhesins such as the type 1 fimbriae induced by the growth culture conditions. More surprisingly, despite the presence of both SPI-1 T3SS and type IV pili that can each independently mediate invasion, deletion of *pagN* impacted both adhesion and invasion of HT-29 cells in a strain of *S.* Typhi [23,24]. Although the culture conditions used might not have activated functionally detectable T3SS expression, type IV pili were still functional, since a *S.* Typhi mutant lacking type IV pili affected invasion as much as the Δ*pagN* mutant [23]. The latter result suggested that both PagN and the type IV pili contribute to *S.* Typhi invasion of cells. In addition, oral challenge of iron-overloaded Swiss Albino mice with wild type and *pagN* mutants of *S.* Typhi indicated that the former strain was more invasive and had increased lethality at an infectious dose of 2×10^7 CFU and in competition assays. Finally, even though no differences were observed between the wild type and *pagN* mutant strains of *S.* Typhimurium [23], use of PagN from each serovar as an immunogen demonstrated some level of immune protection in mice challenged with the wild type strain from the corresponding serovar [23]. Thus, the role of PagN in the invasive properties of *S.* Typhi and *S.* Typhimurium remain somewhat controversial and studies of their function are likely impacted by the confounding effects of additional adhesins/invasins, different levels of PagN expression, and/or variations in the protein sequence of PagN.

Based on these results and our previous findings on FimH adhesin alleles in various *S. enterica* serovars and strains for host cell binding specificities [25,26], we wondered whether allelic variation in PagN [10] modulates bacterial adhesion and invasion. Here we determined that the *S.* Typhi allelic variant of PagN provides significantly better bacterial binding and invasive efficiencies for different enterocytes and the extracellular matrix protein laminin, as compared to the major *S.* Typhimurium allele. To our surprise, PagN from *S. enterica* subsp. *diarizonae* was also significantly more adhesive and invasive than the major *S.* Typhimurium allele. Sequence comparison and functional analysis of substitutions as specific residue positions revealed that amino acids in two of the four PagN surface-exposed loops contributed to these phenotypes. These results further support the role of allelic variation of virulence factors in adjusting the level of pathogenic attributes among *Salmonella* subspecies and serovars.

2. Materials and Methods

2.1. Bacterial Strain and Plasmid Constructions

The bacterial strains and plasmids used in this study are described in Table 1 and all PCR primers are listed in Table S1. Unless stated otherwise, all the reagents were from MilliporeSigma (St. Louis, MO, USA). Bacteria were routinely grown in LB-Lennox media unless otherwise indicated. When appropriate, ampicillin (200 μg/mL) or kanamycin (45 μg/mL) was added to the growth medium. For plasmid constructions, the *pagN* genes were amplified from *S.* Typhimurium, *S.* Typhi and *S. diarizonae* genomic DNA by PCR with the Q5 High-Fidelity DNA Polymerase (New England Biolabs Inc., Ipswich, MA, USA). For PagN expression the allelic genes were cloned into AHT-inducible plasmid pRS1 using Gibson assembly with amplicon prepared from appropriate primers. Three site-directed substitution mutants were prepared by Gibson assembly of pRS1 and amplicons prepared with *pagN* external and internal primers for *S.* Typhimurium or *S.* Typhi, or amplicons prepared with mutagenic primers. A *pagN-his* fusion construct was prepared by insertion of a *Nde*I-*Hind*III restricted amplicon into pET22b. *S.* Typhimurium SL1344 *sipB::aphA-3* mutant was prepared by P22 generalized transduction from strain DMS1507 [27,28] and SL1344 *sipB::aphA-3* ΔpagN was constructed by Gibson assembly and allelic exchange as described [29–31]. All plasmid and strain constructs were confirmed by PCR and sequencing.

Table 1. Strains and plasmids.

Strain	Genus, Species, Serovar and/or Relevant Genotype	Source
AAEC189	*E. coli* MM294 Δ*lac recA endA* Δ*fim* (r_{K-} m_{K+})	[32]
BL21(DE3)	*E. coli* str. B F$^-$ *ompT gal dcm lon hsdS*$_B$($r_B{}^-m_B{}^-$) λ(DE3 [*lacI lacUV5-T7p07 ind1 sam7 nin5*]) [*malB*$^+$]$_{K\text{-}12}$(λ^S)	Novagen
JKE201	*E. coli* MG1655 RP4-2-Tc::[ΔMu1::Δ*aac(3)IV*::*lacI*^{q}-Δ*aphA*-Δ*nic35*-ΔMu2::*zeo*] Δ*dapA*::(*erm-pir*) Δ*recA* Δ*mcrA* Δ(*mrr-hsdRMS-mcrBC*))	[29,33]
SL1344	*S. enterica* subsp. *enterica* serovar Typhimurium	[34]
S. Typhi	*S. enterica* subsp. *enterica* serovar Typhi 9,12,[Vi]:d:[Z66]	*Salmonella* Reference collection C (SARC) no2
S. diarizonae	*S. enterica* subsp. *diarizonae* 50:k:z	SARC no7
DMS1507	*S. enterica* subsp. *enterica* serovar Typhimurium LB5010 *sipB::aphA-3*	[27,28]
DMS1949	SL1344 *sipB* Δ*pagN*	This study
Plasmid	Description	Source
pMG81	Expression plasmid with *tetR* and *tetA* promoter upstream *envZ*, Ap^R	Mark Goulian
pRS1	pMG81Δ*envZ*	This study
pDMS1973	*S.* Typhi *pagN* in pRS1	This study
pDMS1974	SL1344 *pagN* in pRS1	This study
pDMS2062	*S. diarizonae pagN* in pRS1	This study
pDMS2081	SL1344 *pagN*$_{D49E}$ in pRS1	This study
pDMS2082	SL1344 *pagN*$_{D109Q}$ in pRS1	This study
pDMS2083	SL1344 *pagN*$_{D109E}$ in pRS1	This study

2.2. Protein Expression and Antibody Preparation

The histidine-tagged PagN was expressed from the pET22b construct using the IPTG inducer and isolated by metal chelation chromatography as described previously [35]. A specific polyclonal antiserum against PagN-His was prepared in rabbits by using a conventional immunization protocol (Cocalico Biologicals Inc., Reamstown, PA, USA). The antiserum was adsorbed with *E. coli* BL21(DE3)/pET22b before use as described previously [36]. Briefly, 1 mL antiserum with 0.06% sodium azide was incubated with bacterial pellets from 10-mL cultures grown overnight for 18 h at 4 °C. After three adsorption cycles, the antiserum was filtered (0.02 μm-pore-size) before use. PagN expression in *E. coli* AAEC189 for all the binding and invasion studies was induced with AHT by growing the bacteria overnight at 30 °C, or for 2 h at 37 °C, starting with log phase cultures (A_{600} = 0.3). Comparable levels and bacterial surface expression of the three cloned PagN alleles were standardized by using various concentrations of inducers (0.005–2 μg/mL AHT) for Western blot analysis and ELISA, as done previously [25]. Outer membrane proteins were prepared as described previously [37].

2.3. Cell Cultures

The human colonic cell line RKO (ATCC CRL2577) was cultured in Dulbecco's Modified Eagle Medium (DMEM; Invitrogen, Life Technologies) supplemented with 15% (*v*/*v*) heat inactivated fetal bovine serum (FBS) and antibiotics to a final concentration of 100 U/mL penicillin and 100 μg/mL streptomycin (Gibco, Life Technologies) [25]. The porcine cell line IPEC-J2 (DSMZ ACC 701) was cultured with 15% heat inactivated FBS (Sigma-Aldrich), 1% penicillin/streptomycin, 1% insulin/transferrin/selenium (Gibco) and 5 ng/mL epidermal growth factor (Sigma) in DMEM/F-12/HAM (1/1/1, *v*/*v*/*v*; Gibco). The cells were incubated at 37 °C in a humid atmosphere with 5% CO_2.

2.4. Bacterial Binding and Invasion Assays

Both epithelial cell cultures grown to confluence in 24-well plates (Corning, CLS3596) were used for the binding assays with recombinant *E. coli* AAEC189 (*E. coli* Δ*fim*) with pRS1 plasmid constructs s expressing a *Salmonella* PagN allele. Bacteria were grown overnight, diluted 10^{-2} in LB broth with inducers (see above), incubated for 16–17 h, washed three times with PBS and diluted in DMEM to inoculate with a multiplicity of infection of 100 bacteria (in 0.25 mL) to 1 enterocyte. Exact bacterial inoculum numbers were checked by standard CFU counts. The culture plates were centrifuged (600 *g*, 5 min) to initiate contact between the bacteria and the cells and incubated for 1 h at 37 °C in 5% CO_2. To evaluate cell adhesion, the infected monolayers were washed thrice with PBS to remove non-associated bacteria and treated with 0.5% Triton X-100 to release and count the cell-associated bacteria by CFU enumeration. For the invasion assays, a standard gentamicin protection assay was performed [38]. Following a 1 h infection (see above), cells were incubated with medium containing gentamicin (100 μg/mL) for 90 min at 37 °C in 5% CO_2. After three washes with PBS, bacteria were released with Triton X-100 and enumerated as described above. All experiments were done in triplicate wells and repeated at least thrice.

2.5. Microscopy

For fluorescence microscopy, *E. coli* strain AAEC189 carrying plasmids pRS1, pDMS1973 ($pagN_{Ty}$), pDMS1974 ($pagN_{Tm}$) or pDMS2062 ($pagN_{di}$) were grown and induced for PagN expression as described above. The bacterial cells were deposited on slides, dried for 20 min and washed once with PBS. Bacteria were fixed with 4% paraformaldehyde in PBS, pH 7.4, then labeled with adsorbed anti-PagN antisera (1:500), followed by anti-rabbit Alexa Fluor 480 (1:1000; Invitrogen, Life Technologies, Grand Island, NY, USA). Images were captured with a Coolsnap digital camera (Photometrics, Tucson, AZ, USA) mounted onto a Nikon Eclipse E600 microscope with Coolsnap version 1.2.0 software (Roper Scientific, Tucson, Arizona).

2.6. Binding to Extracellular Matrix Proteins

Immuno Maxisorb plates with 96 wells (Nunc; Thermo Fisher Scientific, Rochester, NY, USA) were coated with 10 μg/mL of human collagen I, chicken collagen II, human collagen IV, bovine fibronectin, murine laminin or BSA (Sigma-Aldrich) in PBS at 4 °C overnight and then washed with PBS and blocked with PBS plus 1% BSA for 2 h. Binding of bacteria to laminin coated on plates was studied by using PagN-expressing *E. coli*. Bacteria grown and induced to make PagN were centrifuged, suspended in PBS to 10^7 CFU in 100 μL and added to laminin coated wells. Bacteria harboring empty plasmid pRS1 were used as a control. After incubation for 1 h at 37 °C, unbound bacteria were removed by three washing cycles, anti-PagN antiserum (1:500) was added, followed by wash cycles and incubation with goat anti-rabbit HRP-conjugated antibody (1:2000). After three wash cycles, bound antibodies were detected by using the 1-Step Turbo TMB ELISA substrate (Thermo Fisher Scientific) followed by 2 M sulfuric acid and measuring the absorbance at 450 nm. For the binding inhibition assays, double dilutions of heparin or heparan sulfate (400–0.4 μg/mL) were incubated with bacteria for 1 h and the mixtures were added to the laminin-coated wells for further processing as described above.

2.7. Bacterial Genomes and PagN Sequences

Salmonella genomic sequences from 497 previously studied *S. enterica* from 6 serovars with two biovars (serovars Typhi, Dublin, Choleraesuis, Typhimurium, Enteritidis, Newport and Gallinarum, with biovars Gallinarum and Pullorum for the latter serovar) and from 45 confirmed *S. diarizonae* (Table S2) were obtained from NCBI RefSeq database or assembled from NCBI SRA, EBI ENA and Wellcome Sanger Institute repositories as described [10]. The genomes were used to determine their encoded PagN sequences. The genomes of 13 incorrectly serotyped *S. diarizonae* strains were detected with SISTR (their corrected serovar attribution was added to Table S2) and not analyzed for PagN [39]. Protein alignments were done with Megalign, DNASTAR Lasergene (Madison, WI, USA).

2.8. PagN Structure Analysis

The 3D-structural model of PagN was predicted by using the corresponding sequence from *S.* Typhimurium LT2 and I-TASSER [40,41]. Among the five best predicted models, the 3rd model was chosen to be shown in Figure 1B (Protean 3D, DNASTAR Lasergene), with an overall ERRAT quality factor of 84.4 [42], in agreement with a published model for *S.* Typhi PagN [43]. The five best I-TASSER predicted *S. arizonae* PagN structures essentially overlapped with the ones of *S.* Typhimurium and *S.* Typhi.

2.9. Statistical Analysis

Student's non-paired *t* test (two tailed) was used with Prism 8 (GraphPad Software, San Diego, CA, USA) to calculate statistical significance for all the binding assays (* $p < 0.05$, ** $p < 0.01$, *** $p < 0.001$ and **** $p < 0.0001$).

3. Results and Discussion

PagN of *S.* Typhimurium and *S.* Typhi had similar sequences with two to three substitutions in predicted surface-exposed loops 1 and 2 (Figure 1). Since PagN of both strains act as adhesins and invasins for human intestinal epithelial cells, we wondered whether these allelic variants differentially impacted these properties. To ensure consistent and comparable expression of PagN, we cloned each gene into inducible expression plasmids to make pDMS1973 and pDMS1974 for the expression of PagN from *S.*Typhi ($pagN_{Ty}$) and *S.* Typhimurium ($pagN_{Tm}$) respectively. Western blot analysis of outer membrane preparations from *E. coli* AAEC89 carrying one of these two plasmid constructs detected bands specific for each PagN allele (Figure 2A).

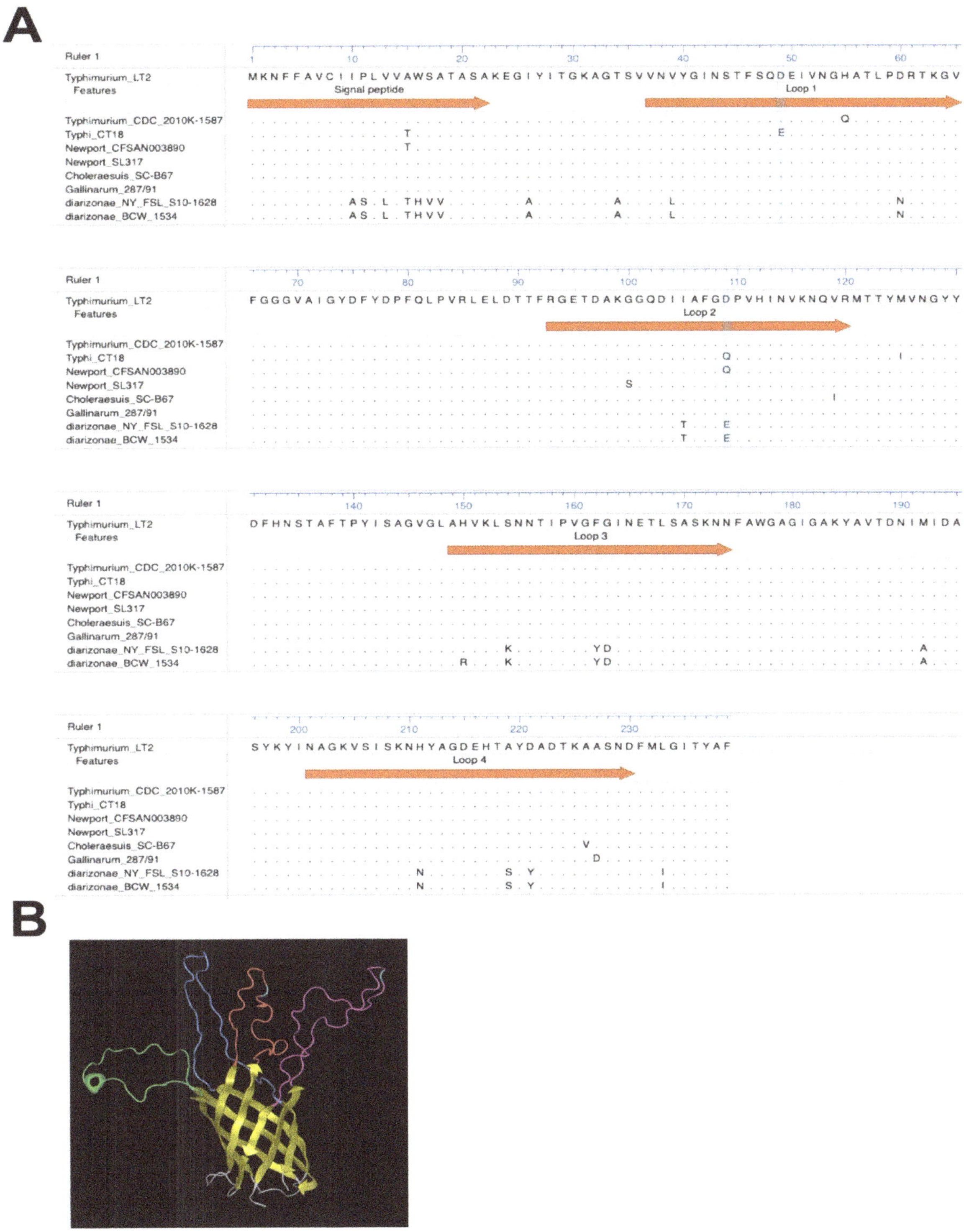

Figure 1. PagN sequences and predicted structure. (**A**) Alignment of PagN alleles from different *Salmonella* strains (Table S3) [10] each representing N strains from one or more serovars, or clusters within serovars or subspecies with the same sequence in the surface loops of mature PagN; *S.* Typhimurium_LT2 ($n = 68$) with same sequence for *S.* Enteritidis ($n = 74$), *S.* Pullorum ($n = 29$), *S.* Dublin ($n = 74$), and a cluster of Newport strains ($n = 25$); *S.* Typhimurium_CDC_2010k-1587 ($n = 7$); *S.* Typhi_CT18 ($n = 75$); *S.* Newport_CFSAN003890 ($n = 23$); *S.* Newport_SL317 ($n = 22$); *S.* Choleraesuis_SC-B67($n = 74$); *S.* Gallinarum 287/91($n = 23$); *S. diarizonae* NY_FSL_S10-1628 ($n = 3$) and *S. diarizonae*_BCW_1534 ($n = 45$). (**B**) *S.* Typhimurium mature PagN model predicted with I-TASSER. Color codes are for the membrane spanning beta-barrel (yellow), the periplasmic loops (grey), surface-exposed loop 1 (purple) with residue 49 (turquoise), loop 2 (red) with residue 109 (turquoise), loop 3 (green) and loop 4 (dark blue).

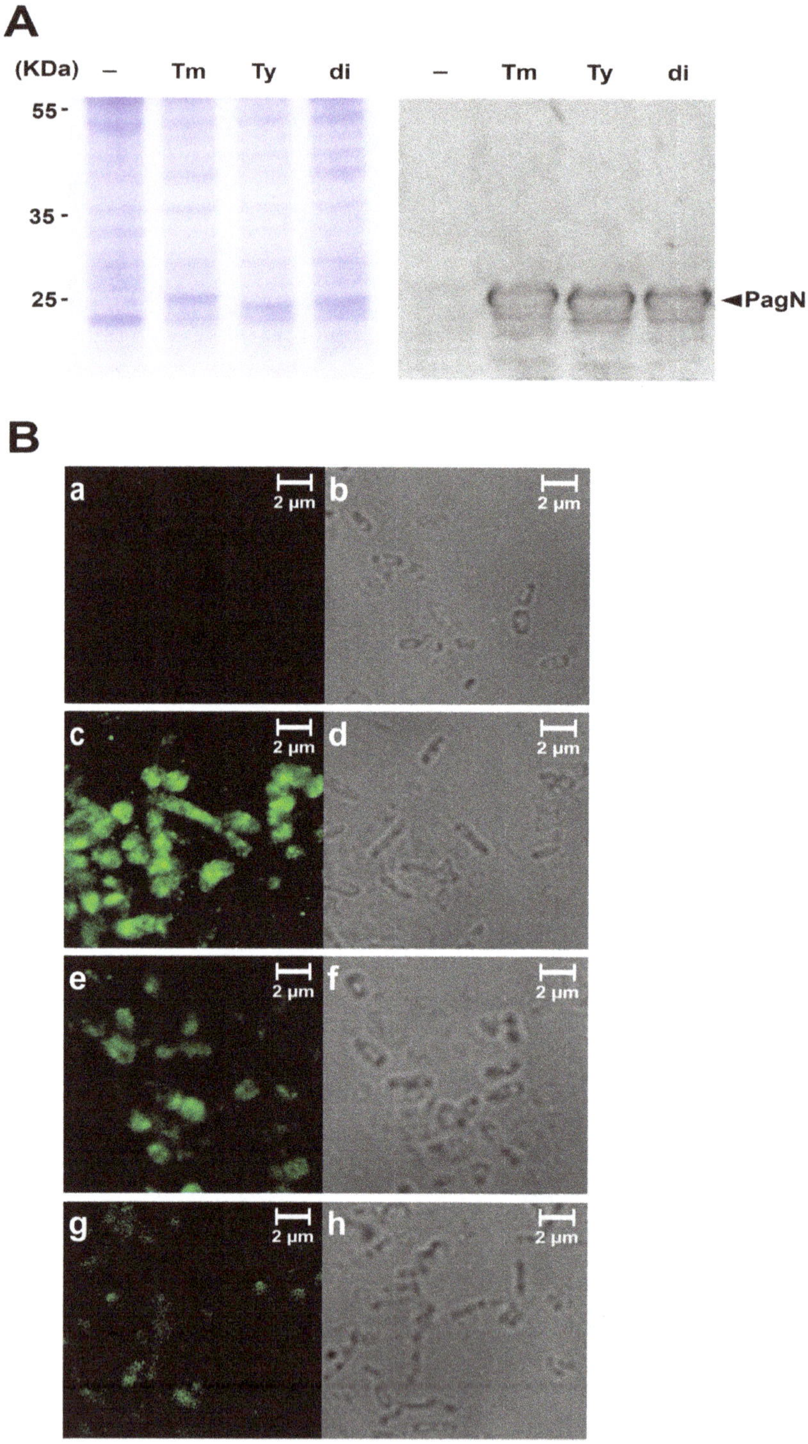

Figure 2. Expression of pagN alleles from *S.* Typhimurium, *S.* Typhi and *S. diarizonae*. (**A**) Expression of PagN in *E. coli* AAEC189 transformed with pRS1 (empty vector, -), pDMS1973 ($pagN_{Ty}$), pDMS1974 ($pagN_{Tm}$) or pDMS2062 ($pagN_{di}$) was induced by AHT (0.2–0.4 µg/mL) for 2 h at 37 °C. Isolated outer membrane proteins analyzed by SDS-PAGE, followed by Coomassie blue staining or western blotting with anti-PagN antisera showed a clear band for PagN expression at 25 kDa. (**B**) Visualization of PagN surface expression in *E. coli* AAEC189 expressing the allele from *S.* Typhimurium (**c**,**d**), *S.* Typhi (**e**,**f**), *S. diarizonae* (**g**,**h**) or empty vector as negative control (**a**,**b**). Phase-contrast microscopy (right) and fluorescence microscopy (left) were used to detect bacteria labeled with anti-PagN antisera, followed by Alexa Fluor 488-conjugated anti-rabbit IgG.

Moreover, both alleles of PagN were detectable on the bacterial surface by immunofluorescence (Figure 2B, panel a to f) and ELISA (not shown). Not surprisingly, the strongest signal was observed for the *S.* Typhimurium PagN allele, as this was the immunogen used to prepare the antiserum.

The *E. coli* strain AAEC189 lacks adhesive type 1 fimbriae, providing us with a bacterial context in which to study PagN-mediated bacterial binding and cellular uptake free of known *Salmonella* adhesins and invasins. Using both RKO and IPEC-J2 enterocytes, we found that both $PagN_{Ty}$ and $PagN_{Tm}$ mediated bacterial binding and invasion, as previously reported for ovarian hamster epithelial-like CHO-K1 cells and human colonic HT-29 cells [12,23]. More importantly, comparisons of the two alleles indicated that $PagN_{Ty}$ was more efficient than $PagN_{Tm}$ for both cell adhesion and invasion (Figure 3A), supporting an allelic variant effect on a virulence property. Additional studies with a *S.* Typhimurium *pagN* and *sipB* (essential SPI-1 translocon subunit) deletion mutant complemented with different PagN-expressing plasmids did not show significant different levels of adhesion/invasion of RKO cells (data not shown), suggesting a dominant phenotype due to the expression of one or more other *Salmonella* adhesin(s) and invasin(s) under the used growth conditions. Thus, the use of *E. coli* with a controlled expression system allowed us to bypass the masking effect of additional *Salmonella* adhesins/invasins differentially expressed in different serovars and environmental growth conditions and identify functional differences due only to sequence variations of PagN alleles [44,45].

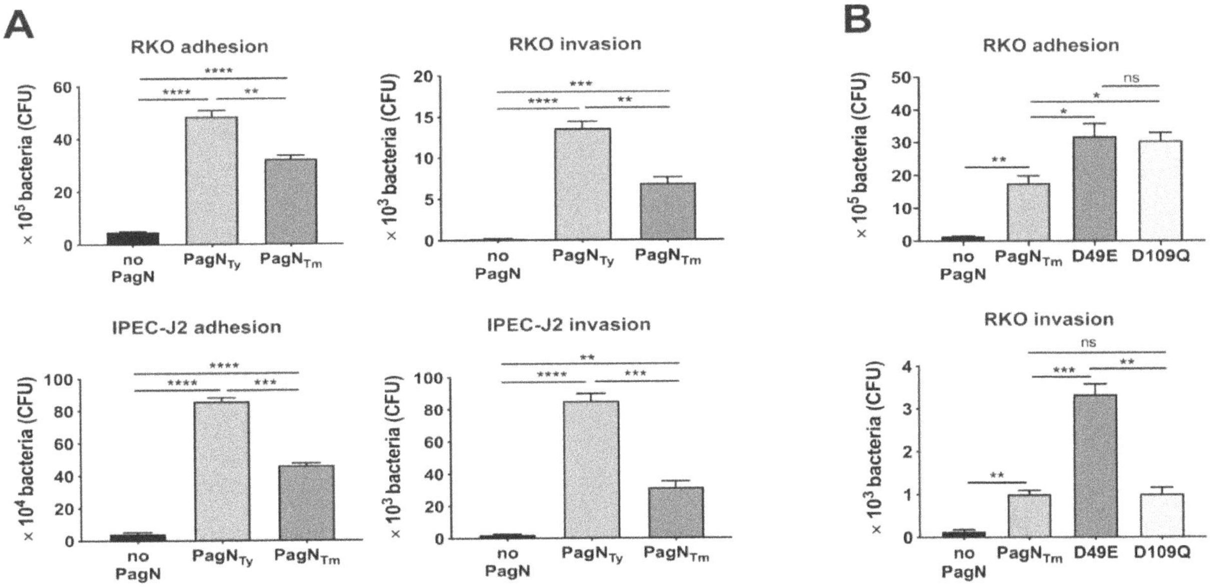

Figure 3. Binding and uptake of *E. coli* AAEC189 to intestinal epithelial cells mediated by PagN expression. (**A**) Adherence and invasion of *E. coli* AAEC189 with empty vector pRS1 (no pagN), pDMS1973 or pDMS1974 to express $PagN_{Ty}$ or $PagN_{Tm}$ respectively, to human (RKO) and porcine (IPEC-J2) was analyzed by incubating 3×10^7 CFU/mL bacteria at a MOI of 100 for 60 min for adherence and another 90 min for invasion assays. Bacteria expressing $PagN_{Ty}$ bound and invaded significantly better than the bacteria expressing $PagN_{Tm}$ ($p < 0.01$–0.001). (**B**) Adherence of *E. coli* AAEC189 expressing $PagN_{Tm}$ to RKO cells was significantly enhanced ($p < 0.05$) when $PagN_{Tm}$ was mutated from aspartate to glutamate (at site 49, D49E) with pDMS2081 or to glutamine (at site 109, D109Q) with pDMS2082, whereas invasion of epithelial cells was affected only by the D49E substitution ($p < 0.001$), but not by the D109Q substitution. Data represent one of three separate and reproducible experiments each with triplicate data expressed as mean ± SEM (ns is for not significant, * $p < 0.05$, ** $p < 0.01$, *** $p < 0.001$ and **** $p < 0.0001$).

PagN sequence alignments for 52–75 strains for each of the seven *S. enterica* serovars, including *S.* Typhimurium [10], highlighted that all PagN had aspartic acid residues at position 49 and 109, with the exceptions of *S.* Typhi that had a glutamic acid at position 49, and a group of *S.* Newport strains that had a glutamine at position 109 (Figure 1A). Since the allelic PagN proteins of all strains of

S. Typhi and *S.* Typhimurium varied at these two positions and were each predicted to be located in a different bacterial surface loop (Figure 1B), we investigated their relative involvement in bacterial adhesion and invasion. For this, we generated $PagN_{Tm}$ with a D49E or a D109Q substitution and expressed them in *E. coli* strain AAEC189. Although both mutated PagN mediated better bacterial binding to RKO cells than did $PagN_{Tm}$, only the D49E substitution in PagN had a significantly stronger effect on bacterial invasion (Figure 3B). This result highlighted the contribution of the *S.* Typhi glutamic acid at position 49 for the improved interaction of PagN with a host cell receptor to promote bacterial uptake. This result is consistent with a role for the PagN allele in the increased pathogenicity of *S.* Typhi relative to *S.* Typhimurium pathogenesis following human infection, in agreement with the former serovar's hematogenous bacterial spreading in humans resulting frequently in sepsis, in contrast to the latter serovar and its pathogenesis that is usually contained in the gastro-intestinal organs.

Other than subsp. *enterica*, most subsp. of *S. enterica* are associated with cold-blooded animals. Therefore, we expected that a construct expressing the PagN allele of these non-*enterica* subspecies would neither bind nor efficiently invade human RKO cells and therefore would serve as a negative control. Thus, we cloned the *S. diarizonae* PagN ($PagN_{di}$) in the same inducible expression plasmid used for the two other PagN alleles to make pDMS2062 and confirmed protein production (Figure 2A) and surface expression (Figure 2B, panels g and h). To our surprise, *E. coli* making $PagN_{di}$ were significantly more adhesive and invasive than the ones expressing $PagN_{Tm}$ (Figure 4A).

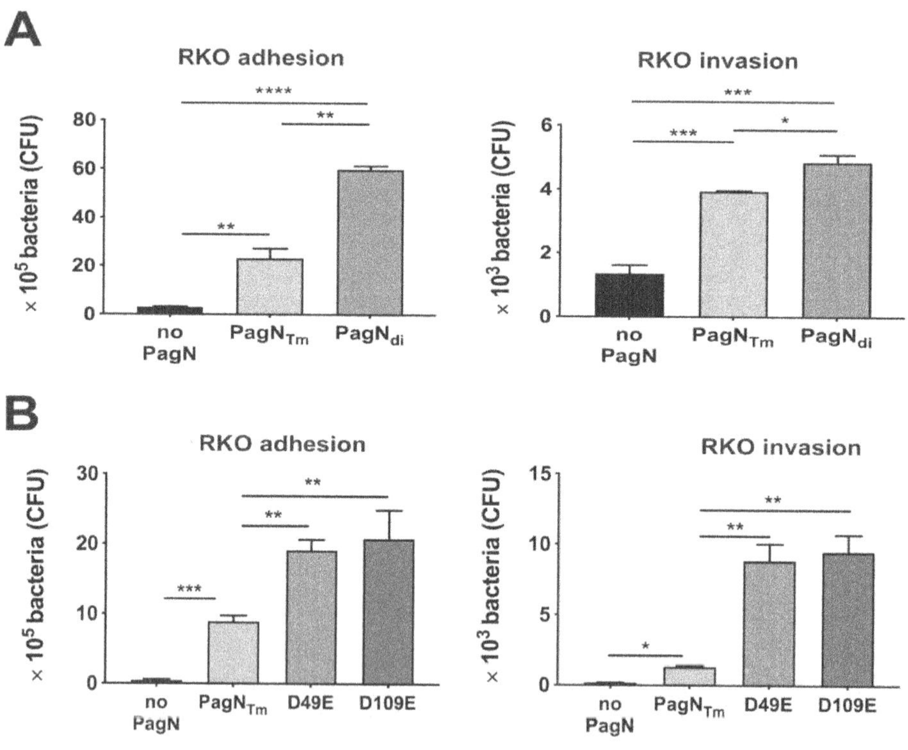

Figure 4. Binding and uptake of *E. coli* expressing PagN from non-*enterica* allelic variants. (**A**) Adhesion and invasion of *E. coli* AAEC189 expressing *pagN* allele from *S. diarizonae* PagN ($PagN_{di}$) and *S.* Typhimurium PagN ($PagN_{Tm}$) to RKO cells showed the bacteria expressing $PagN_{di}$ binds significantly better than $PagN_{Tm}$ ($p < 0.01$) and was slightly more invasive ($p < 0.05$). (**B**) A substitution of aspartate to glutamate at site 109 in *S.* Typhimurium PagN (D109E) increased both binding and invasion of *E. coli* into RKO cells as compared to the bacteria expressing $PagN_{Tm}$ ($p < 0.01$). Data represent one of three separate and reproducible experiments, each with triplicate data expressed as mean ± SEM (* $p < 0.05$, ** $p < 0.01$, *** $p < 0.001$ and **** $p < 0.0001$).

PagN alignments of 48 available strains of *S. diarizonae* highlighted that they all had an aspartic acid at position 49, like most evaluated subsp. *enterica* serovars (Typhi being the exception, Figure 1A).

In contrast, unlike the subsp. *enterica* serovars, all $PagN_{di}$ carried a glutamic acid at position 109, suggesting that a D109E substitution at this position would be functionally significant. In support, a D109E substitution in the *S.* Typhimurium PagN (pDMS 2083) improved not only bacterial binding, but also bacterial uptake by RKO cells (Figure 4B), indicating that glutamic acid in this position optimizes the function of PagN as both an adhesin and invasin. Whether other substitutions in $PagN_{di}$, such as the arginine or lysine at position 150 and 154 in loop 3 (Figure 1) modulate bacterial invasion remains to be determined. Like *S.* Typhi, *S. diarizonae* have type IVB pili involved in intestinal cell invasion, raising the possibility that the concomitant increased binding property of the *S. diarizonae* PagN allele contributes to the reported increased bacterial virulence in humans under specific conditions [5]. Taken together, the results showed that PagN alleles with a glutamic acid residue at either 49 or 109 improves bacterial binding and/or invasiveness, possibly due to the more ionizable and long chain characteristics of glutamic acid relative to aspartic acid and glutamine.

In addition to promoting bacterial attachment to cells, many bacterial adhesins interact with various host glycoprotein of the extracellular matrix, as exemplified by the ability of $PagN_{Ty}$ to bind to laminin [23,46–48]. *S. enterica* may encounter laminin either on intestinal areas denuded of epithelial cells (e.g., extrusion zones at villi tips) or in the subepithelial space after invading enterocytes and crossing the intestinal epithelial layer. Notably, the low pH and magnesium concentrations in *Salmonella*-containing vacuoles (SCV) of invaded cells induce the PhoPQ two-component system responsible for PagN expression [49–51]. Thus, whereas the *S. enterica* SPI-1 system is induced in the intestinal environment and used for enterocyte invasion, expression of PagN in SCV (where SPI-1 is largely repressed) may prepare *Salmonella* for future cycles of cell invasion after escape from intestinal epithelial cells. Our side-by side comparison of $PagN_{Ty}$-, $PagN_{Tm}$- and $PagN_{di}$-expressing *E. coli* showed that all three bacteria adhered significantly to laminin, albeit the former better than the latter two (Figure 5A). None of the bacteria bound to collagen I, II or IV or fibronectin (not shown).

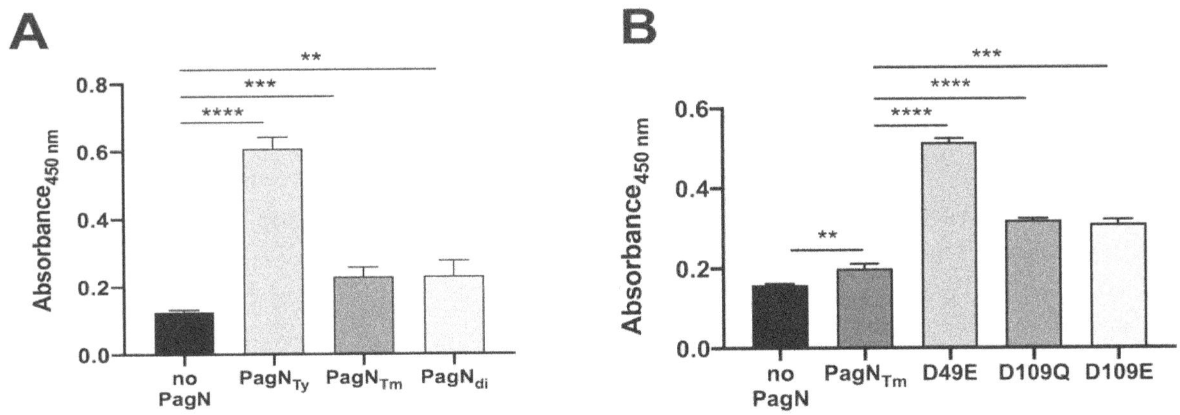

Figure 5. Binding of PagN allelic variants to murine laminin. (**A**) The $PagN_{Ty}$-expressing bacteria bound best to laminin. *E. coli* AAEC189 expressing $PagN_{Tm}$, $PagN_{Ty}$, $PagN_{di}$ or containing empty vector (no *pagN*) were incubated with microtiter wells coated with murine laminin. Bacterial binding was detected by an ELISA-method with anti-PagN antiserum. (**B**) All substitution mutants bound better to laminin than bacteria expressing $PagN_{Tm}$, with the mutant expressing glutamic acid at position 49 of $PagN_{Tm}$ (D49E) binding best ($p < 0.0001$). Data represent one of three separate and reproducible experiments, each with triplicate data expressed as mean ± SEM (** $p < 0.01$, *** $p < 0.001$ and **** $p < 0.0001$).

To determine the potential role of PagN residue 49 and 109 in $PagN_{Ty}$ binding to laminin, we tested the three mutants described above. As for the intestinal epithelial cell binding results, bacteria with a glutamic acid at position 49 of $PagN_{Tm}$ (D49E) bound significantly better to laminin than did bacteria with $PagN_{Tm}$ (Figure 5B). Glutamic acid or glutamine at position 109 of $PagN_{Tm}$ (D109E and D109Q) also increased binding, albeit less efficiently.

Since both PagN and heparin bind to laminin [52], we next determined whether heparin or heparan sulfate could inhibit PagN-mediated bacterial binding to laminin. In contrast to the reported inhibitory effect of heparin on PagN-mediated invasion of CHO-K1 cells [53], neither heparin nor heparan sulfate at concentrations as high as 400 µg/mL interfered with the binding of $PagN_{Ty}$-expressing bacteria to laminin (data not shown). These combined results suggested that PagN and heparin bind to different laminin sites and that the invasion of CHO-K1 cells by PagN-expressing bacteria is laminin-independent. Thus, our studies highlight the independent adhesive properties of PagN in binding to either intestinal cells or the extracellular matrix protein laminin, two relevant targets for *Salmonella* host invasion.

In summary and together with our previous studies on variants of fimbrial adhesins [25,26,54], this study on PagN, a *Salmonella* adhesin/invasin, further supports the importance of protein sequence allelic variants in virulence properties [55], including pathogenic properties such as adhesion and invasion [4].

Author Contributions: Conceptualization, D.M.S. and I.N.O.; methodology, D.M.S. and I.N.O.; software, A.V.R. and D.M.S.; validation, D.M.S. and R.D.; formal analysis, Y.W., Q.H., R.D., N.G.; investigation, Y.W., Q.H., R.D., N.G., E.C.C. and J.H.; resources, D.M.S. and I.N.O.; data curation, R.D. and D.M.S.; writing—original draft preparation, D.M.S.; writing—review and editing, D.M.S.; visualization, R.D., Y.W., Q.H.; supervision, D.M.S. and I.N.O.; project administration, D.M.S. and I.N.O.; funding acquisition, D.M.S. and I.N.O. All authors have read and agreed to the published version of the manuscript.

Acknowledgments: We thank all the contributors for publicly sharing their *Salmonella* genomic data through the National Center for Biotechnology Information, European Bioinformatics Institute and Wellcome Sanger Institute *Salmonella* genome projects. We thank Mark Goulian for plasmid pMG81, Olivier Cunrath and Dirk Bumann for *E. coli* strain JKE201 and Gibson assembly protocols, and Leslie King for proofreading the manuscript. The opinions expressed in this manuscript are solely the responsibility of the authors and do not necessarily represent the official views and policy of the National Institutes of Health.

References

1. Tsolis, R.M.; Xavier, M.N.; Santos, R.L.; Baumler, A.J. How to become a top model: Impact of animal experimentation on human *Salmonella* disease research. *Infect. Immun.* **2011**, *79*, 1806–1814. [CrossRef]
2. Alikhan, N.F.; Zhou, Z.; Sergeant, M.J.; Achtman, M. A genomic overview of the population structure of *Salmonella*. *PLoS Genet.* **2018**, *14*, e1007261. [CrossRef]
3. Grimont, P.A.D.; Weill, F.-X. *Antigenic Formulae of the Salmonella Serovars*; WHO Collaborating Center for Reference and Research on *Salmonella*; Institut Pasteur, 28 rue du Dr. Roux: Paris, France, 2007; pp. 1–166.
4. Yue, M.; Schifferli, D.M. Allelic variation in *Salmonella*: An underappreciated driver of adaptation and virulence. *Front. Microbiol.* **2014**, *4*, 419. [CrossRef]
5. Giner-Lamia, J.; Vinuesa, P.; Betancor, L.; Silva, C.; Bisio, J.; Soleto, L.; Chabalgoity, J.A.; Puente, J.L.; Salmonella, C.N.; Garcia-Del Portillo, F. Genome analysis of *Salmonella enterica* subsp. diarizonae isolates from invasive human infections reveals enrichment of virulence-related functions in lineage ST1256. *BMC Genomics* **2019**, *20*, 99. [CrossRef]
6. Uelze, L.; Borowiak, M.; Deneke, C.; Jacobs, C.; Szabo, I.; Tausch, S.H.; Malorny, B. First complete genome sequence and comparative analysis of *Salmonella enterica* subsp. diarizonae serovar 61:k:1,5,(7) indicates host adaptation traits to sheep. *Gut Pathog.* **2019**, *11*, 48. [CrossRef]
7. Bäumler, A.J.; Tsolis, R.M.; Ficht, T.A.; Adams, L.G. Evolution of host adaptation in *Salmonella enterica*. *Infect. Immun.* **1998**, *66*, 4579–4587. [CrossRef]
8. Hopkins, K.L.; Threlfall, E.J. Frequency and polymorphism of sopE in isolates of *Salmonella enterica* belonging to the ten most prevalent serotypes in England and Wales. *J. Med. Microbiol.* **2004**, *53*, 539–543. [CrossRef]

9. Heffron, F.; Niemann, G.; Yoon, H.; Kidwai, A.; Brown, R.N.E.; McDermott, J.D.; Smith, R.; Adlkins, J.N. *Salmonella*-Secreted Virulence Factors. In *Salmonella: From Genome to Function*; Porwollik, S., Ed.; Caister Academic Press: Norfolk, UK, 2011; pp. 187–223.
10. Rakov, A.V.; Mastriani, E.; Liu, S.L.; Schifferli, D.M. Association of Salmonella virulence factor alleles with intestinal and invasive serovars. *BMC Genom.* **2019**, *20*, 429. [CrossRef]
11. Elhadad, D.; Desai, P.; Grassl, G.A.; McClelland, M.; Rahav, G.; Gal-Mor, O. Differences in Host Cell Invasion and *Salmonella* Pathogenicity Island 1 Expression between *Salmonella enterica* Serovar Paratyphi A and Nontyphoidal *S.* Typhimurium. *Infect. Immun.* **2016**, *84*, 1150–1165. [CrossRef]
12. Lambert, M.A.; Smith, S.G. The PagN protein of *Salmonella enterica* serovar Typhimurium is an adhesin and invasin. *BMC Microbiol.* **2008**, *8*, 142. [CrossRef]
13. Cirillo, D.M.; Heffernan, E.J.; Wu, L.; Harwood, J.; Fierer, J.; Guiney, D.G. Identification of a domain in Rck, a product of the Salmonella typhimurium virulence plasmid, required for both serum resistance and cell invasion. *Infect. Immun.* **1996**, *64*, 2019–2023. [CrossRef] [PubMed]
14. Velge, P.; Wiedemann, A.; Rosselin, M.; Abed, N.; Boumart, Z.; Chausse, A.M.; Grepinet, O.; Namdari, F.; Roche, S.M.; Rossignol, A.; et al. Multiplicity of *Salmonella* entry mechanisms, a new paradigm for *Salmonella* pathogenesis. *Microbiologyopen* **2012**, *1*, 243–258. [CrossRef] [PubMed]
15. Wiedemann, A.; Mijouin, L.; Ayoub, M.A.; Barilleau, E.; Canepa, S.; Teixeira-Gomes, A.P.; Le Vern, Y.; Rosselin, M.; Reiter, E.; Velge, P. Identification of the epidermal growth factor receptor as the receptor for *Salmonella* Rck-dependent invasion. *FASEB J.* **2016**, *30*, 4180–4191. [CrossRef] [PubMed]
16. Heffernan, E.J.; Wu, L.; Louie, J.; Okamoto, S.; Fierer, J.; Guiney, D.G. Specificity of the complement resistance and cell association phenotypes encoded by the outer membrane protein genes rck from *Salmonella typhimurium* and ail from *Yersinia enterocolitica*. *Infect. Immun.* **1994**, *62*, 5183–5186. [CrossRef]
17. Ho, D.K.; Jarva, H.; Meri, S. Human complement factor H binds to outer membrane protein Rck of Salmonella. *J. Immunol.* **2010**, *185*, 1763–1769. [CrossRef]
18. Glaubman, J.; Hofmann, J.; Bonney, M.E.; Park, S.; Thomas, J.M.; Kokona, B.; Ramos Falcon, L.I.; Chung, Y.K.; Fairman, R.; Okeke, I.N. Self-association motifs in the enteroaggregative Escherichia coli heat-resistant agglutinin 1. *Microbiology* **2016**, *162*, 1091–1102. [CrossRef]
19. Bhargava, S.; Johnson, B.B.; Hwang, J.; Harris, T.A.; George, A.S.; Muir, A.; Dorff, J.; Okeke, I.N. Heat-resistant agglutinin 1 is an accessory enteroaggregative *Escherichia coli* colonization factor. *J. Bacteriol.* **2009**, *191*, 4934–4942. [CrossRef]
20. Fleckenstein, J.M.; Kopecko, D.J.; Warren, R.L.; Elsinghorst, E.A. Molecular characterization of the tia invasion locus from enterotoxigenic Escherichia coli. *Infect. Immun.* **1996**, *64*, 2256–2265. [CrossRef]
21. Fagan, R.P.; Lambert, M.A.; Smith, S.G. The hek outer membrane protein of Escherichia coli strain RS218 binds to proteoglycan and utilizes a single extracellular loop for adherence, invasion, and autoaggregation. *Infect. Immun.* **2008**, *76*, 1135–1142. [CrossRef]
22. Mancini, J.; Weckselblatt, B.; Chung, Y.K.; Durante, J.C.; Andelman, S.; Glaubman, J.; Dorff, J.D.; Bhargava, S.; Lijek, R.S.; Unger, K.P.; et al. The heat-resistant agglutinin family includes a novel adhesin from enteroaggregative *Escherichia coli* strain 60A. *J. Bacteriol.* **2011**, *193*, 4813–4820. [CrossRef]
23. Ghosh, S.; Chakraborty, K.; Nagaraja, T.; Basak, S.; Koley, H.; Dutta, S.; Mitra, U.; Das, S. An adhesion protein of *Salmonella enterica* serovar Typhi is required for pathogenesis and potential target for vaccine development. *Proc. Natl. Acad. Sci. USA* **2011**, *108*, 3348–3353. [CrossRef] [PubMed]
24. Zhang, X.L.; Tsui, I.S.; Yip, C.M.; Fung, A.W.; Wong, D.K.; Dai, X.; Yang, Y.; Hackett, J.; Morris, C. *Salmonella enterica* serovar typhi uses type IVB pili to enter human intestinal epithelial cells. *Infect. Immun.* **2000**, *68*, 3067–3073. [CrossRef] [PubMed]
25. Yue, M.; Han, X.; Masi, L.D.; Zhu, C.; Ma, X.; Zhang, J.; Wu, R.; Schmieder, R.; Kaushik, R.S.; Fraser, G.P.; et al. Allelic variation contributes to bacterial host specificity. *Nat. Commun.* **2015**, *6*, 8754. [CrossRef] [PubMed]
26. Guo, A.; Cao, S.; Tu, L.; Chen, P.; Zhang, C.; Jia, A.; Yang, W.; Liu, Z.; Chen, H.; Schifferli, D.M. FimH alleles direct preferential binding of *Salmonella* to distinct mammalian cells or to avian cells. *Microbiology* **2009**, *155*, 1623–1633. [CrossRef]
27. Hersh, D.; Monack, D.M.; Smith, M.R.; Ghori, N.; Falkow, S.; Zychlinsky, A. The Salmonella invasin SipB induces macrophage apoptosis by binding to caspase-1. *Proc. Natl. Acad. Sci. USA* **1999**, *96*, 2396–2401. [CrossRef]

28. Hermant, D.; Menard, R.; Arricau, N.; Parsot, C.; Popoff, M.Y. Functional Conservation of the Salmonella and Shigella Effectors of Entry into Epithelial-Cells. *Mol. Microbiol.* **1995**, *17*, 781–789. [CrossRef]
29. Cunrath, O.; Meinel, D.M.; Maturana, P.; Fanous, J.; Buyck, J.M.; Saint Auguste, P.; Seth-Smith, H.M.B.; Korner, J.; Dehio, C.; Trebosc, V.; et al. Quantitative contribution of efflux to multi-drug resistance of clinical Escherichia coli and Pseudomonas aeruginosa strains. *EBio Med.* **2019**, *41*, 479–487. [CrossRef]
30. Gibson, D.G.; Young, L.; Chuang, R.Y.; Venter, J.C.; Hutchison, C.A., 3rd; Smith, H.O. Enzymatic assembly of DNA molecules up to several hundred kilobases. *Nat. Methods* **2009**, *6*, 343–345. [CrossRef]
31. Edwards, R.A.; Keller, L.H.; Schifferli, D.M. Improved allelic exchange vectors and their use to analyze 987P fimbria gene expression. *Gene* **1998**, *207*, 149–157. [CrossRef]
32. Blomfield, I.C.; McClain, M.S.; Eisenstein, B.I. Type 1 fimbriae mutants of *Escherichia coli* K12: Characterization of recognized afimbriate strains and construction of new *fim* deletion mutants. *Mol. Microbiol.* **1991**, *5*, 1439–1445. [CrossRef]
33. Harms, A.; Liesch, M.; Korner, J.; Quebatte, M.; Engel, P.; Dehio, C. A bacterial toxin-antitoxin module is the origin of inter-bacterial and inter-kingdom effectors of Bartonella. *PLoS Genet.* **2017**, *13*, e1007077. [CrossRef] [PubMed]
34. Hoiseth, S.K.; Stocker, B.D. Aromatic-dependent *Salmonella typhimurium* are nonvirulent and effective as live vaccines. *Nature* **1981**, *291*, 238–239. [CrossRef] [PubMed]
35. Cao, J.; Khan, A.S.; Bayer, M.E.; Schifferli, D.M. Ordered translocation of 987P fimbrial subunits through the outer membrane of *Escherichia coli*. *J. Bacteriol.* **1995**, *177*, 3704–3713. [CrossRef] [PubMed]
36. Nair, M.K.; De Masi, L.; Yue, M.; Galvan, E.M.; Chen, H.; Wang, F.; Schifferli, D.M. Adhesive properties of YapV and paralogous autotransporter proteins of *Yersinia pestis*. *Infect. Immun.* **2015**, *83*, 1809–1819. [CrossRef]
37. Schifferli, D.M.; Alrutz, M.A. Permissive linker insertion sites in the outer membrane protein of 987P fimbriae of *Escherichia coli*. *J. Bacteriol.* **1994**, *176*, 1099–1110. [CrossRef]
38. Liu, F.; Chen, H.; Galván, E.M.; Lasaro, M.A.; Schifferli, D.M. Effects of Psa and F1 on the adhesive and invasive interactions of *Yersinia pestis* with human respiratory tract epithelial cells. *Infect. Immun.* **2006**, *74*, 5636–5644. [CrossRef]
39. Yoshida, C.E.; Kruczkiewicz, P.; Laing, C.R.; Lingohr, E.J.; Gannon, V.P.; Nash, J.H.; Taboada, E.N. The *Salmonella* In Silico Typing Resource (SISTR): An Open Web-Accessible Tool for Rapidly Typing and Subtyping Draft *Salmonella* Genome Assemblies. *PLoS ONE* **2016**, *11*, e0147101. [CrossRef]
40. Zhang, C.; Freddolino, P.L.; Zhang, Y. COFACTOR: Improved protein function prediction by combining structure, sequence and protein-protein interaction information. *Nucleic Acids Res.* **2017**, *45*, W291–W299. [CrossRef]
41. Yang, J.; Zhang, Y. I-TASSER server: New development for protein structure and function predictions. *Nucleic Acids Res.* **2015**, *43*, W174–W181. [CrossRef]
42. Colovos, C.; Yeates, T.O. Verification of protein structures: Patterns of nonbonded atomic interactions. *Protein Sci.* **1993**, *2*, 1511–1519. [CrossRef]
43. Goswami, N.; Hussain, M.I.; Borah, P. Molecular dynamics approach to probe the antigenicity of PagN—An outer membrane protein of *Salmonella* Typhi. *J. Biomol. Struct. Dyn.* **2018**, *36*, 2131–2146. [CrossRef] [PubMed]
44. Yue, M.; Rankin, S.C.; Blanchet, R.T.; Nulton, J.D.; Edwards, R.A.; Schifferli, D.M. Diversification of the *Salmonella* fimbriae: A model of macro- and microevolution. *PLoS ONE* **2012**, *7*, e38596. [CrossRef] [PubMed]
45. Hansmeier, N.; Miskiewicz, K.; Elpers, L.; Liss, V.; Hensel, M.; Sterzenbach, T. Functional expression of the entire adhesiome of Salmonella enterica serotype Typhimurium. *Sci. Rep.* **2017**, *7*, 10326. [CrossRef] [PubMed]
46. Su, Y.C.; Halang, P.; Fleury, C.; Jalalvand, F.; Morgelin, M.; Riesbeck, K. Haemophilus Protein F Orthologs of Pathogens Infecting the Airways: Exploiting Host Laminin at Heparin-Binding Sites for Maximal Adherence to Epithelial Cells. *J. Infect. Dis.* **2017**, *216*, 1303–1307. [CrossRef]
47. Izquierdo, M.; Navarro-Garcia, F.; Nava-Acosta, R.; Nataro, J.P.; Ruiz-Perez, F.; Farfan, M.J. Identification of cell surface-exposed proteins involved in the fimbria-mediated adherence of enteroaggregative Escherichia coli to intestinal cells. *Infect. Immun.* **2014**, *82*, 1719–1724. [CrossRef]

48. Samadder, P.; Xicohtencatl-Cortes, J.; Saldana, Z.; Jordan, D.; Tarr, P.I.; Kaper, J.B.; Giron, J.A. The Escherichia coli ycbQRST operon encodes fimbriae with laminin-binding and epithelial cell adherence properties in Shiga-toxigenic E. coli O157:H7. *Environ. Microbiol.* **2009**, *11*, 1815–1826. [CrossRef]
49. Gunn, J.S.; Belden, W.J.; Miller, S.I. Identification of PhoP-PhoQ activated genes within a duplicated region of the Salmonella typhimurium chromosome. *Microb. Pathog.* **1998**, *25*, 77–90. [CrossRef]
50. Park, S.Y.; Groisman, E.A. Signal-specific temporal response by the *Salmonella* PhoP/PhoQ regulatory system. *Mol. Microbiol.* **2014**, *91*, 135–144. [CrossRef]
51. Golubeva, Y.A.; Ellermeier, J.R.; Cott Chubiz, J.E.; Slauch, J.M. Intestinal Long-Chain Fatty Acids Act as a Direct Signal To Modulate Expression of the *Salmonella* Pathogenicity Island 1 Type III Secretion System. *mBio* **2016**, *7*, e02170-15. [CrossRef]
52. Kouzi-Koliakos, K.; Koliakos, G.G.; Tsilibary, E.C.; Furcht, L.T.; Charonis, A.S. Mapping of three major heparin-binding sites on laminin and identification of a novel heparin-binding site on the B1 chain. *J. Biol. Chem.* **1989**, *264*, 17971–17978.
53. Lambert, M.A.; Smith, S.G. The PagN protein mediates invasion via interaction with proteoglycan. *FEMS Microbiol. Lett.* **2009**, *297*, 209–216. [CrossRef] [PubMed]
54. De Masi, L.; Yue, M.; Hu, C.; Rakov, A.V.; Rankin, S.C.; Schifferli, D.M. Cooperation of Adhesin Alleles in *Salmonella*-Host Tropism. *mSphere* **2017**, *2*. [CrossRef] [PubMed]
55. Hayden, H.S.; Matamouros, S.; Hager, K.R.; Brittnacher, M.J.; Rohmer, L.; Radey, M.C.; Weiss, E.J.; Kim, K.B.; Jacobs, M.A.; Sims-Day, E.H.; et al. Genomic Analysis of *Salmonella enterica* Serovar Typhimurium Characterizes Strain Diversity for Recent U.S. Salmonellosis Cases and Identifies Mutations Linked to Loss of Fitness under Nitrosative and Oxidative Stress. *MBio* **2016**, *7*, e00154. [CrossRef] [PubMed]

7

Salmonella Extracellular Polymeric Substances Modulate Innate Phagocyte Activity and Enhance Tolerance of Biofilm-Associated Bacteria to Oxidative Stress

Mark M. Hahn [1,2] and John S. Gunn [1,2,3,*]

1 Center for Microbial Pathogenesis, Abigail Wexner Research Institute at Nationwide Children's Hospital, Columbus, OH 43205, USA; mark.hahn@nationwidechildrens.org
2 Infectious Diseases Institute, The Ohio State University, Columbus, OH 43210, USA
3 Department of Pediatrics, College of Medicine, The Ohio State University, Columbus, OH 43210, USA
* Correspondence: John.Gunn@nationwidechildrens.org

Abstract: *Salmonella enterica* serovar Typhi causes 14.3 million acute cases of typhoid fever that are responsible for 136,000 deaths each year. Chronic infections occur in 3%–5% of those infected and *S.* Typhi persists primarily in the gallbladder by forming biofilms on cholesterol gallstones, but how these bacterial communities evade host immunity is not known. *Salmonella* biofilms produce several extracellular polymeric substances (EPSs) during chronic infection, which are hypothesized to prevent pathogen clearance either by protecting biofilm-associated bacteria from direct humoral attack or by modulating innate phagocyte interaction with biofilms. Using wild-type and EPS-deficient planktonic and biofilm *Salmonella*, the direct attack hypothesis was tested by challenging biofilms with human serum and antimicrobial peptides. Biofilms were found to be tolerant to these molecules, but these phenotypes were independent of the tested EPSs. By examining macrophage and neutrophil responses, new roles for biofilm-associated capsular polysaccharides and slime polysaccharides were identified. The *S.* Typhi Vi antigen was found to modulate innate immunity by reducing macrophage nitric oxide production and neutrophil reactive oxygen species (ROS) production. The slime polysaccharides colanic acid and cellulose were found to be immune-stimulating and represent a key difference between non-typhoidal serovars and typhoidal serovars, which do not express colanic acid. Furthermore, biofilm tolerance to the exogenously-supplied ROS intermediates hydrogen peroxide (H_2O_2) and hypochlorite (ClO^-) indicated an additional role of the capsular polysaccharides for both serovars in recalcitrance to H_2O_2 but not ClO^-, providing new understanding of the stalemate that arises during chronic infections and offering new directions for mechanistic and clinical studies.

Keywords: *Salmonella*; biofilm; innate immunity; extracellular polymeric substances

---

1. Introduction

Salmonella enterica subspecies *enterica* serovar Typhi (*S.* Typhi) is a chronic pathogen of the gallbladder, where it forms biofilms anchored to cholesterol gallstones and encased in self-produced extracellular polymeric substances (EPSs) [1–5]. The conditions and location of these recalcitrant infections is both perplexing and problematic. Bile is rich in bile acids and bile salts with extensive immune-stimulating, antimicrobial, and detergent-like properties that can disrupt bacterial membranes, halt proton gradients, and induce redox stress [6,7]. How and why *S.* Typhi establishes chronic infections in such a repressive environment is not well understood [7]. Furthermore, bile is an important environmental signal that causes opposite effects between non-typhoidal and typhoidal *Salmonella*, the most prominent being those involved in host cell invasion [6–9]. The chronic biofilm lifecycle of *S.* Typhi is also problematic as it presents unique challenges for diagnosing infections [10–13], providing efficacious treatment [5,14], and the eradication of endemic disease [15–17]. However, these issues must be addressed because chronic carriers are the only known reservoir of *S.* Typhi and eradication of these infections will be an essential step in preventing the 136,000 deaths caused by 14.3 million cases of acute typhoid fever each year [15].

S. Typhi is a human-restricted pathogen. An important aspect that sets *S.* Typhi apart from *Salmonella enterica* subspecies *enterica* serovar Typhimurium (*S.* Typhimurium) and other non-typhoidal serovars is rampant genomic decay with pseudogenes representing roughly 5% of its genome, as well as specific gene acquisitions [18–20]. These adaptions resulted in host specialization and the ability to cause systemic disease, which begins primarily by the infection of M cells in the distal ileum. Subsequent invasion and persistence inside macrophages of Peyer's Patches allows *S.* Typhi to disseminate to deep tissues, such as the liver [21,22]. From the liver, *S.* Typhi descends the hepatobiliary duct to the gallbladder and establishes acute or chronic infection [1,4]. Throughout this process, planktonic *S.* Typhi exhibit anti-inflammatory properties to avoid immune detection [23–30]. However, the intracellular lifecycle is a major factor in immune evasion, and biofilms—existing extracellularly—must have additional mechanisms to elicit immune modulation.

Many chronic pathogens are known to inhibit immune cell functions with a well-established link between biofilms and cellular suppression [31–35]. Specific EPSs are often attributed to these abilities, as EPSs have been found to be fundamental to recalcitrance to host immunity and pharmaceutical approaches. One of the most prominent examples of this phenomenon comes from *Pseudomonas aeruginosa* biofilms, which commonly infect cystic fibrosis and burn wound patients. Alginate, the major exopolysaccharide of *P. aeruginosa* biofilms, scavenges hypochlorite and inhibits innate immunity at multiple processes, including complement activation, polymorphonuclear chemotaxis, and phagocytosis by neutrophils and macrophages [36]. *Salmonella* biofilms produce various EPSs in vitro, and biofilm formation during chronic infection has been directly observed in vivo [3,4]. The asymptomatic nature of chronic biofilm infections suggests that *S.* Typhi EPSs have a role in altering innate immune activities to avoid detection. Therefore, we hypothesized that one or more of the EPSs are crucial for biofilm tolerance and contribute to the chronic pathogenicity of *S.* Typhi biofilms by skewing innate immune function(s). Broadly, this prediction presented two functional categories: (a) EPSs that protect biofilm-associated bacteria from innate immune functions that are otherwise inhibitory to planktonic *Salmonella* or (b) EPSs that have immune-modulating function(s) and thus alter the host response to biofilms. We have previously defined the major EPSs of *Salmonella* biofilms (curli fimbriae, colanic acid, cellulose, extracellular DNA, O antigen capsule, and Vi antigen) and characterized the role of each component for biofilm development in vitro [37]. Although these EPSs (particularly curli fimbriae) account for 90% of the biofilm biomass [38], the contribution of each EPS to resisting innate immune functions has not been thoroughly studied.

To test our hypothesis, we compared the outcomes of planktonic and biofilm-associated *Salmonella* when challenged with soluble innate immune molecules (normal human serum and antimicrobial peptides [AMPs]) and tested neutrophils and macrophages for functional responses to planktonic and biofilm *Salmonella*. Furthermore, by comparing wild-type (WT) and EPS-deficient biofilms, we present new evidence that *Salmonella* biofilm tolerance to the host oxidative burst is dependent on the Vi antigen, the O antigen capsule, and colanic acid.

2. Materials and Methods

2.1. Bacterial Strains and Growth Conditions

The *Salmonella* strains used in this study were the parental WT strains or derivatives of *S.* Typhimurium ATCC 14028 (JSG210) and *S.* Typhi Ty2 (JSG698, JSG4383) (Table 1). The latter WT *S.* Typhi was substituted when appropriate to correct for a known *rpoS* mutation in this strain [39]. At times, clinical isolates were also tested (Table 2). All clinical *S.* Typhi isolates tested positive for Vi antigen by serum agglutination tests. The O antigen capsule mutant does not alter the LPS structure. All planktonic and biofilm cultures were grown in tryptic soy broth (TSB). Planktonic cells were collected from 16-hour overnight broth cultures. Biofilms were cultured in 96-well polypropylene microtiter plates coated with 500 μg of cholesterol. To initiate biofilm growth, overnight planktonic bacteria were normalized to OD_{490} = 0.65 in TSB and then diluted 1:6 in TSB and incubated at 37 °C for 3 hours in a static 12-well polypropylene plate. After 3 hours, static cultures were diluted 1:2500 in TSB and distributed (200 μL/well) to the aforementioned cholesterol-coated wells and transferred to 30 °C. Biofilms were cultured on a nutator at 30 °C for 96 hours. Supernatants were replaced with fresh TSB once every 24 hours. Prior to experimental use, mature biofilms were washed with phosphate-buffered saline (PBS) to remove unattached and planktonic bacteria.

Table 1. Strains used in this study. EPS: extracellular polymeric substances.

Strain	Genotype	EPS Deficiency	Reference Source
JSG210	WT *S.* Typhimurium	-	ATCC14028
JSG3736	Δ*csgA*	Curli fimbriae	[37]
JSG3742	Δ*wcaM*	Colanic acid	[37]
JSG3672	Δ*yihO*	O antigen capsule	[37]
JSG3838	Δ*bcsE*	Cellulose	[37]
JSG3790	Δ*csgA*Δ*wcaM*	Curli fimbriae, Colanic acid	[37]
JSG3829	Δ*csgA*Δ*wcaM*Δ*yihO*	Curli fimbriae, Colanic acid, O antigen capsule	[37]
JSG3841	Δ*csgA*Δ*wcaM*Δ*yihO*Δ*bcsE*	Curli fimbriae, Colanic acid, O antigen capsule, Cellulose	[37]
JSG3738	*S.* Typhimurium + pTH170 (*viaB*)	Vi antigen$^+$ (ViAg$^+$)	[24]
JSG698	WT *S.* Typhi	-	Ty2
JSG4383	WT *S.* Typhi *rpoS*$^+$	-	[40]
JSG1213	*S.* Typhi Δ*tviB*	Vi antigen	[41]
JSG4123	*S.* Typhi Ch-1 Δ*tviB*	Vi antigen	This study

Table 2. Clinical isolates used in this study.

Strain	Designation	Geographic Source	Isolation Site
JSG3074	Ch-1	Mexico City	Gallstone
JSG3076	Ch-2	Mexico City	Gallbladder tissue
JSG3979	Ch-3	Vietnam	Gallbladder
JSG3980	Ch-4	Vietnam	Gallbladder
JSG3981	Ch-5	Vietnam	Gallbladder
JSG3982	Ch-6	Vietnam	Gallbladder
JSG3983	Ch-7	Vietnam	Gallbladder
JSG3984	Ch-8	Vietnam	Gallbladder
JSG3985	Ac-1	Vietnam	Unspecified
JSG3986	Ac-2	Vietnam	Unspecified
JSG3987	Ac-3	Vietnam	Unspecified
JSG3988	Ac-4	Vietnam	Unspecified
JSG3989	Ac-5	Vietnam	Unspecified
JSG3990	Ac-6	Vietnam	Unspecified
JSG3395	Ac-7	Ohio Department of Health	Blood
JSG3400	Ac-8	Ohio Department of Health	Bile

2.2. Mutant Generation

The Vi antigen was eliminated from a *S.* Typhi clinical isolate (JSG3074) by λ-Red mutagenesis [42]. The primer designs are detailed in Table 3. The marked Δ*tviB* gene deletion was transformed into *S.* Typhi JSG3074 carrying the λ-Red recombinase (creating strain JSG4097), and the antibiotic resistance marker was subsequently removed using pCP20 [43]. The final mutant (JSG4123) was verified by PCR and analysis by gel electrophoresis.

Table 3. Oligonucleotide primers used in this study.

Primer	Sequence	Purpose
JG2934	5′—ATAAAATTTTAGTAAAGGATTAATAAGAGT GTTCGGTATAGTGTAGGCTGGAGCTGCTTC—3′	Forward *tviB*
JG2935	5′—GTCCGTAGTTCTTCGTAAGCCGTCATGATT ACAATCTCACCATATGAATATCCTCCTTAG—3′	Reverse *tviB*
JG2936	5′—TCAGCGACTTCTGTTCTATTCAAGTAAGAAAGGGGTACGG—3′	Forward verification *tviB*
JG2937	5′—GCTCCTCACTGACGGACGTGCGAACGTCGTCTAGATTATG—3′	Reverse verification *tviB*

2.3. Sensitivity and Tolerance to Human Serum

Sensitivity to normal human serum was determined using WT planktonic *Salmonella* spp. Overnight broth cultures were normalized to 1.0×10^7 colony forming units per milliliter (CFUs/mL) in 30% Human AB serum pooled from healthy male donors (Mediatech Inc.; Manassas, VA, USA). Heat-inactivated serum (56 °C for 30 minutes) was included as the negative control. Cultures were incubated at 37 °C for 3 hours on a nutator and then quantified by dilution platting and colony forming unit (CFU) enumeration.

After washing 2× with PBS, biofilms were challenged with 30% normal human serum or heat-inactivated serum. Serum-exposed biofilms were incubated at 37 °C for 3 hours on a nutator and then washed with PBS to remove residual serum. Viable bacteria remaining in the biofilm were enumerated by serial dilution platting.

2.4. Sensitivity and Tolerance to Antimicrobial Peptides

WT planktonic *Salmonella* spp. normalized to approximately 2.0×10^6 CFUs/mL in TSB were used to determine the minimum inhibitory concentration (MIC) of the AMPs polymyxin B sulfate (Gibco; Billings, MT, USA) and melittin (Sigma-Aldrich; St. Louis, MO, USA). Concentrations were assayed in two-fold serial dilution series, and growth at 37 °C was monitored by OD_{600} on a SpectraMax M3 plate reader. The MICs for each AMP were determined by the lowest concentration tested that prevented detectable growth. Mature biofilms were washed and exposed to each AMP at concentrations 10× that of the WT planktonic MIC. Biofilms were incubated with each AMP at 37 °C for 2 hours on a nutator before PBS washing to remove trace peptides and enumeration by mechanical collection and serial dilution platting.

2.5. Biofilm Aggregate Collection

Mature biofilms aggregates were used for all host–response experiments and subsequent pathway analysis investigation. Aggregates were mechanically collected by scraping microtiter plate biofilms and normalized by total protein quantification (Bradford method). The reported multiplicity of infection (MOI) values refer to the biofilm aggregate protein equivalent (MOI_{eq}) to that of planktonic bacteria at the reported MOI. Normalized aggregates were analyzed for size and granularity characteristics by flow cytometry (assay optimization only) using a BD FACSCanto II flow cytometer (BD Biosciences; San Jose, CA, USA).

2.6. Macrophage Nitric Oxide Response to Salmonella

The THP-1 cell line was maintained in Roswell Park Memorial Institute (RPMI) media supplemented with 10% fetal bovine serum (FBS) and 2 mM of L-glutamine. Prior to infection, THP-1 cells were washed and normalized in equivalent media lacking phenol red. Then, the cell line was infected with planktonic or biofilm samples ($MOI_{eq} = 100$, 4.0×10^5 THP-1 cells total), and infections were synchronized by centrifugation. Cultures were incubated for 3 hours at 37 °C, 5% CO_2. Supernatant nitric oxide (NO) was measured each hour by the Griess diazotization reaction, and viable extracellular CFUs remaining in the supernatant were quantified by serial dilution platting.

2.7. *Neutrophil Reactive Oxygen Species Response to Salmonella*

PLB-985 cells [44,45] were differentiated to a neutrophil-like phenotype [46,47] by 6-day incubation in Advanced RPMI supplemented with 0.5% N, N-Dimethylformamide, 0.5% FBS, 1% Nutridoma-SP (Roche; Mannheim, Germany), 2 mM L-glutamine, and 1× penicillin/streptomycin. Media was replaced on day 3. Differentiated PLB-985 cells were infected with planktonic or biofilm samples ($MOI_{eq} = 50$, 6.0×10^6 PLB-985 cells total) that had been opsonized in 20% normal human serum for 20 minutes prior to infection. Uninfected PLB-985 cells were stimulated with phorbol 12-myristate 13-acetate (PMA) (final concentration of 1.0×10^{-4} mg/mL). All samples were supplied with luminol (final concentration of 500 μM); then, infections were synchronized by centrifugation. Reactive oxygen species (ROS) production at 37 °C was monitored in triplicate by luminol-dependent chemiluminescence measured every 2 minutes for 1 hour using a SpectraMax M3 plate reader. Area under the curve (AUC) was calculated for each condition and normalized to the AUC calculated for PMA-stimulated PLB-985 cells. Parallel infections were conducted to determine total CFUs remaining at 80 minutes post-infection. Gentamicin was not added to the media, and the PLB-985 cells were lysed by 0.1% sodium dodecyl sulfate treatment prior to serial dilution platting; thus, the reported CFUs represent total bacteria remaining from input after 80 minutes.

2.8. *Sensitivity and Tolerance to Oxidative Species*

Overnight cultures were normalized to approximately 2.0×10^6 CFUs/mL in TSB and incubated at 37 °C on a rolling drum. Planktonic sensitivity to hydrogen peroxide (H_2O_2) and hypochlorite (ClO^-) was initially assayed using WT *S.* Typhimurium or *S.* Typhi exposed to 0 mM, 5 mM, or 10 mM H_2O_2 or 0 μg/mL, 250 μg/mL, or 1000 μg/mL ClO^-. Viable cells remaining after 30- and 60-minute exposure were enumerated by dilution platting.

The MIC of each oxidative species against planktonic *Salmonella* was determined by 16-hour growth curves (OD_{600}). Starting cultures contained approximately 2.0×10^6 CFUs/mL in TSB with H_2O_2 or ClO^- supplied at final concentrations ranging from 10 mM to 0.3125 mM or 1000 μg/mL to 15 μg/mL (respectively) in two-fold serial dilutions. Microtiter plates were incubated at 37 °C for 16 hours and growth was monitored by OD_{600}. Readings were recorded every 30 minutes using a SpectraMax M3 plate reader. The MICs for each oxidative species were determined by the lowest concentration that prevented detectable growth.

Biofilm aggregates were challenged with H_2O_2 or ClO^- supplied at 1×, 10×, 25×, of 50× the experimentally-determined planktonic cell MIC and incubated at 37 °C for 2 hours on an orbital shaker. Viable biofilm aggregates were disrupted and enumerated before and after exposure by serial dilution platting.

3. Results

3.1. *Biofilm Tolerance to Innate Immunity*

3.1.1. Each of the Four Major *Salmonella* Biofilm EPSs Contribute to Tolerance to Innate Immunity

Cytolytic activity of the complement system membrane attack complex and of AMPs is dependent on direct cell contact. Therefore, these soluble innate immune factors readily target planktonic bacterial surfaces (Figure 1A, Figure 2A) but could be functionally inhibited by EPSs. To address the hypothesis that EPSs are responsible for biofilm tolerance to soluble innate immune factors that successfully target planktonic bacteria, WT and EPS-deficient *S.* Typhimurium (Δ*csgA*Δ*wcaM*Δ*yihO*Δ*bcsE*) and *S.* Typhi biofilms were challenged with normal human serum and AMPs with the expectation that viable CFUs in EPS-deficient biofilms would be reduced compared to WT biofilms.

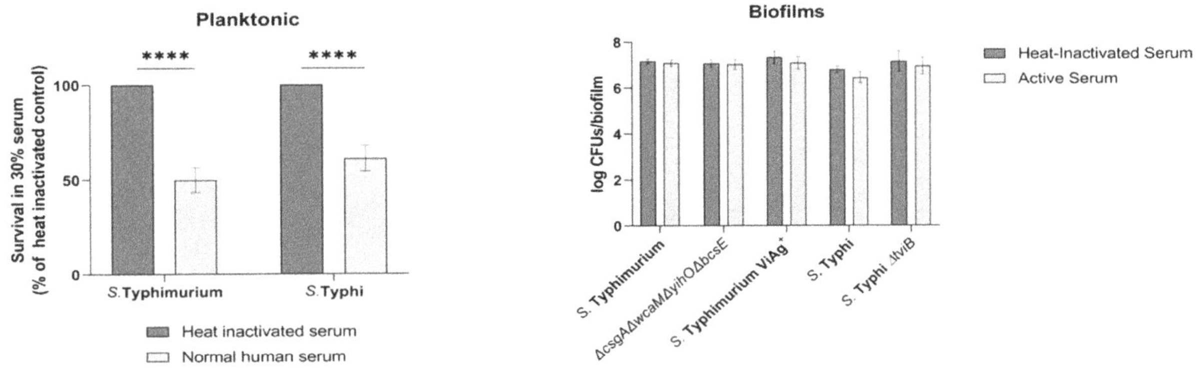

(**A**) (**B**)

Figure 1. Sensitivity and tolerance to human serum. JSG698 was used for wild-type (WT) *S.* Typhi. (**A**) Growth from input of WT planktonic *Salmonella* following challenge with 30% normal human serum or heat-inactivated serum determined by colony forming unit (CFU) enumeration (data are normalized to heat-inactivated control) ($n = 5$). Significance between conditions was identified by multiple t tests using the Holm–Sidak method ($\alpha = 0.05$) to correct for multiple comparisons (****, $p < 0.000001$). (**B**) CFU enumeration of biofilms following the same conditions as planktonic bacteria. Significance difference were tested for using two-way analysis of variance (ANOVA) and the Sidak method to correct for multiple comparisons ($n = 4$, daily experiments conducted in quintuplicate). Error bars indicate standard deviation (SD).

WT planktonic *Salmonella* were significantly inhibited by 30% serum, with *S.* Typhimurium 50% inhibited and *S.* Typhi inhibited by 39% (Figure 1A). The same concentration of serum was unable to significantly reduce the viability of WT *Salmonella* biofilm-associated bacteria after 3 hours, even when the four major EPSs (*S.* Typhimurium) or the Vi antigen (*S.* Typhi) had been genetically eliminated (Figure 1B). Further analysis of individual EPS mutants was not conducted because their combined elimination did not produce an altered phenotype. The addition of Vi antigen to *S.* Typhimurium also did not significantly affect serum resistance (Figure 1B). These data suggest that *S.* Typhimurium maintains intrinsic tolerance to complement due to the biofilm lifestyle by unidentified EPSs or other multicellular behaviors.

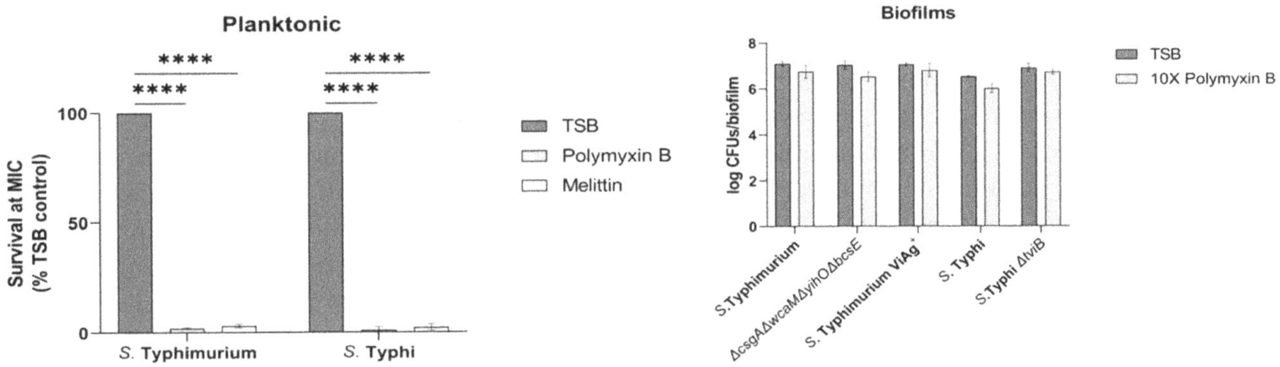

(**A**) (**B**)

Figure 2. *Cont.*

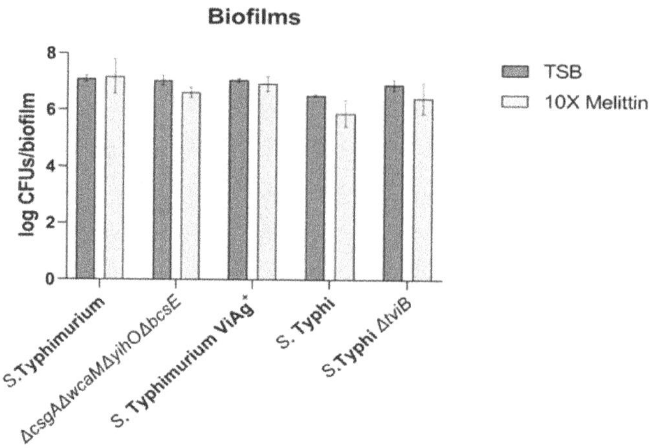

(C)

Figure 2. Sensitivity and tolerance to antimicrobial peptides (AMPs). JSG698 used for WT *S.* Typhi. (**A**) Growth from input of WT planktonic *Salmonella* after 2-hour exposure to each AMP at the minimum inhibitory concentration (MIC) determined by CFU enumeration (data are normalized to AMP-free control) ($n = 3$). *S.* Typhimurium challenged with 0.49 μg/mL polymyxin B and 10 μg/mL melittin. *S.* Typhi challenged with 0.24 μg/mL polymyxin B and 10 μg/mL melittin. Significance calculated by two-way ANOVA with Dunnett's multiple comparison test (***, $p < 0.0005$; ****, $p < 0.0001$). (**B**,**C**) Biofilm tolerance to AMPs supplied at 10× the WT planktonic MIC. Significance was tested for by two-way ANOVA with a Sidak multiple comparison correction ($n = 3$, daily experiments conducted in triplicate). Error bars indicate SD.

To test the activity of AMPs, the WT planktonic MIC was experimentally determined by assaying for growth inhibition. For *S.* Typhimurium, the MIC for polymyxin B and melittin was 0.49 μg/ml and 10 μg/ml (respectively). *S.* Typhi had the same melittin MIC but was twice as susceptible to polymyxin B with an MIC of 0.24 μg/ml (Figure 2A). Similar to the serum sensitivity results, the viability of biofilm-associated bacteria was not reduced by challenge with polymyxin B or melittin supplied at 10× the WT planktonic MIC (Figure 2B,C). This result was consistent for WTs from both serovar and for each of the EPS mutants (*S.* Typhimurium *ΔcsgAΔwcaMΔyihOΔbcsE*, *S.* Typhimurium Vi antigen^{+}, and *S.* Typhi *ΔtviB*), so further analysis of individual EPS mutants was not conducted. Once again, these data indicate that there may be additional EPSs or biofilm behaviors responsible tolerance to soluble immune components.

3.1.2. Laboratory *S.* Typhi is Representative of Clinical Isolates from Both Acute and Chronic Patients

The majority of EPS mutants were generated and tested in the *S.* Typhimurium serovar because *S.* Typhimurium generates a chronic typhoid-like disease in mice similar to *S.* Typhi in humans and allows for in vivo modeling of a human-restricted pathogen. Since biofilm tolerance data (Figures 1 and 2) indicate that tolerance mechanisms exist beyond the EPS components that were tested, a panel of *S.* Typhi clinical isolates acquired from acute and chronic patients were surveyed to know if the laboratory strain of *S.* Typhi under scrutiny is representative of acute versus chronic patient isolates. When cultured under biofilm-inducing conditions and challenged with 10× polymyxin B, biofilm-associated CFUs were not significantly reduced for any of the 8 acute or 8 chronic isolates (supplemental data; Figure S1A). Similar results were obtained by challenge with 10× melittin, although one acute isolate (Ch-1) did exhibit reduced biofilm-associated CFUs (supplemental data; Figure S1B). Interestingly, when the Vi antigen was eliminated from this isolate, no inhibition from polymyxin B or melittin was observed (supplemental data; Figure S1A,B). Additionally, no major distinctions were evident between the acute patient isolates, the chronic patient isolates, and the laboratory *S.* Typhi WT.

3.2. The Innate Immune Response to Salmonella Biofilms

After determining that the four major *Salmonella* EPSs do not play a role in resisting attack by the tested innate immune factors, the possibility that biofilms somehow regulate host immunity was investigated. Given the prominent published anti-inflammatory role of the Vi antigen for planktonic cells [48] compared to the relative lack of phenotypes detected for the other major EPSs in vitro, the Vi antigen was predicted to have a significant role in biofilm inhibition of innate phagocytic cell function.

Conducting these experiments required the collection and normalization of biofilm aggregate populations of similar physical characteristics. The system developed to achieve this goal (scraped biofilms from 96-well plates) was validated by flow cytometry quantifying the size and granularity distribution of the normalized aggregates. While the biofilm aggregates were distinct from planktonic controls, among the biofilm aggregates, no major differences were observed between either serovar or EPS mutants in terms of predominant size, distribution of sizes, or granularity (supplemental data; Figure S2). Using aggregate populations of consistent size and granularity limits the possibility that subsequent experimental outcomes are due to differences in physical interactions between the aggregates and host cells.

3.2.1. Vi Antigen Has a Direct Effect on Macrophage Nitric Oxide Production

Dendritic cells and macrophages are responsible for the delivery of *S.* Typhi from the gut to the liver, and tissue-resident macrophages are presumably the first innate immune cell to interact with *S.* Typhi after it arrives at the gallbladder [21,22,49,50]. Due to these extensive and early interactions between *S.* Typhi and macrophages, *S.* Typhi would be predicted to benefit from the ability to inhibit NO production in vivo. Both planktonic and biofilm infections of macrophages induced peak NO production 2 hours post infection. At these early time points, extracellular planktonic bacteria and biofilm aggregates resisted killing by macrophages equally (Figure 3A). While the four major EPSs did not influence NO production, addition of the Vi antigen to *S.* Typhimurium planktonic and biofilm cultures significantly reduced macrophage NO (Figure 3B,C). Interestingly, elimination of the Vi antigen from both planktonic and biofilm *S.* Typhi cultures showed a similar reduction of NO as was observed with *S.* Typhimurium, instead of the expected increase.

3.2.2. Vi Antigen Inhibition of Neutrophil ROS is Dependent on the Growth State

Upon infiltration, neutrophils have the potential to inflict extensive damage through ROS production and other antimicrobial activities. Preventing these functions would enhance biofilm survival in the gallbladder. To determine if EPSs altered neutrophil ROS production, neutrophils were challenged with planktonic bacteria and biofilm aggregates of WT *Salmonella* and EPS-deficient mutants. Similar to the experiments in macrophages, planktonic bacteria and biofilms resisted early killing by neutrophils (Figure 4A,B) with the total CFUs (bacteria inside and outside neutrophils) not different from control conditions, yet the ROS response from neutrophils varied markedly by the microbial growth state (biofilm or planktonic) and EPS mutation (Figure 4C,D). Consistent with studies of planktonic *Salmonella* indicating anti-inflammatory functions of Vi antigen [23,27,29,48,51–53], less ROS was produced in response to planktonic *S.* Typhi (Vi antigen present) compared to planktonic *S.* Typhimurium (Vi antigen absent). However, for biofilm aggregates, ROS levels were similar between neutrophils infected with *S.* Typhi and *S.* Typhimurium. As expected, loss of the Vi antigen in both planktonic and biofilm *S.* Typhi resulted in a ROS increase upon infection, although the increase was much higher in planktonic than biofilm infections (Figure 4C). For *S.* Typhimurium producing the Vi antigen (versus *S.* Typhimurium), a decrease in ROS production was expected, but it was only observed with biofilm aggregates and not planktonic bacteria. Thus in most, but not all conditions, Vi antigen suppressed ROS production.

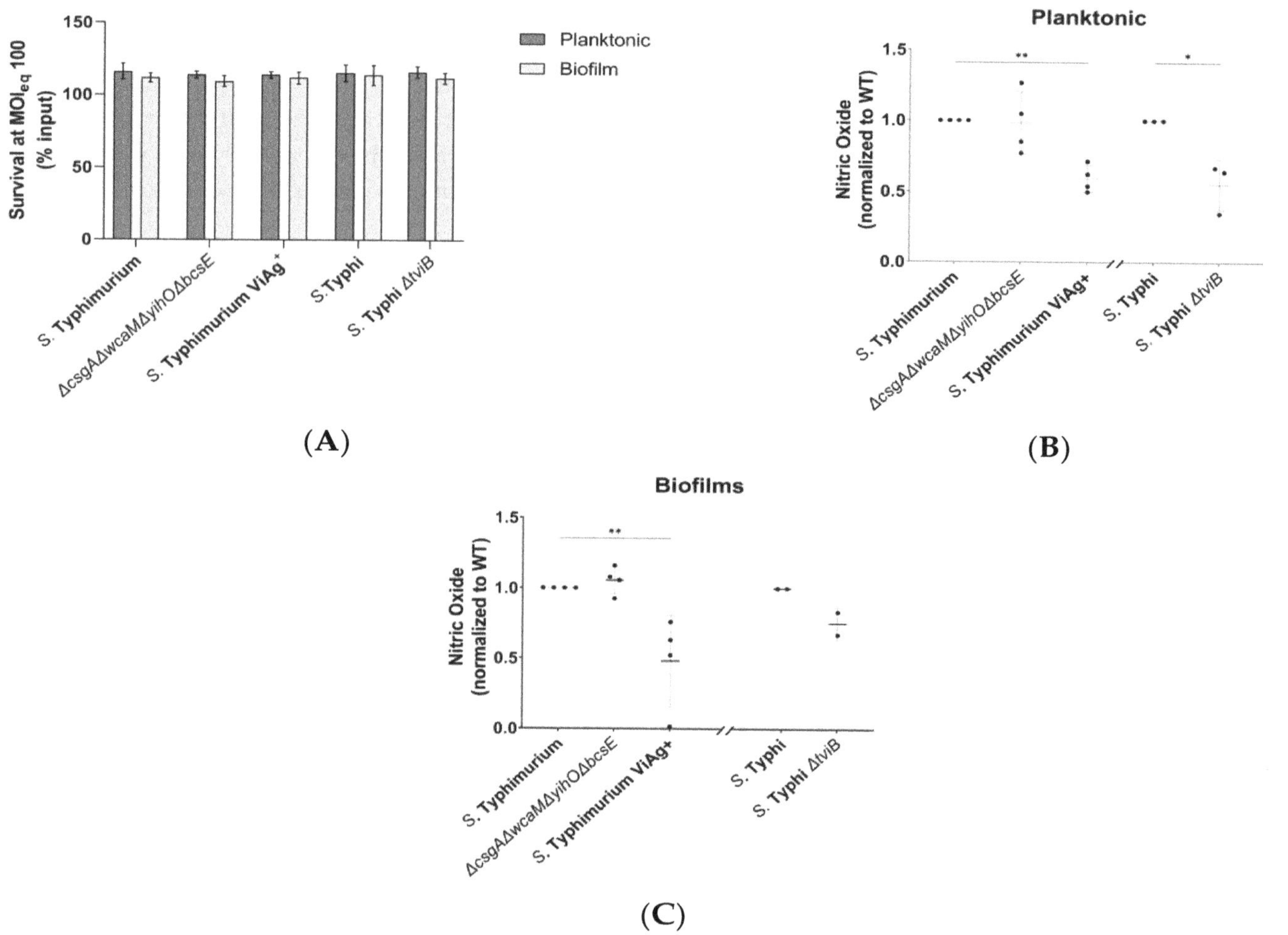

Figure 3. Effect of planktonic and biofilm-associated *Salmonella* on macrophage nitric oxide (NO) production. JSG4383 used for WT *S.* Typhi. (**A**) Planktonic and biofilm aggregate survival determined by CFU enumeration after 2-hour incubation with THP-1 macrophages. Analysis by two-way ANOVA with Sidak correction for multiple comparisons demonstrated no difference in CFU viability between growth states ($n = 4$, daily enumeration conducted in triplicate). (**B**,**C**) NO production by THP-1 macrophages after 2-hour infection with planktonic or biofilm-aggregate *Salmonella*. Significance for *S.* Typhimurium experiments was determined by ordinary one-way ANOVA with Dunnett correction for multiple comparisons (**, $p < 0.005$). *S.* Typhi significant differences were identified by unpaired t test (*, $p < 0.05$) ($n = 4$, daily experiments conducted in duplicate). Error bars indicate SD.

3.2.3. Slime Polysaccharides Have a Role in ROS Stimulation

Surprisingly, a precipitous drop in ROS production was observed with the *S.* Typhimurium *ΔcsgAΔwcaMΔyihOΔbcsE* strain in the biofilm state (Figure 4C). These data indicated a need to investigate individual EPSs that may be responsible for this observation. Loss of curli fimbriae or the O antigen capsule from biofilm aggregates of *S.* Typhimurium eliminated this phenotype and resulted in a ROS response equivalent to infections with their planktonic counterparts (Figure 4D), thus implicating these two EPS components, along with Vi antigen, in the regulation of ROS production in neutrophils.

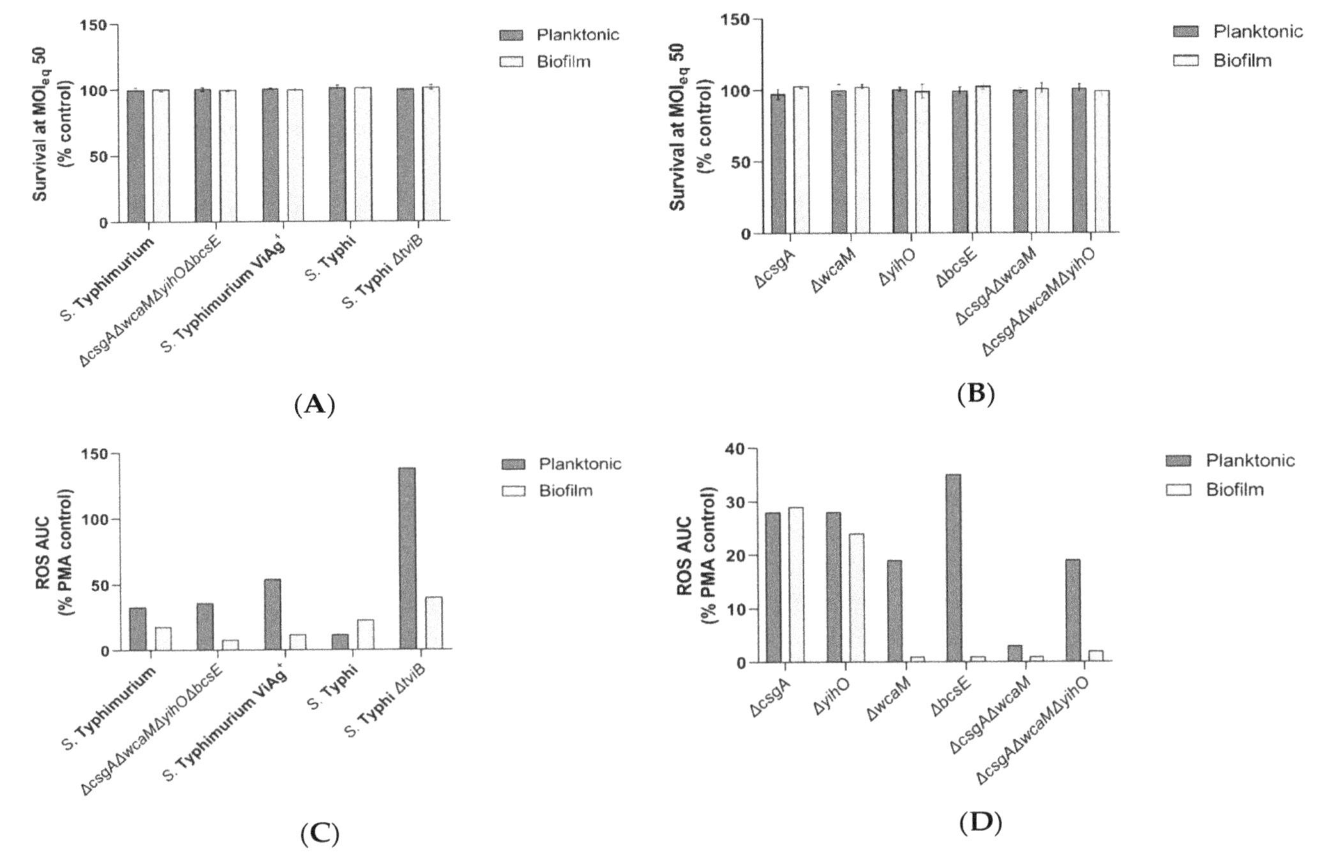

Figure 4. Effect of planktonic and biofilm-associated *Salmonella* on neutrophil ROS production. JSG4383 used for WT *S.* Typhi. (**A**,**B**) CFU enumeration of total (intracellular and extracellular) planktonic and biofilm aggregate survival for each WT and all mutants 80 minutes post-infection. No significant differences in survival were identified by two-way ANOVA with Sidak's method for multiple comparisons ($n = 3$, enumerated in triplicate). Error bars indicate SD. (**C**,**D**) Reactive oxygen species (ROS) production from neutrophils challenged with planktonic or biofilm aggregates of WT and all EPS mutants. Daily experiments were normalized by a phorbol 12-myristate 13-acetate (PMA)-stimulated control and the data shown are representative of three independent experiments, each with similar trends.

3.2.4. Biofilms Are Tolerant to H_2O_2 but Provide no Protection to ClO^-

Having identified the Vi antigen as a crucial regulatory component used by *S.* Typhi during both planktonic and biofilm infections, we investigated if mechanisms other than the reported blocking of complement-fixing antibodies [53] might be in play, hypothesizing that the capsule enhances bacterial detoxification pathways and/or inhibits host toxicity pathways. Briefly, host neutrophils produce superoxide through the NADPH oxidase + cytochrome B complex. Bacterial superoxide dismutase converts superoxide to H_2O_2, which can be further detoxified to water by catalase or converted to ClO^- by myeloperoxidase. ClO^- is a precursor for singlet oxygen, peroxynitrites, and chloramines, all of which are potent antimicrobial compounds. By supplying H_2O_2 or ClO^- independent of host and bacterial functions, the following experiments aimed to identify if one of these divergent pathways in the ROS antimicrobial response was mitigated by *Salmonella*.

Initial concentration ranges of H_2O_2 and ClO^- where *Salmonella* demonstrate stratified sensitivity were determined using planktonic bacteria. A challenge was conducted with 5–10 mM H_2O_2 or 250–1000 µg/mL ClO^- for 60 minutes to determine the best experimental range (supplemental data; Figure S3A,B). Using this data in new experiments, WT planktonic bacteria from both serovars were found to have the same MICs for H_2O_2 and ClO^-: 2.5 mM and 500 µg/mL, respectively (Figure 5A–D). Interestingly, the planktonic MIC to H_2O_2 was reduced in *S.* Typhi Δ*tviB* (1.25 mM) and enhanced for

S. Typhimurium Vi antigen$^+$ (4.25 mM), but it remained unchanged in *S.* Typhimurium lacking other EPSs (supplemental data; Figures S4 and S5), suggesting the involvement of Vi antigen in planktonic tolerance to H_2O_2. The planktonic sensitivity of both serovars to ClO^- was unchanged in EPS mutants versus their parental WT, suggesting the involvement of Vi antigen in planktonic tolerance to H_2O_2.

To determine if EPSs afforded protection to biofilm-resident bacteria, biofilm aggregates were challenged with H_2O_2 or ClO^- at the WT planktonic MIC or at 10×, 25×, or 50× the MIC concentrations of each compound. Surprisingly, biofilms were as sensitive as planktonic cultures to ClO^- as no viable CFUs could be detected beyond challenge at the WT planktonic MIC for either serovar (Figure 5E–I). On the contrary, biofilms of *S.* Typhimurium challenged with H_2O_2 at planktonic-lethal doses demonstrated remarkable tolerance. This tolerance was in part due to EPS, as the *S.* Typhimurium *ΔcsgAΔwcaMΔyihOΔbcsE* EPS mutant was more sensitive to H_2O_2 (Figure 5E–I). Since a H_2O_2 tolerance defect was detected in *S.* Typhimurium *ΔcsgAΔwcaMΔyihOΔbcsE* biofilms (Figure 5G), further analysis of EPS single mutants was conducted (Figure 6) and revealed that the primary EPSs involved in the tolerance phenotype were the O antigen capsule (*ΔyihO*) and colanic acid (*ΔwcaM*). As observed in *S.* Typhimurium, *S.* Typhi biofilms were tolerant to H_2O_2 compared to planktonic, although this serovar was notably less tolerant than *S.* Typhimurium (Figure 5E,F,I). Consistent with planktonic data, *S.* Typhi *ΔtviB* biofilms were less tolerant to H_2O_2 than WT and survived only at the WT planktonic MIC (Figure 5I).

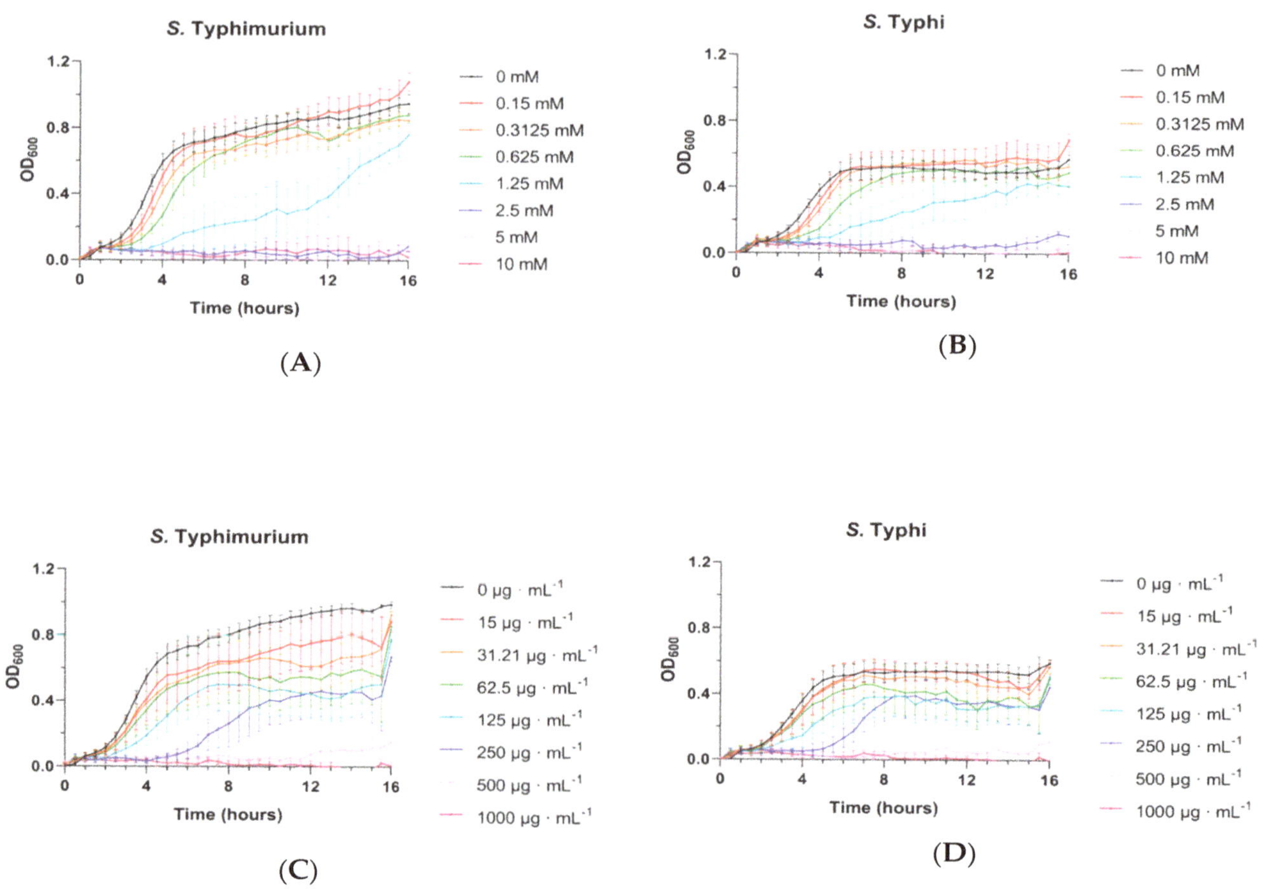

Figure 5. *Cont.*

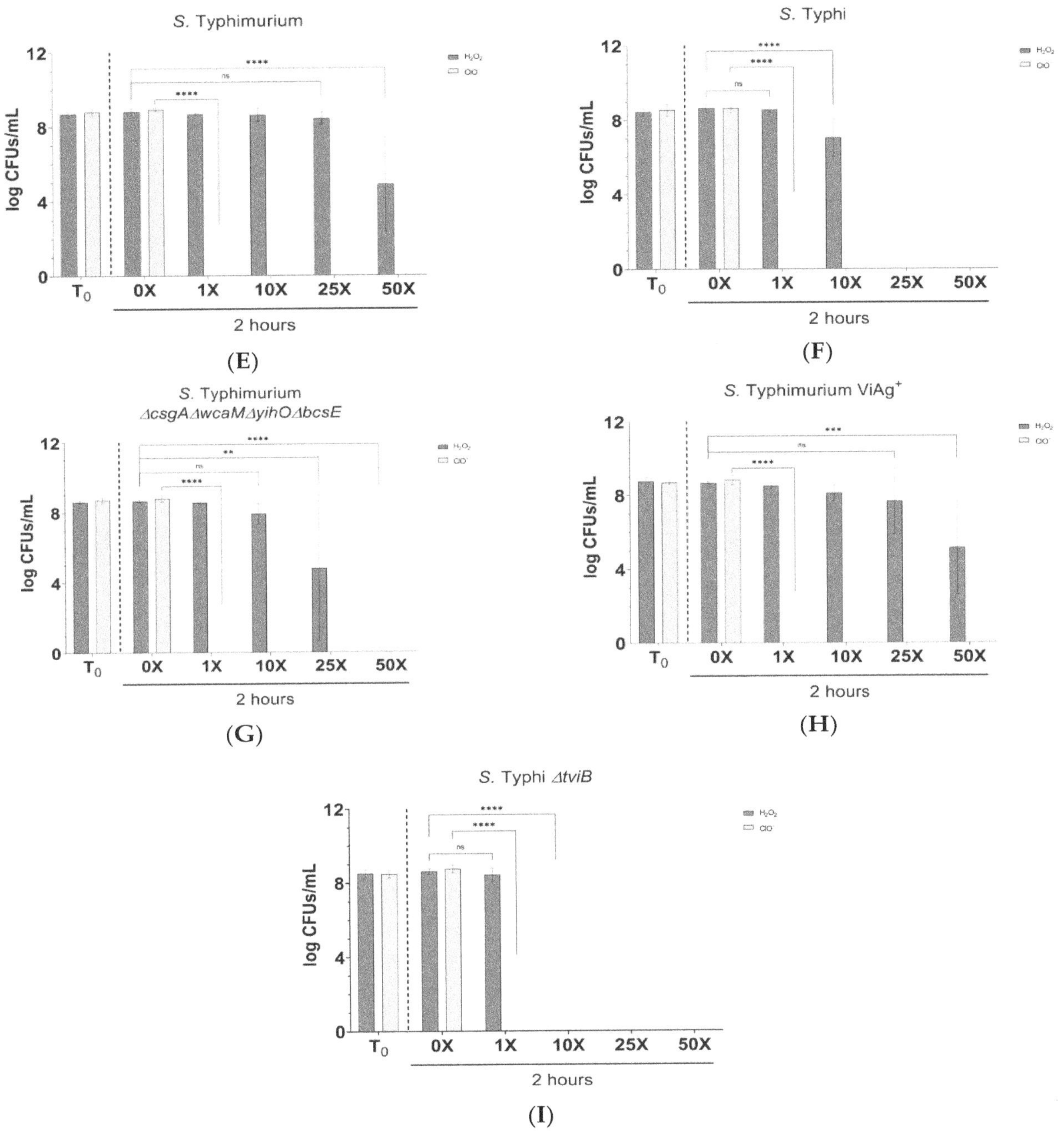

Figure 5. Sensitivity and tolerance to oxidative species. JSG4383 used for WT *S.* Typhi. (**A**,**B**) Growth of WT planktonic *Salmonella* in the presence of H_2O_2 demonstrating a minimum inhibitory concentration (MIC) of 2.5 mM for both serovars. (**C**,**D**) Growth of WT planktonic *Salmonella* in the presence of ClO^- demonstrating a MIC of 500 µg/ml for both serovars. (**E–I**) CFU enumeration of biofilm aggregates challenged with H_2O_2 supplied at 1× (2.5 mM), 10× (25 mM), 25× (62.5 mM), or 50× (125 mM) the WT planktonic MIC or ClO^- supplied at 1× (0.50 mg/mL), 10× (5 mg/mL), 25× (12.5 mg/mL), or 50× (25 mg/mL) the WT planktonic MIC. Significant reductions in tolerance were identified by comparing control (0×) CFUs with the CFUs of each concentration tested by two-way ANOVA with Tukey's multiple correction method (**, $p < 0.01$; ***, $p < 0.0005$; ****, $p < 0.0001$). All experiments were conducted in triplicate and the data are the averages of three independent experiments. Error bars indicate SD.

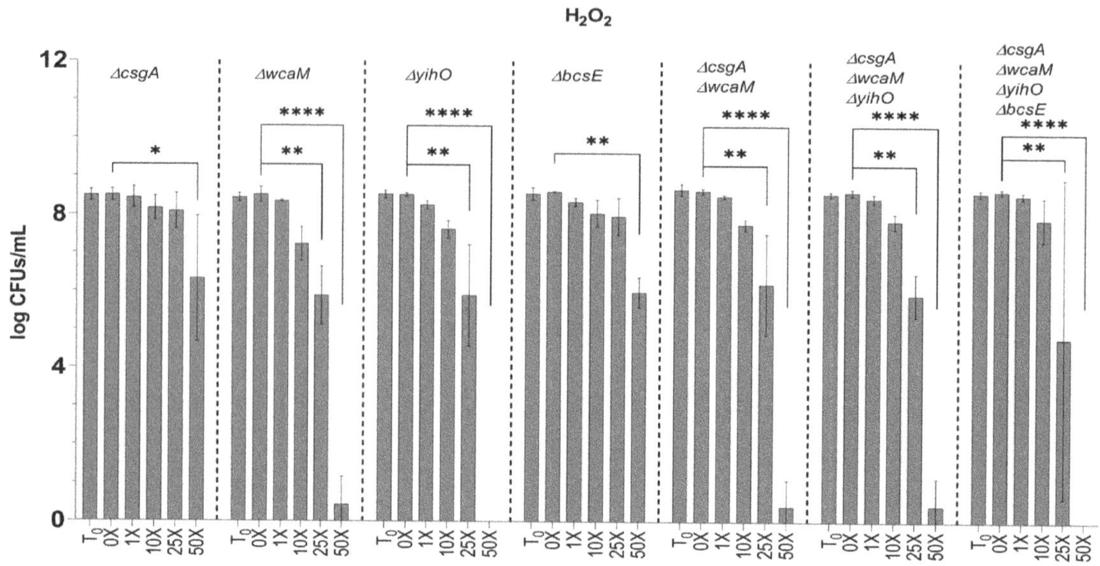

Figure 6. Tolerance of EPS mutants to H_2O_2. Biofilm aggregates deficient in one or more EPS(s) were challenged with H_2O_2 at the same concentrations detailed above. *S.* Typhimurium Δ*csgA*Δ*wcaM*Δ*yihO*Δ*bcsE* data were used from Figure 5 for comparative purposes. Significance between CFUs determined by two-way ANOVA with Tukey multiple correction (*, $p < 0.05$; **, $p < 0.01$; ****, $p < 0.0001$). Error bars indicate SD.

4. Discussion

Our analysis probed for phenotypic differences caused by EPS mutations with two unique perspectives: differences in bacterial survival versus differences in host response. Experiments to determine EPSs that enhance biofilm recalcitrance to selected soluble innate immune factors demonstrated that while the biofilm lifestyle did provide tolerance, an EPS that is solely responsible for inhibiting the bactericidal activities of human serum and AMPs was not identified (Figures 1 and 2). It was hypothesized that EPSs would physically protect biofilm-associated *Salmonella* by preventing diffusion into the biofilm and contact with bacterial membranes, or that they may sequester these molecules through means including electrostatic attraction. However, while EPSs may provide a shield to some innate immune factors, the sensitivity of planktonic cells but robust survival by biofilms deficient for all four major EPSs (*S.* Typhimurium Δ*csgA*Δ*wcaM*Δ*yihO*Δ*bcsE*, Figures 1 and 2) supports the notion that unknown EPSs or other biofilm-induced surface alterations can result in recalcitrance to humoral immunity.

Dendritic cells and macrophages generate NO via the upregulation of inducible nitric oxide synthase (iNOS) [54–56], which is positively stimulated by the pro-inflammatory mediators interleukin-12, interferon-γ, and tumor necrosis factor-α as well as bacterial pathogen-associated molecular patterns [54]. Given the early interaction of dendritic cells and macrophages with planktonic *S.* Typhi and the continued presence of both cell types (planktonic and biofilm) during chronic infection [57], it would be beneficial for the pathogen to limit iNOS activity during the acute and chronic stages of disease. The macrophage NO response to *Salmonella* is independent of curli fimbriae, colanic acid, O antigen capsule, and cellulose (Figure 3B,C). However, we found that the presence of Vi antigen inhibits the NO response to both planktonic and biofilm *Salmonella*, as the addition of Vi antigen to *S.* Typhimurium had an anti-inflammatory effect (Figure 3B,C). Failure by macrophages to exhibit a hyper-inflammatory response to *S.* Typhi Δ*tviB* suggests that *S.* Typhi possesses additional mechanisms for controlling the host response. It is reasonable to expect such a stealthy pathogen to have redundant mechanisms in order to not only control but also fine-tune iNOS activity. The ability to reduce, but not abrogate, iNOS activity would benefit the long-term survival of *S.* Typhi in the gallbladder and fits emerging models for the transition from Th1 to Th2 immunity characteristic of chronic *S.* Typhi infections [57–60]. Although several studies have demonstrated NO to be a potent and early defense mechanism to many intracellular infections [54–56,61–63], the global stationary-phase regulator *rpoS* confers *S.* Typhi with a high degree of resistance [55], and a recent study [64] of persistent *Salmonella* found abundant expression of genes for the sensing and detoxification of reactive nitrogen species (RNS) even when the bacteria were in a dormant state. The *S.* Typhi used in our study is *rpoS*$^+$ and therefore was expected to be resistant to NO. Furthermore, NO is highly diffusible and has immunosuppressive effects on T and B cell activity [54]. It has long been known that iNOS-deficient macrophages are more likely to become apoptotic when infected by *S.* Typhi [55] and that NO has potent anti-apoptotic activity [55,65,66]. By permitting some NO production, *S.* Typhi may limit the production of RNS to a tolerable concentration while preventing an interferon-driven apoptotic response that would lead to Th1 immunity. While some amount of iNOS activity does lead to an initial Th1 response to gallbladder biofilms, control by *S.* Typhi aids in the development of M2 polarization and the transition to Th2 immunity in the gallbladder.

RAW-264 mouse macrophages treated with the iNOS inhibitor N^{ω}-monomethyl L-arginine (L-NMMA) and iNOS$^{-/-}$ mice are still able to resist *S.* Typhi infection [55]. In these cases, the antimicrobial activity is mediated by superoxide activity as ROS production occurs independent of iNOS. We chose to examine neutrophil ROS activity because it has been reported that iNOS enhances neutrophil rolling, adhesion, and migration (diapedesis) [67,68], and we have previously found neutrophils in the gallbladder of chronically-infected mice [57]. Although expression of the Vi antigen from planktonic *S.* Typhi has previously been shown to inhibit neutrophil chemotaxis and ROS production [48], it was unknown if this function also occurs in biofilms. Addition of the Vi antigen to planktonic *S.* Typhimurium failed to reduce ROS production from neutrophils, but the presence of Vi antigen in biofilms did cause a decrease in ROS production (Figure 4C). As expected, planktonic *S.* Typhi Δ*tviB* elicited a robust response from neutrophils. Although the response to biofilms from the same mutant was also greater than the response to WT biofilms, the increase in ROS production was surprisingly less dramatic (Figure 4C). These data indicate that while the planktonic inhibition of neutrophil ROS is dependent on the Vi antigen, ROS inhibition by biofilms is dependent on a combination of Vi antigen and other biofilm functions. This biofilm-dependent enhancement demonstrates how neutrophil recruitment may prevent *S.* Typhi from causing systemic disease (which would require the release of planktonic bacteria) but simultaneously is unable to clear biofilm infections. This type of stalemate is in line with many persistent infections that are restricted but not sterilized by the host.

Infections with *S.* Typhimurium EPS mutants indicated that the slime polysaccharides cellulose and colanic acid are required for neutrophil recognition of *S.* Typhimurium biofilms (Figure 4D). Considering that *S.* Typhimurium elicits early neutrophil recruitment and inflammatory disease in humans (to a point of self-limiting infection in the gut) and the fact that *S.* Typhi lacks colanic acid, this discovery highlights one way that *S.* Typhi has undergone host specialization and has an advantage in biofilm recalcitrance to innate immunity. On the other hand, both serovars possess cellulose, which presents an interesting question to investigate further. Since we found cellulose to be immune-stimulating, we predict that the localization of cellulose to the host–biofilm interface would reduce biofilm stealth but the presence of other EPS components in vivo prevents this interaction from occurring.

Consistent with a stalemate infection, our data indicated planktonic and biofilm *Salmonella* resisted killing by oxidative species (Figure 4A,B). To determine the degree to which this phenotype is intrinsic to *Salmonella* versus the biofilm lifestyle, we challenged planktonic and biofilm *Salmonella* with exogenously supplied (chemical) oxidative species. We demonstrated that 500 μg/ml ClO^- readily kills planktonic and biofilm-associated *Salmonella* alike (Figure 5C–I), indicating that the presence of EPSs does not afford protection to peroxynitrites, chloramines, or singlet oxygen (downstream ROS molecules produced by ClO^-). However, the survival of biofilm-associated bacteria in conditions with 50-fold more H_2O_2 than the WT planktonic MIC (Figure 5A,B,E–I) indicates that EPSs augment biofilm tolerance to the ROS precursor of ClO^-. We predict that EPSs slow the diffusion of H_2O_2 into the biofilm to a rate that permits the effective detoxification of H_2O_2 by catalase enzymes expressed by *Salmonella* [69–71]. The H_2O_2 tolerance defect detected in S. Typhimurium Δ*csgA*Δ*wcaM*Δ*yihO*Δ*bcsE* biofilms (Figure 5E,G) can be attributed specifically to the O antigen capsule and colanic acid (Figure 6). Interestingly, S. Typhi Δ*tviB* biofilms also demonstrated a tolerance defect, as they only survived H_2O_2 challenge at the planktonic MIC (Figure 5F,I). Consistently, the MIC of planktonic S. Typhi Δ*tviB* was reduced to 1.25 mM H_2O_2 (supplemental data; Figure S4A); the growth of planktonic S. Typhimurium expressing the Vi antigen was reduced—but not inhibited—by the WT H_2O_2 MIC, and complete inhibition required 4.25 mM H_2O_2 (1.7-fold the WT MIC) (supplemental data; Figure S5). Together, these data implicate biofilm Vi antigen as well as S. Typhimurium O antigen capsule and colanic acid in tolerance to oxidative killing.

In our view, it is no coincidence that S. Typhi has dispensed colanic acid; even though the polysaccharide augments S. Typhimurium tolerance to H_2O_2, the ability of S. Typhi to outright prevent or reduce oxidative pathways by eliminating this immunostimulatory EPS pays far greater dividends. Furthermore, the other S. Typhimurium EPS that was identified as important for tolerance to H_2O_2 (O antigen capsule) is analogous to the Vi antigen in typhoidal serovars in that it drives H_2O_2 tolerance. The discovery that each capsule is responsible for H_2O_2 tolerance in its respective serovar fits with our other evidence and highlights how S. Typhi relies on the Vi antigen to establish and maintain chronic infections. While S. Typhimurium biofilms depend on the O antigen capsule to reduce ROS production and for tolerance to H_2O_2, the O antigen capsule was unable to reduce NO production in the same manner that the Vi antigen and S. Typhi succeed in reducing NO production. Overall, the evolution of the Vi antigen in typhoidal serovars and the ability to fine-tune iNOS activity sets these human-adapted pathogens apart from other *Salmonella*, as the Vi antigen has a prominent role in regulating the host NO and ROS responses to biofilm infections as well as enhancing biofilm recalcitrance during chronic infections that are bound to be exposed to some level of antimicrobial defenses. We have shown how the Vi antigen represents a key EPS of S. Typhi biofilms and that it likely elicits modulation of the innate immune system of chronic carriers.

5. Conclusions

We have provided strong evidence that S. Typhi inhibits innate immunity, but also acknowledge that host functions can ultimately prevail. Adaptive immunity has been documented in chronic carriers in the form of *Salmonella*-specific circulating antibodies and *Salmonella*-specific T cells [61,64,72,73]. Yet the inability to clear infections by innate or adaptive means indicates a true stalemate infection. From the perspective of the infected individual, a chronic stalemate infection is beneficial in the sense that it is preventing systemic disease. Of course, from a public health standpoint, chronic disease is the apex issue and must be mitigated, but in a manner that does not target biofilms so effectively that they rapidly disburse and cause systemic morbidity. By studying the innate immune interactions of *Salmonella* biofilms, we have demonstrated one potential pathway in which innate immunity could potentially be enhanced to help achieve this goal and believe that activating myeloperoxidase activity in vivo in response to Vi antigen would benefit the natural ability of host clearance.

Author Contributions: Conceptualization, M.M.H. and J.S.G.; methodology, M.M.H. and J.S.G.; formal analysis, M.M.H. and J.S.G.; investigation, M.M.H.; data curation, M.M.H.; writing—original draft preparation, M.M.H.; writing—review and editing, J.S.G.; visualization, M.M.H.; supervision, J.S.G.; funding acquisition, J.S.G. All authors have read and agreed to the published version of the manuscript.

Acknowledgments: We thank Bradley Eichar for mutant generation and Evan Bernard for experimental support.

References

1. Gonzalez-Escobedo, G.; Marshall, J.M.; Gunn, J.S. Chronic and acute infection of the gall bladder by *Salmonella* Typhi: understanding the carrier state. *Nat. Rev. Microbiol.* **2010**, *9*, nrmicro2490. [CrossRef] [PubMed]
2. Crawford, R.W.; Reeve, K.E.; Gunn, J.S. Flagellated but Not Hyperfimbriated *Salmonella enterica* Serovar Typhimurium Attaches to and Forms Biofilms on Cholesterol-Coated Surfaces. *J. Bacteriol.* **2010**, *192*, 2981–2990. [CrossRef] [PubMed]
3. Crawford, R.W.; Rosales-Reyes, R.; Ramirez-Aguilar Mde, L.; Chapa-Azuela, O.; Alpuche-Aranda, C.; Gunn, J.S. Gallstones play a significant role in *Salmonella* spp. gallbladder colonization and carriage. *Proc. Natl. Acad. Sci. U.S.A.* **2010**, *107*, 4353. [CrossRef]
4. Gunn, J.S.; Marshall, J.M.; Baker, S.; Dongol, S.; Charles, R.C.; Ryan, E.T. *Salmonella* chronic carriage: epidemiology, diagnosis, and gallbladder persistence. *Trends Microbiol.* **2014**, *22*, 648. [CrossRef] [PubMed]
5. Gunn, J.S.; Bakaletz, L.O.; Wozniak, D.J. What's on the Outside Matters: The Role of the Extracellular Polymeric Substance of Gram-negative Biofilms in Evading Host Immunity and as a Target for Therapeutic Intervention. *J. Biol. Chem.* **2016**, *291*, 12538. [CrossRef] [PubMed]
6. Johnson, R.; Ravenhall, M.; Pickard, D.; Dougan, G.; Byrne, A.; Frankel, G. Comparison of *Salmonella enterica* serovars Typhi and Typhimurium reveals typhoidal serovar-specific responses to bile. *Infect. Immun.* **2018**, *86*, e00490-17. [CrossRef]
7. Hay, A.; Zhu, J. In Sickness and in Health: The relationships between bacteria and bile in the human gut. In *Advances in applied microbiology*; Elsevier: Amsterdam, The Netherlands, 2016; Volume 96, pp. 43–64.
8. González, J.F.; Tucker, L.; Fitch, J.; Wetzel, A.; White, P.; Gunn, J.S. Human bile-mediated regulation of *Salmonella* curli fimbriae. *J. Bacteriol.* **2019**, *201*, e00055-19. [CrossRef]
9. Chin, K.C.J.; Taylor, T.D.; Hebrard, M.; Anbalagan, K.; Dashti, M.G.; Phua, K.K. Transcriptomic study of *Salmonella enterica* subspecies *enterica* serovar Typhi biofilm. *BMC Genom.* **2017**, *18*, 836. [CrossRef] [PubMed]
10. Deksissa, T.; Gebremedhin, E.Z. A cross-sectional study of enteric fever among febrile patients at Ambo hospital: Prevalence, risk factors, comparison of Widal test and stool culture and antimicrobials susceptibility pattern of isolates. *BMC Infect. Dis.* **2019**, *19*, 288. [CrossRef]
11. Mawazo, A.; Bwire, G.M.; Matee, M.I. Performance of Widal test and stool culture in the diagnosis of typhoid fever among suspected patients in Dar es Salaam, Tanzania. *BMC Res. Notes* **2019**, *12*, 316. [CrossRef]
12. Arora, P.; Thorlund, K.; Brenner, D.R.; Andrews, J.R. Comparative accuracy of typhoid diagnostic tools: A Bayesian latent-class network analysis. *Plos Negl. Trop. Dis.* **2019**, *13*, e0007303. [CrossRef] [PubMed]
13. Chang, M.S.; Woo, J.H.; Kim, S. Management of Typhoid Fever–Clinical and Historical Perspectives in Korea. *Infect. Chemother.* **2019**, *51*, 330–335. [CrossRef] [PubMed]
14. González, J.F.; Alberts, H.; Lee, J.; Doolittle, L.; Gunn, J.S. Biofilm Formation Protects *Salmonella* from the Antibiotic Ciprofloxacin In Vitro and In Vivo in the Mouse Model of chronic Carriage. *Sci. Rep.* **2018**, *8*, 222. [CrossRef] [PubMed]
15. Stanaway, J.D.; Reiner, R.C.; Blacker, B.F.; Goldberg, E.M.; Khalil, I.A.; Troeger, C.E.; Andrews, J.R.; Bhutta, Z.A.; Crump, J.A.; Im, J. The global burden of typhoid and paratyphoid fevers: a systematic analysis for the Global Burden of Disease Study 2017. *Lancet Infect. Dis.* **2019**, *19*, 369–381. [CrossRef]
16. Crump, J.A.; Luby, S.P.; Mintz, E.D. The global burden of typhoid fever. *Bull. World Health Organ.* **2004**, *82*, 346.
17. Kirk, M.D.; Pires, S.M.; Black, R.E.; Caipo, M.; Crump, J.A.; Devleesschauwer, B.; Döpfer, D.; Fazil, A.; Fischer-Walker, C.L.; Hald, T. World Health Organization estimates of the global and regional disease burden of 22 foodborne bacterial, protozoal, and viral diseases, 2010: a data synthesis. *Plos Med.* **2015**, *12*, e1001921.
18. Bäumler, A.; Fang, F.C. Host specificity of bacterial pathogens. *Cold Spring Harb Perspect. Med.* **2013**, *3*, a010041. [CrossRef]
19. Wain, J.; House, D.; Parkhill, J.; Parry, C.; Dougan, G. Unlocking the genome of the human typhoid bacillus. *Lancet Infect. Dis.* **2002**, *2*, 163–170. [CrossRef]

20. Langridge, G.C.; Fookes, M.; Connor, T.R.; Feltwell, T.; Feasey, N.; Parsons, B.N.; Seth-Smith, H.M.; Barquist, L.; Stedman, A.; Humphrey, T. Patterns of genome evolution that have accompanied host adaptation in *Salmonella*. *Proc. Natl. Acad. Sci.* **2015**, *112*, 863–868. [CrossRef]
21. Kurtz, J.R.; Goggins, J.A.; McLachlan, J.B. *Salmonella* infection: Interplay between the bacteria and host immune system. *Immunol. Lett.* **2017**, *190*, 42. [CrossRef]
22. Hurley, D.; McCusker, M.P.; Fanning, S.; Martins, M. *Salmonella*–host interactions–modulation of the host innate immune system. *Front. Immunol.* **2014**, *5*, 481. [CrossRef] [PubMed]
23. Raffatellu, M.; Santos, R.L.; Chessa, D.; Wilson, R.P.; Winter, S.E.; Rossetti, C.A.; Lawhon, S.D.; Chu, H.; Lau, T.; Bevins, C.L.; et al. The capsule encoding the *viaB* locus reduces interleukin-17 expression and mucosal innate responses in the bovine intestinal mucosa during infection with *Salmonella enterica* serotype Typhi. *Infect. Immun.* **2007**, *75*, 4342. [CrossRef] [PubMed]
24. Haneda, T.; Winter, S.E.; Butler, B.P.; Wilson, R.P.; Tükel, Ç.; Winter, M.G.; Godinez, I.; Tsolis, R.M.; Bäumler, A.J. The capsule-encoding *viaB* locus reduces intestinal inflammation by a *Salmonella* pathogenicity island 1-independent mechanism. *Infect. Immun.* **2009**, *77*, 2932–2942. [CrossRef] [PubMed]
25. Winter, S.E.; Raffatellu, M.; Wilson, R.P.; Rüssmann, H.; Bäumler, A.J. The *Salmonella enterica* serotype Typhi regulator TviA reduces interleukin-8 production in intestinal epithelial cells by repressing flagellin secretion. *Cell. Microbiol.* **2008**, *10*, 247. [CrossRef] [PubMed]
26. Crawford, R.W.; Keestra, A.M.; Winter, S.E.; Xavier, M.N.; Tsolis, R.M.; Tolstikov, V.; Bäumler, A.J. Very long O-antigen chains enhance fitness during *Salmonella*-induced colitis by increasing bile resistance. *Plos Pathog.* **2012**, *8*, e1002918. [CrossRef]
27. Wilson, R.P.; Winter, S.E.; Spees, A.M.; Winter, M.G.; Nishimori, J.H.; Sanchez, J.F.; Nuccio, S.P.; Crawford, R.W.; Tukel, C.; Baumler, A.J. The Vi capsular polysaccharide prevents complement receptor 3-mediated clearance of *Salmonella enterica* serotype Typhi. *Infect. Immun.* **2011**, *79*, 830. [CrossRef]
28. Tükel, Ç.; Raffatellu, M.; Humphries, A.D.; Wilson, R.P.; Andrews-Polymenis, H.L.; Gull, T.; Figueiredo, J.F.; Wong, M.H.; Michelsen, K.S.; Akçelik, M. CsgA is a pathogen-associated molecular pattern of *Salmonella enterica* serotype Typhimurium that is recognized by Toll-like receptor 2. *Mol. Microbiol.* **2005**, *58*, 289–304. [CrossRef]
29. Raffatellu, M.; Chessa, D.; Wilson, R.P.; Dusold, R.; Rubino, S.; Baumler, A.J. The Vi capsular antigen of *Salmonella enterica* serotype Typhi reduces Toll-like receptor-dependent interleukin-8 expression in the intestinal mucosa. *Infect. Immun.* **2005**, *73*, 3367. [CrossRef]
30. Parween, F.; Yadav, J.; Qadri, A. The virulence polysaccharide of *Salmonella* Typhi suppresses activation of Rho family GTPases to limit inflammatory responses from epithelial cells. *Front. Cell. Infect. Microbiol.* **2019**, *9*, 141. [CrossRef]
31. Leid, J.G. Bacterial biofilms resist key host defenses. *Microbe* **2009**, *4*, 66.
32. Valentini, M.; Filloux, A. Biofilms and Cyclic di-GMP (c-di-GMP) Signaling: Lessons from *Pseudomonas aeruginosa* and Other Bacteria. *J. Biol. Chem.* **2016**, *291*, 12547. [CrossRef] [PubMed]
33. Van Acker, H.; Coenye, T. The Role of Efflux and Physiological Adaptation in Biofilm Tolerance and Resistance. *J. Biol. Chem.* **2016**, *291*, 12565. [CrossRef] [PubMed]
34. Keestra-Gounder, A.M.; Tsolis, R.M.; Bäumler, A.J. Now you see me, now you don't: The interaction of *Salmonella* with innate immune receptors. *Nat. Rev. Microbiol.* **2015**, *13*, 206. [CrossRef] [PubMed]
35. Pestrak, M.J.; Chaney, S.B.; Eggleston, H.C.; Dellos-Nolan, S.; Dixit, S.; Mathew Steiner, S.S.; Roy, S.; Parsek, M.R.; Sen, C.K.; Wozniak, D.J. *Pseudomonas aeruginosa* rugose small-colony variants evade host clearance, are hyper-inflammatory, and persist in multiple host environments. *Plos Pathog.* **2018**, *14*, e1006842. [CrossRef]
36. Leid, J.G.; Willson, C.J.; Shirtliff, M.E.; Hassett, D.J.; Parsek, M.R.; Jeffers, A.K. The exopolysaccharide alginate protects *Pseudomonas aeruginosa* biofilm bacteria from IFN-γ-mediated macrophage killing. *J. Immunol.* **2005**, *175*, 7512–7518. [CrossRef]
37. Adcox, H.E.; Vasicek, E.M.; Dwivedi, V.; Hoang, K.V.; Turner, J.; Gunn, J.S. *Salmonella* Extracellular Matrix Components Influence Biofilm Formation and Gallbladder Colonization. *Infect. Immun.* **2016**, *84*, 3243. [CrossRef]
38. Kostakioti, M.; Hadjifrangiskou, M.; Hultgren, S.J. Bacterial biofilms: development, dispersal, and therapeutic strategies in the dawn of the postantibiotic era. *Cold Spring Harb Perspect.Med.* **2013**, *3*, a010306. [CrossRef]

39. Coynault, C.; Robbe-Saule, V.; Norel, F. Virulence and vaccine potential of *Salmonella* typhimurium mutants deficient in the expression of the RpoS (σs) regulon. *Mol. Microbiol.* **1996**, *22*, 149–160. [CrossRef]
40. Santander, J.; Wanda, S.-Y.; Nickerson, C.A.; Curtiss, R. Role of RpoS in fine-tuning the synthesis of Vi capsular polysaccharide in *Salmonella enterica* serotype Typhi. *Infect. Immun.* **2007**, *75*, 1382–1392. [CrossRef]
41. Virlogeux, I.; Waxin, H.; Ecobichon, C.; Popoff, M.Y. Role of the *viaB* locus in synthesis, transport and expression of *Salmonella* typhi Vi antigen. *Microbiology* **1995**, *141*, 3039–3047. [CrossRef]
42. Datsenko, K.A.; Wanner, B.L. One-step inactivation of chromosomal genes in *Escherichia coli* K-12 using PCR products. *Proc. Natl. Acad. Sci. USA* **2000**, *97*, 6640. [CrossRef] [PubMed]
43. Cherepanov, P.P.; Wackernagel, W. Gene disruption in *Escherichia coli*: TcR and KmR cassettes with the option of Flp-catalyzed excision of the antibiotic-resistance determinant. *Gene* **1995**, *158*, 9–14. [CrossRef]
44. Tucker, K.A.; Lilly, M.B.; Heck, L., Jr.; Rado, T.A. Characterization of a new human diploid myeloid leukemia cell line (PLB-985) with granulocytic and monocytic differentiating capacity. *Blood* **1987**, *70*, 372. [CrossRef] [PubMed]
45. Drexler, H.G.; Dirks, W.G.; Matsuo, Y.; MacLeod, R.A.F. False leukemia–lymphoma cell lines: an update on over 500 cell lines. *Leukemia* **2003**, *17*, 416. [CrossRef] [PubMed]
46. Pedruzzi, E.; Fay, M.; Elbim, C.; Gougerot-Pocidalo, M.A. Differentiation of PLB-985 myeloid cells into mature neutrophils, shown by degranulation of terminally differentiated compartments in response to N-formyl peptide and priming of superoxide anion production by granulocyte–macrophage colony-stimulating factor. *Br. J. Haematol.* **2002**, *117*, 719. [PubMed]
47. Pivot-Pajot, C.; Chouinard, F.C.; El Azreq, M.A.; Harbour, D.; Bourgoin, S.G. Characterisation of degranulation and phagocytic capacity of a human neutrophilic cellular model, PLB-985 cells. *Immunobiology* **2010**, *215*, 38. [CrossRef]
48. Hiyoshi, H.; Wangdi, T.; Lock, G.; Saechao, C.; Raffatellu, M.; Cobb, B.A.; Bäumler, A.J. Mechanisms to evade the phagocyte respiratory burst arose by convergent evolution in typhoidal *Salmonella* serovars. *Cell Rep.* **2018**, *22*, 1787–1797. [CrossRef]
49. Bravo-Blas, A.; Utriainen, L.; Clay, S.L.; Kästele, V.; Cerovic, V.; Cunningham, A.F.; Henderson, I.R.; Wall, D.M.; Milling, S.W. *Salmonella enterica* serovar typhimurium travels to mesenteric lymph nodes both with host cells and autonomously. *J. Immunol.* **2019**, *202*, 260–267. [CrossRef]
50. Hume, P.J.; Singh, V.; Davidson, A.C.; Koronakis, V. Swiss army pathogen: The *Salmonella* entry toolkit. *Front. Cell. Infect. Microbiol.* **2017**, *7*, 348. [CrossRef]
51. Jansen, A.M.; Hall, L.J.; Clare, S.; Goulding, D.; Holt, K.E.; Grant, A.J.; Mastroeni, P.; Dougan, G.; Kingsley, R.A. A *Salmonella* Typhimurium-Typhi genomic chimera: A model to study Vi polysaccharide capsule function in vivo. *Plos Pathog.* **2011**, *7*, e1002131. [CrossRef]
52. Sharma, A.; Qadri, A. Vi polysaccharide of *Salmonella* typhi targets the prohibitin family of molecules in intestinal epithelial cells and suppresses early inflammatory responses. *Proc. Natl. Acad. Sci.* **2004**, *101*, 17492–17497. [CrossRef] [PubMed]
53. Wangdi, T.; Lee, C.-Y.; Spees, A.M.; Yu, C.; Kingsbury, D.D.; Winter, S.E.; Hastey, C.J.; Wilson, R.P.; Heinrich, V.; Bäumler, A.J. The Vi capsular polysaccharide enables *Salmonella enterica* serovar Typhi to evade microbe-guided neutrophil chemotaxis. *Plos Pathog.* **2014**, *10*, e1004306. [CrossRef] [PubMed]
54. BIEDZKA-SAREK, M.; El Skurnik, M. How to outwit the enemy: dendritic cells face *Salmonella*. *Apmis* **2006**, *114*, 589–600. [CrossRef] [PubMed]
55. Alam, M.S.; Zaki, M.H.; Yoshitake, J.; Akuta, T.; Ezaki, T.; Akaike, T. Involvement of *Salmonella enterica* serovar Typhi RpoS in resistance to NO-mediated host defense against serovar Typhi infection. *Microb. Pathog.* **2006**, *40*, 116–125. [CrossRef] [PubMed]
56. Jiang, P.; Yang, W.; Jin, Y.; Huang, H.; Shi, C.; Jiang, Y.; Wang, J.; Kang, Y.; Wang, C.; Yang, G. *Lactobacillus reuteri* protects mice against *Salmonella* typhimurium challenge by activating macrophages to produce nitric oxide. *Microb. Pathog.* **2019**, *137*, 103754. [CrossRef] [PubMed]
57. González, J.F.; Kurtz, J.; Bauer, D.L.; Hitt, R.; Fitch, J.; Wetzel, A.; La Perle, K.; White, P.; McLachlan, J.; Gunn, J.S. Establishment of Chronic Typhoid Infection in a Mouse Carriage Model Involves a Type 2 Immune Shift and T and B Cell Recruitment to the Gallbladder. *MBio* **2019**, *10*, e02262-19. [CrossRef]
58. Muraille, E.; Leo, O.; Moser, M. TH1/TH2 paradigm extended: macrophage polarization as an unappreciated pathogen-driven escape mechanism? *Front. Immunol.* **2014**, *5*, 603. [CrossRef]

59. Eisele, N.A.; Ruby, T.; Jacobson, A.; Manzanillo, P.S.; Cox, J.S.; Lam, L.; Mukundan, L.; Chawla, A.; Monack, D.M. *Salmonella* require the fatty acid regulator PPARδ for the establishment of a metabolic environment essential for long-term persistence. *Cell Host Microbe* **2013**, *14*, 171–182. [CrossRef]
60. McCoy, M.W.; Moreland, S.M.; Detweiler, C.S. Hemophagocytic macrophages in murine typhoid fever have an anti-inflammatory phenotype. *Infect. Immun.* **2012**, *80*, 3642–3649. [CrossRef]
61. Monack, D.M.; Bouley, D.M.; Falkow, S. *Salmonella* typhimurium persists within macrophages in the mesenteric lymph nodes of chronically infected Nramp1+/+ mice and can be reactivated by IFNγ neutralization. *J. Exp. Med.* **2004**, *199*, 231–241. [CrossRef]
62. Frawley, E.R.; Karlinsey, J.E.; Singhal, A.; Libby, S.J.; Doulias, P.-T.; Ischiropoulos, H.; Fang, F.C. Nitric oxide disrupts zinc homeostasis in *Salmonella enterica* serovar Typhimurium. *MBio* **2018**, *9*, e01040-18. [CrossRef] [PubMed]
63. Khan, S.; Fujii, S.; Matsunaga, T.; Nishimura, A.; Ono, K.; Ida, T.; Ahmed, K.A.; Okamoto, T.; Tsutsuki, H.; Sawa, T. Reactive persulfides from *Salmonella* Typhimurium downregulate autophagy-mediated innate immunity in macrophages by inhibiting electrophilic signaling. *Cell Chem. Biol.* **2018**, *25*, 1403–1413.e4. [CrossRef] [PubMed]
64. Goldberg, M.F.; Roeske, E.K.; Ward, L.N.; Pengo, T.; Dileepan, T.; Kotov, D.I.; Jenkins, M.K. *Salmonella* Persist in Activated Macrophages in T Cell-Sparse Granulomas but Are Contained by Surrounding CXCR3 Ligand-Positioned Th1 Cells. *Immunity* **2018**, *49*, 1090–1102.e7. [CrossRef] [PubMed]
65. Alam, M.S.; Akaike, T.; Okamoto, S.; Kubota, T.; Yoshitake, J.; Sawa, T.; Miyamoto, Y.; Tamura, F.; Maeda, H. Role of nitric oxide in host defense in murine salmonellosis as a function of its antibacterial and antiapoptotic activities. *Infect. Immun.* **2002**, *70*, 3130–3142. [CrossRef]
66. Akaike, T. Role of free radicals in viral pathogenesis and mutation. *Rev. Med Virol.* **2001**, *11*, 87–101. [CrossRef]
67. Nolan, S.; Dixon, R.; Norman, K.; Hellewell, P.; Ridger, V. Nitric oxide regulates neutrophil migration through microparticle formation. *Am. J. Pathol.* **2008**, *172*, 265–273. [CrossRef]
68. Hossain, M.; Qadri, S.M.; Liu, L. Inhibition of nitric oxide synthesis enhances leukocyte rolling and adhesion in human microvasculature. *J. Inflamm.* **2012**, *9*, 28. [CrossRef]
69. Walawalkar, Y.D.; Vaidya, Y.; Nayak, V. Response of *Salmonella* Typhi to bile-generated oxidative stress: implication of quorum sensing and persister cell populations. *Pathog. Dis.* **2016**, *74*.
70. Tsolis, R.M.; Bäumler, A.J.; Heffron, F. Role of *Salmonella* typhimurium Mn-superoxide dismutase (SodA) in protection against early killing by J774 macrophages. *Infect. Immun.* **1995**, *63*, 1739–1744. [CrossRef]
71. Farr, S.B.; Kogoma, T. Oxidative stress responses in *Escherichia coli* and *Salmonella* typhimurium. *Microbiol. Mol. Biol. Rev.* **1991**, *55*, 561–585. [CrossRef]
72. Ravindran, R.; Foley, J.; Stoklasek, T.; Glimcher, L.H.; McSorley, S.J. Expression of T-bet by CD4 T cells is essential for resistance to *Salmonella* infection. *J. Immunol.* **2005**, *175*, 4603–4610. [CrossRef] [PubMed]
73. Nauciel, C.; Espinasse-Maes, F. Role of gamma interferon and tumor necrosis factor alpha in resistance to *Salmonella* typhimurium infection. *Infect. Immun.* **1992**, *60*, 450–454. [CrossRef] [PubMed]

8

Genetic Markers in *S.* Paratyphi C Reveal Primary Adaptation to Pigs

Satheesh Nair [1], Maria Fookes [2], Craig Corton [2], Nicholas R. Thomson [2], John Wain [3,4,*] and Gemma C. Langridge [4]

1 Gastrointestinal Bacteria Reference Unit, Public Health England, Colindale, London NW9 5EQ, UK; satheesh.nair@phe.gov.uk
2 Wellcome Trust Sanger Institute, Hinxton, Cambridge CB10 1SA, UK; mcf@sanger.ac.uk (M.F.); chc@sanger.ac.uk (C.C.); nrt@sanger.ac.uk (N.R.T.)
3 Norwich Medical School, University of East Anglia, Norwich NR4 7UQ, UK
4 Microbes in the Food Chain, Quadram Institute, Norwich Research Park, Norwich NR4 7UQ, UK; Gemma.Langridge@quadram.ac.uk
* Correspondence: john.wain@quadram.ac.uk

Abstract: *Salmonella enterica* with the identical antigenic formula 6,7:c:1,5 can be differentiated biochemically and by disease syndrome. One grouping, *Salmonella* Paratyphi C, is currently considered a typhoidal serovar, responsible for enteric fever in humans. The human-restricted typhoidal serovars (*S.* Typhi and Paratyphi A, B and C) typically display high levels of genome degradation and are cited as an example of convergent evolution for host adaptation in humans. However, *S.* Paratyphi C presents a different clinical picture to *S.* Typhi/Paratyphi A, in a patient group with predisposition, raising the possibility that its natural history is different, and that infection is invasive salmonellosis rather than enteric fever. Using whole genome sequencing and metabolic pathway analysis, we compared the genomes of 17 *S.* Paratyphi C strains to other members of the 6,7:c:1,5 group and to two typhoidal serovars: *S.* Typhi and Paratyphi A. The genome degradation observed in *S.* Paratyphi C was much lower than *S.* Typhi/Paratyphi A, but similar to the other 6,7:c:1,5 strains. Genomic and metabolic comparisons revealed little to no overlap between *S.* Paratyphi C and the other typhoidal serovars, arguing against convergent evolution and instead providing evidence of a primary adaptation to pigs in accordance with the 6,7:c:1.5 strains.

Keywords: host adaptation; convergent evolution; genome degradation; genomic lesions

---

1. Introduction

Standardisation in the classification and fine typing of *Salmonella* in the mid-20th century led to a revolution in our understanding of the biological properties, particularly host associations, of this heterogenous group of animal pathogens [1,2]. For *Salmonella enterica* there are six defined subspecies. Nearly all isolates from humans are from subspecies I, in which more than 1500 serotypes can be distinguished by their cell wall (O) and flagella (H) antigens [3]. The combination of O:H1:H2 is known as the antigenic formula and each unique combination is given a name. For example (using the simplified antigenic formulae used by front line diagnostic laboratories) 9:d:- (where "-" means no antigen) identifies *S.* Typhi isolates and 2:a:1,5 is *S.* Paratyphi A. Both of these serovars are human-restricted and cause enteric fever. The situation, however, is more complex for *S.* Paratyphi B where its antigenic formula, 4:b:1,2 is shared by several *Salmonella* capable of causing mild to severe disease [4]. The 4:b:1,2 group can be split into subtypes using metabolic ability (e.g., tartrate utilisation), but these groups do not map to specific host species. For example, the human restricted *S.* Paratyphi B *sensu stricto* is always tartrate negative, but other 4:b:1,2 tartrate negative strains are highly diverse and are collectively known as *S.* Java. To date, only sequence typing has been able to define the phylogroup of tartrate negative strains that are human restricted [4]. Currently all *Salmonella* with the antigenic formula 4:b:1,2 are categorised as dangerous pathogens [5], but this may change as evidence linking the sub-types to clinical phenotypes accumulates.

The fourth *Salmonella* serotype considered to be a human restricted enteric fever pathogen is *S.* Paratyphi C; this belongs to a highly variable group with the antigenic formula 6,7:c:1,5, for which subtyping has never been fully resolved [6,7]. The most commonly isolated member of this group, *S.* Choleraesuis, has been divided into biotypes (Table 1): *sensu stricto* and Kunzendorf have a limited ability to grow using single sugars as a carbon source and differ only in their ability to produce H_2S from sulphates—a test which is difficult to standardise for routine diagnostic use.

Table 1. Differentiation by biochemistry of 6,7:c:1,5 *Salmonella.*

	Dulcitol	H2S	Mucate
Paratyphi C	+	+	−
Choleraesuis var. sensu stricto	−	−	−
Choleraesuis var. Kunzendorf	−	+	−
Choleraesuis var. Decatur	+	+	+
Typhisuis *	−	−	−

Adapted from the Kauffman White scheme [3]. * Typhisuis is *d*-tartrate negative in contrast to the other four.

S. Choleraesuis var. Decatur, on the other hand, has a greater metabolic capacity but is also far more genetically diverse [8]. Current biotyping schemes often lead to errors in identification [8], and so molecular tests have been developed using multi locus sequence typing (MLST) [6]. However, the mapping of these sequence types to phylogenetically related clusters is not clean and the association with animal hosts even less so [8]. The utility of these biotypes is therefore disputed.

The host restricted biotypes within the 6,7:c:1,5 group, (*S.* Paratyphi C to humans and *S.* Typhisuis to pigs) are clearly distinguishable from *S.* Choleraesuis; this has led to the hypothesis that the adaptation of salmonellae to humans by *S.* Typhi, Paratyphi A, B and C, is the result of convergent evolution of a diverse set of *Salmonella* adapting to survive and transmit between human hosts [7]. Comparative genomic studies on *S.* Typhi and Paratyphi A support this theory [9,10], but for *S.* Paratyphi B and C the evolutionary trajectory is less clear. Sequencing of ancient DNA from humans suggests that the 6,7:c:1,5 group of *Salmonella* were far more common in the past than now and were part of a historic clade (Ancient Eurasian Super Branch) which falls within the much larger extant *S. enterica* diversity. The early members of this clade cluster with their pig-adapted modern counterparts [11].

Clinically, the disease caused by *S.* Typhi and Paratyphi A is indistinguishable [12], but the evidence from a search of the accessible published literature that *S.* Paratyphi C causes only enteric fever is less clear. Rather, the clinical descriptions range from opportunistic infection resembling sepsis [13–16] to classic enteric fever [17]. This presentation, in some cases, is very similar to the infection caused in humans by the pig-adapted *S.* Choleraesuis [18]. The clinical picture is confused by difficulties in identifying *S.* Paratyphi C in the laboratory, but it is possible that this human restricted pathogen has undergone very different selective pressures to *S.* Typhi and Paratyphi A. If *S.* Paratyphi C has evolved convergently with *S.* Typhi and Paratyphi A, then the genome sequence should reveal this through the accumulation, across serotypes, of genetic changes that cause lesions in the pathways associated with host adaptation [19]. Here, we investigate this by describing the genomic lesions present in the genomes of 58 isolates from the 6,7:c:1,5 group, and comparing the evolutionary dynamics of this important group with those reported for *S.* Typhi and Paratyphi A.

2. Materials and Methods

2.1. Isolates

All 6,7:c1,5 strains used in the study are listed in Table 1, along with accession numbers for the raw sequence data. We assembled a collection of 6,7:c1,5 isolates for genome sequencing and supplemented these with publicly available sequences where necessary.

2.2. DNA Preparation

All isolates were cultured on non-selective agar (LB agar, Difco, Oxford, United Kingdom) for purity checking, and in non-selective broth (LB broth, Difco) for DNA extraction. DNA was extracted using a genomic DNA extraction (Sigma, Gillingham, United Kingdom) and sequenced using the Illumina Genome Analyzer II (Cambridge, United Kingdom), as previously described [20].

2.3. Genomes from Databases

A search was performed in Enterobase [21] for entries with the antigenic formula 6,7:c:1,5. An additional 2 genome sequences were identified and included in this study, *S.* Choleraesuis var. Decatur SARB70 (ERR3482081) and *S.* Paratyphi C RKS4594 (CP000857). 21 *S.* Typhi genomes, CT18 (accession AL513382), Ty2 (AE014613) and 19 from [22], and 2 *S.* Paratyphi A genomes, ATCC 9150 (CP000026) and AKU_12601 (FM200053) were also used.

2.4. Reference Genome Assembly

For the *S.* Typhisuis 61-6 and *S.* Paratyphi C 66-8 reference genomes, a high-quality sequence was assembled using data from two sequencing platforms. DNA was sequenced on both 454 Roche GS FLX Titanium (paired end library with 3kb insert; Connecticut, United States) and the Illumina Genome Analyzer II (200–300bp standard paired end library run in one lane for 37 cycles). Illumina sequences were assembled using Velvet [23] and combined with 454 sequences using Newbler (Roche). The combined assemblies were converted to Gap4 databases [24], to guide gap closure based upon 454 read pair information. ABACAS [25] was used to order and orient the fragmented assemblies against the complete genomes of *S.* Enteritidis P125109 (accession AM933172) and *S.* Choleraesuis SC-B67 (AE017220), enabling many small repeat regions to be correctly assembled. Finally, iCORN [26] was used to correct the assembled sequences using the Illumina data and checked in the Gap4 database. Initial genome annotation was carried out using annotation transfer via RATT [27] from *S.* Choleraesuis SC-B67. Genome assemblies are available under the project accession PRJEB37271.

2.5. Sequence QC

Where necessary, sequence data were trimmed using Trimmomatic (Galaxy v0.38.0) [28] with sliding window trimming of 4;20, leading and trailing trimming at quality 3 and appropriate adapter clipping (GAII or HiSeq).

2.6. Comparative Genomics

The identification of genomic lesions (mutations resulting in premature stop codons, frameshifts or insertion/deletions relative to an intact version of the gene), and comparison between genomes, was carried out using Artemis Comparison Tool (v10) [29]. For each identified lesion, the appropriate reference genome annotation was amended to accurately reflect the mutation, and therefore allow inclusion of these genomic features in downstream analysis. Velvet assemblies were generated for all isolates sequenced in this study. Per cluster, all mutations leading to genomic lesions in the reference genome were checked for their presence in at least 2 other draft genome assemblies from that cluster. The comparators (*S.* Choleraesuis, RKS1235 and RKS1249; *S.* Paratyphi C, 6610 and 664; *S.* Typhisuis, 38K and 871997) were chosen for their divergent positions within the phylogeny. Genomic lesions were deemed core if the same mutation was present in both, or variable if the mutation was absent in one or both sequences. OrthoMCL [30] with default parameters was used to determine orthologues between the three 6,7:c:1,5 genomes, *S.* Typhi CT18 and *S.* Paratyphi A AKU_12601. *S.* Enteritidis P125109 was also used as a comparator. All core disrupted genes were compared via orthology to identify which were shared or unique to each cluster. Core genomic lesions were also identified for *S.* Typhi across 19 genomes and *S.* Paratyphi A across the 2 publicly available genomes at the time.

2.7. Pathway Comparison

Lists of disrupted genes were overlaid onto the metabolic pathway overview of the *S.* Typhi CT18 pathway/genome database [31] to identify disrupted pathways and transport reactions. Disrupted pathways were compared between the 5 *Salmonella* to produce an UpSet plot [32].

3. Results and Discussion

3.1. Reductive Evolution and Genome Degradation

We generated a core SNP phylogeny from the genomes of 58 isolates to investigate the relationship between related 6,7:c:1,5 biotypes of *S. enterica* subspecies I (Figure 1). These included 17 isolates of *S.* Paratyphi C which spanned a range of 57 years and were collected from Europe, Africa and the Middle East (Table S1).

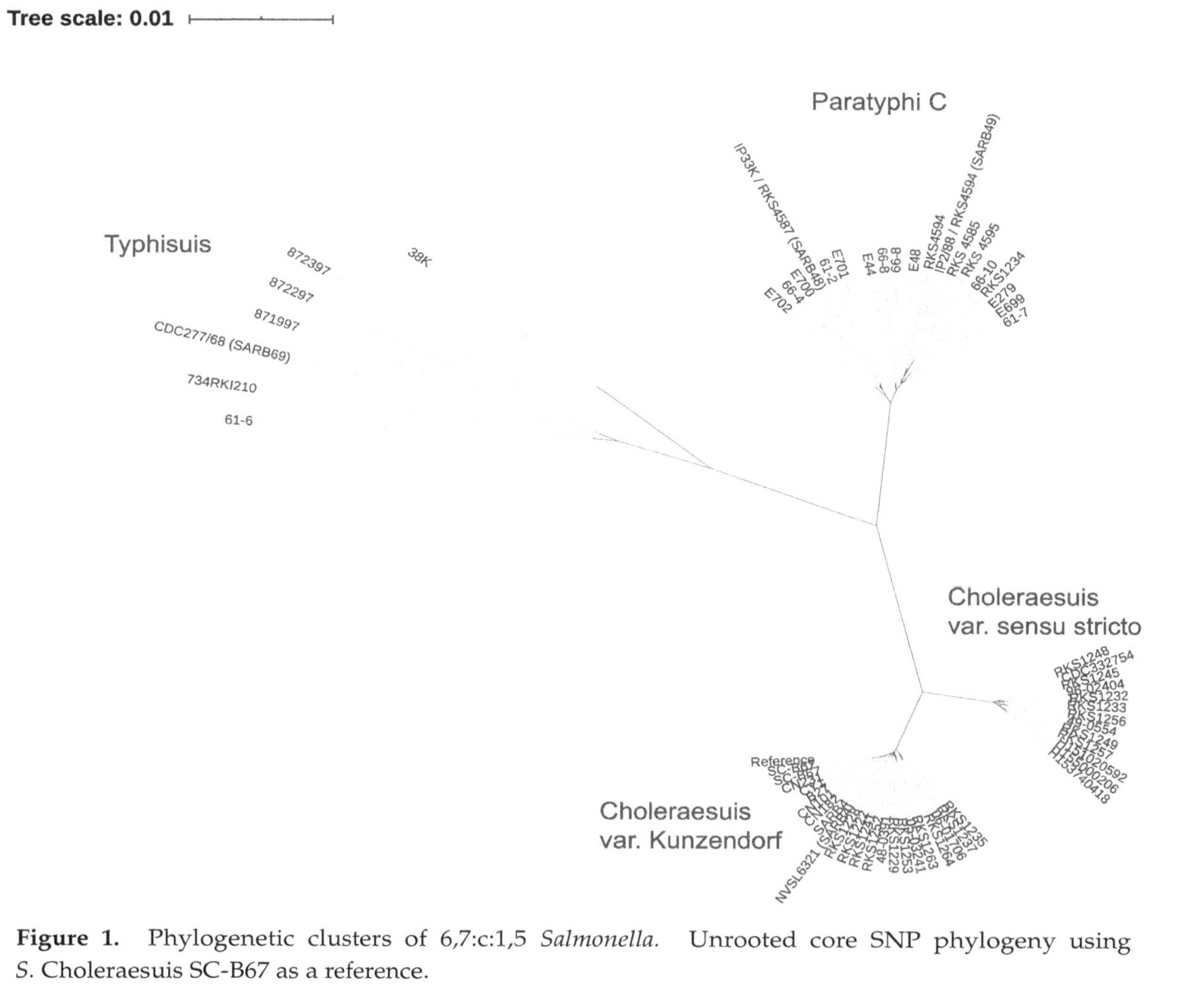

Figure 1. Phylogenetic clusters of 6,7:c:1,5 *Salmonella.* Unrooted core SNP phylogeny using *S.* Choleraesuis SC-B67 as a reference.

The two *S*. Decatur genomes showed more SNP variation between them than was found across all of the remaining biotypes (Figure S1), and so they were removed from the phylogeny. It is generally accepted that organisms classified as *S*. Decatur represent a very diverse group which should be considered separate from other 6,7:c:1,5 *Salmonella*. The remaining strains grouped into four phyloclusters (Figure 1, supported by hierBAPS analysis, Table S1). We also prepared an extended phylogeny, including an additional 116 assemblies from Enterobase, which confirmed the phylogenetic relationships were robust (Figure S1). The separation of these clusters was matched to the currently accepted classification scheme: 1, *S*. Typhisuis; 2, *S*. Paratyphi C; 3, *S*. Choleraesuis var. *sensu stricto;* 4, *S*. Choleraesuis var. Kunzendorf. This phylogeny confirmed that the isolates included in this study were typical of the 6,7:c:1,5 group, and also allowed us to select representative genomes for comparative analyses. For this analysis, the two biotypes of *S*. Choleraesuis were considered together because the core variation across the two groups was similar to that seen across the *S*. Typhisuis group, and this study focused on the human adaptation of *S*. Paratyphi C, *S*. Choleraesuis var. *sensu stricto* and var. Kunzendorf are both associated with pigs.

In bacteria restricted to a niche, such as infection of the human host, the accumulation of mutations that disrupt gene sequences (termed "pseudogenes") is well described [10]. The term pseudogene typically infers a loss of gene function but that is not always accurate, as many of these changes (deletions, insertions or major amino acid substitutions) can cause a change of function [33,34], and so here we use the term genomic lesion (GL) to infer changes that are predicted to have an impact on phenotype but do not necessarily cause loss of function. The association of genomic lesions with host adaptation is an active research area [35]; however, grouping genomic lesions by functional impact remains challenging. We have therefore treated all GLs (mutations resulting in premature stop codons, frameshifts or insertion/deletions relative to an intact version of the gene) as equal. We found that the number of GLs per serotype was much greater for *S*. Paratyphi A and *S*. Typhi than for *S*. Paratyphi C, suggesting a potentially shorter evolutionary time period for accumulation. However, the presence of *S*. Paratyphi C DNA found in ancient human samples [36,37], coupled with the descriptions of *S*. Paratyphi C as being very common in more ancient periods of human history suggests that the effective population size was at least as large as *S*. Typhi. This, in turn, suggests a different selective pressure driving the preservation of metabolic diversity, by the removal of genomic lesions from the population. For *S*. Paratyphi C then, a history of colonisation and transmission between varied environments seems more likely than one of being restricted to the human host. However, it is possible that *S*. Paratyphi C is at an early point along the pathway to human restriction, and so we looked for signs of early adaptation to the human host.

We performed comparative genomics within and between multiple genome sequences of *S*. Paratyphi C, *S*. Typhisuis and *S*. Choleraesuis, to determine if genome degradation was evident. At the time of sequencing, a high-quality contiguous reference genome only existed for *S*. Choleraesuis SCB67; we therefore generated references for both *S*. Paratyphi C and *S*. Typhisuis (Table S1). Within each biotype, a core set of genomic lesions was identified by comparison of the reference with two other members of that group, selected to represent the diversity within the group (Table S2). Any lesion that was absent from one or more of the sequences was considered variable and not included. All the 6,7:c:1,5 biotypes sequenced here, showed similar levels of genome degradation, with just over 100 genomic lesions seen in each genome representative (Figure 2). When compared with the core genomic lesions of the human restricted serotypes, it was evident that the scale of genome degradation was much greater in the two classic human restricted serotypes *S*. Typhi (186 lesions) and Paratyphi A (144 lesions). To understand the impact of these differences in genome degradation, we investigated the possible functional consequences of these genomic lesions.

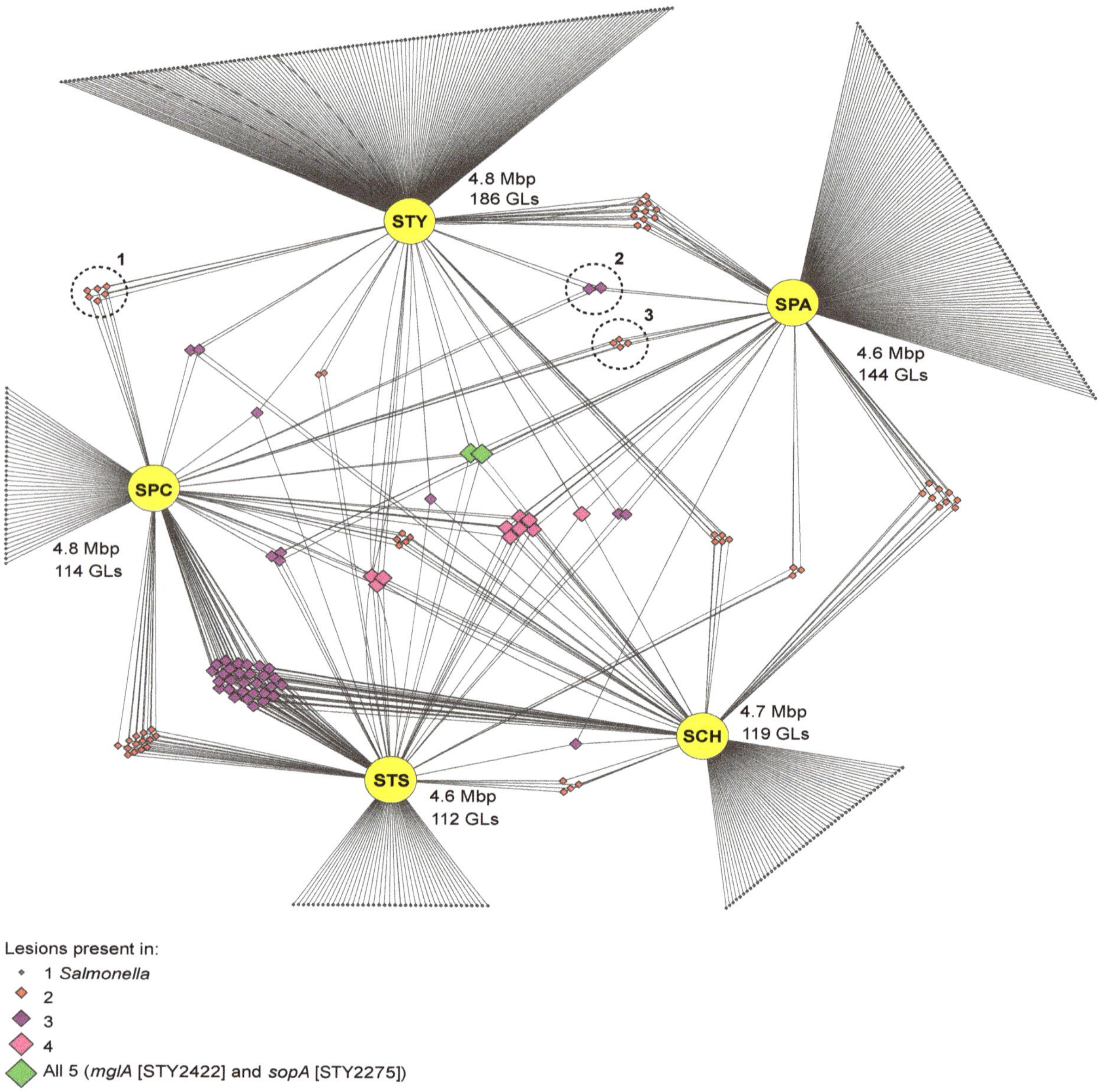

Figure 2. Distribution of disrupted genes. Network of shared and unique disrupted genes in *S.* Paratyphi C (SPC), *S.* Typhisuis (STS), *S.* Choleraesuis (SCH), *S.* Paratyphi A (SPA) and *S.* Typhi (STY). Yellow circles are false nodes representing each *Salmonella*. Diamonds indicate a single genomic lesion; size and colour indicate how many *Salmonella* share that lesion. Black lines connect *Salmonella* to genomic lesions. Lesions unique to each *Salmonella* are shown as fans around the false nodes. Mbp, megabase pairs; GL, genomic lesion. Dashed circles indicate lesions shared between SPC and STY and/or SPC and SPA. 1: *torC*, *ratC*, STY4541, STY2432, STY1834, STY1781; 2: *slrP* and *fliB*; 3: STY4472, STY4044, STY1408, STY1353.

3.2. Genomic Lesions are Functionally Distinct

Genomic lesions were located in metabolic pathways according to a pathway/genome database generated for *S.* Typhi (Table S3). This enabled us to determine which (potentially different) lesions affected the same pathways or transporters between the three 6,7:c1,5 representatives and *S.* Typhi/Paratyphi A (Figure 3). The intersection of affected pathways and transporters revealed that *S.* Paratyphi C had no lesions in pathways/transporters that were also degraded in *S.* Typhi or Paratyphi A (Figure S2). However, there were two genomic lesions that were common to all three 6,7:c1,5 representatives and *S.* Typhi/Paratyphi A: *sopA* and *mglA*. The former encodes a Type Three secretion system (T3SS) effector protein secreted by the T3SS encoded on *Salmonella* Pathogenicity

Island 1 (SPI-1), and the latter encodes a galactoside transporter. SPI-1 effectors are associated with the invasion of host intestinal cells and subsequent enteritis [38], and so the disruption of SopA through genomic lesion in all of the *Salmonella* investigated here is not surprising. Disruption of *mglA* has previously been reported in other host-adapted *Salmonella* [39], which combined with our findings suggests that the gene is linked to the former generalist lifestyle of all of these adapted salmonellae.

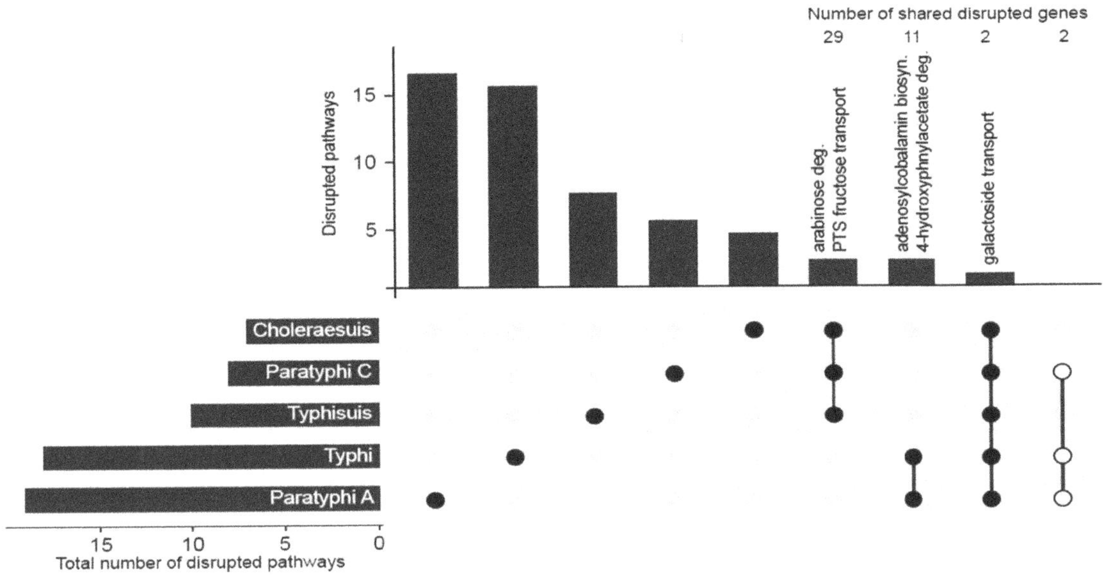

Figure 3. Distribution of disrupted pathways. Annotated UpSet plot of shared and unique disrupted pathways. Number of genes disrupted in pathways given above the columns (includes multiple genes disrupted in same pathway). Open circles: no disrupted pathways are shared between *S.* Typhi, *S.* Paratyphi A and *S.* Paratyphi C.

For the 6,7:c:1,5 biotypes we saw 29 genomic lesions, two of which impacted two shared pathways/transporters: arabinose degradation and a PTS fructose transport system, which have not been linked to bacterial colonisation of pigs previously. This most likely reflects their shared ancestry but may be the result of selection for colonisation of a shared habitat. We therefore examined the exact nature of the mutations causing these genomic lesions: the same base pair change at the same site was considered to be inheritance whereas a different mutation in the same gene (or pathway) was considered to show selection indicative of convergent evolution. The lesions affecting arabinose degradation and PTS fructose transport were identical and thus considered inheritance. This leaves open the possibility that the ancestor of *S.* Paratyphi C evolved as a pig pathogen, which then crossed the species barrier into humans. If this was the case, it seems likely that *S.* Paratyphi C has crossed from pigs to become an opportunistic human pathogen that has subsequently become restricted to the human host. *S.* Paratyphi C and *S.* Choleraesuis cause a similar pathology in humans but *S.* Paratyphi C has lost the ability to infect pigs. This hypothesis is supported by the reporting of *Salmonella* genomes in ancient DNA studies [11]. The genomes of *Salmonella* from 400 to 900 years ago cluster with modern *S.* Paratyphi C, but the older genomes (1600–5000 years old) cluster more closely with the pig-adapted *S.* Choleraesuis. This supports the hypothesis that the ancestor of *S.* Paratyphi C was adapted to pigs and that host restriction in humans actually represents an evolutionary dead end, explaining why *S.* Paratyphi C is so rare today.

Five pathways/transporters were found to be disrupted in both *S.* Typhi and Paratyphi A, of which two were shared by them alone. For *S.* Typhi/Paratyphi A, approximately 25% of their genome is shared through a recombination event, and the mutations causing GLs in this region of the genome accordingly have identical base pair changes [9]. However, outside of this shared region there are many mutations casing GLs that are clearly the result of convergent evolution: independent mutations linked to the disruption of the same metabolic pathways. Our analysis agrees with this finding, we identified genomic lesions in 11 genes and two pathways present only in S. Typhi and Paratyphi A, once all shared lesions with the 6,7:c:1,5 biotypes had been considered. Of these lesions, some were identical mutations and some were independent [9], suggesting convergent evolution by both selection for independent mutations and horizontally acquired characteristics.

3.3. Anaerobic Respiration Intact in S. Paratyphi C

The link between host adaptation (leading towards restriction) in *Salmonella* is perhaps best described for the metabolic functions associated with tetrathionate. Tetrathionate reduction allows the bacterial cell to carry out anaerobic respiration, this in turn increases the growth rate in the anaerobic environment of the animal gut and generates specific metabolic end products which stimulate inflammatory diarrhoea and in turn transmission between hosts [40]. The loss of anaerobic metabolism through the disruption of tetrathionate reduction is a hallmark of host adaptation, where a balance between pathogenicity and long-term colonisation of the host is the evolutionary strategy, rather than population expansion through rapid transmission. In Salmonella, disruption of anaerobic respiration is seen in S. Typhi, S. Paratyphi A and the S. Gallinarum/Pullorum group (restricted to birds) [10,19]. For S. Paratyphi C no such disruption was seen, the anaerobic respiration pathways were intact. In fact, only two genomic lesions were shared solely between S. Paratyphi C, S. Typhi and S. Paratyphi A (*slrP* and *fliB*), and these did not map to metabolic functions.

4. Conclusions

For S. Typhi and Paratyphi A, there is a clear genomic signal that suggests convergent evolution during adaptation and eventual restriction to the human host. In this study of 17 S. Paratyphi C genomes, we found: (i) the level of genome degradation caused by mutational disruption was much lower than in other host-restricted *Salmonella*, (ii) the metabolic pathways involved did not match the pathways disrupted in the human restricted *Salmonella*, and (iii) the acquisition of mutations appeared to be through inheritance from the ancestor with S. Choleraesuis, rather than by the selection of randomly occurring errors of DNA replication. In short, this suggests that convergent evolution does not explain the host restriction of S. Paratyphi C. Indeed, since anaerobic respiration is intact in S. Paratyphi C, we hypothesise that pathogenicity would be more similar to non-typhoidal *Salmonella* than to the enteric fever group. This has implications for both biological understanding and risk assessment for safety in clinical laboratories.

Supplementary Materials:
Figure S1. Extended phylogeny. Strains in red indicate those sequenced as part of this study. Strains in black are from Enterobase assemblies with > 60x coverage from Illumina sequencing. All S. Typhisuis and S. Paratyphi C genome assemblies from Enterobase with >60x coverage (representing 10 and 41 strains, respectively). We then selected a diverse geographical and temporal range of assemblies from Choleraesuis Kunzendorf (25), sensu stricto (15) and those defined only as Choleraesuis (25), all with > 60x coverage. 14 strains appear to be distantly related, possibly indicating misclassification. All other strains conform to the same phylogenetic relationship demonstrated by the strains sequenced in this study. **Figure S2.** Network of disrupted pathways and transporters. Yellow circles are false nodes representing each *Salmonella*. Diamonds indicate a single disrupted pathway (connected by straight lines) or transporters (connected by wavy lines); size and colour indicate how many *Salmonella* share that disrupted pathway/transporter. Disrupted pathways/transporters unique to each *Salmonella* are shown as fans around the false nodes. Table S1. 6,7:c1,5 strains in this paper. Table S2. Genomic lesions affecting genes: S. Paratyphi C (SPC), S. Typhisuis (STS), S. Choleraesuis (SCH), S. Paratyphi A (SPA) and S. Typhi (STY). Table S3. Genomic lesions affecting pathways: S. Paratyphi C (SPC), S. Typhisuis (STS), S. Choleraesuis (SCH), S. Paratyphi A (SPA) and S. Typhi (STY).

Author Contributions: Concept and study design: S.N., N.R.T., J.W. and G.C.L.; data analysis: M.F., C.C. and G.C.L.; drafting and revision of the manuscript: S.N., J.W. and G.C.L. All authors have read and agreed to the published version of the manuscript.

Acknowledgments: We thank Ken Sanderson, Wolfgang Rabsch, Reiner Helmuth, Sam Kariuki and Cheng-Hsun Chiu for their kind donation of strains.

References

1. Su, L.; Chiu, C. Salmonella: Clinical importance and evolution of nomenclature. *Chang. Gung Med. J.* **2007**, *30*, 210.
2. Langridge, G.C.; Wain, J.; Nair, S. Invasive salmonellosis in humans. *EcoSal Plus* **2012**, *5*. [CrossRef] [PubMed]
3. Grimont, P.A.; Weill, F.-X. Antigenic formulae of the Salmonella serovars. *WHO Collab. Cent. Ref. Res. Salmonella* **2007**, *9*, 1–166.
4. Connor, T.R.; Owen, S.V.; Langridge, G.; Connell, S.; Nair, S.; Reuter, S.; Dallman, T.J.; Corander, J.; Tabing, K.C.; Le Hello, S.; et al. What's in a name? Species-wide whole-genome sequencing resolves invasive and noninvasive lineages of salmonella enterica serotype paratyphi B. *mBio* **2016**, *7*. [CrossRef] [PubMed]
5. Health and Safety Executive: Advisory Committee on Dangerous Pathogens. *The Approved List of Biological Agents*; Health and Safety Executive: Advisory Committee on Dangerous Pathogens: London, UK, 2013.
6. Uzzau, S.; Hovi, M.; Stocker, B.A. Application of ribotyping and IS200 fingerprinting to distinguish the five Salmonella serotype O6, 7:c:1, 5 groups: Choleraesuis sensu stricto, Choleraesuis var. Kunzendorf, Choleraesuis var. Decatur, Paratyphi C, and Typhisuis. *Epidemiol. Infect.* **1999**, *123*, 37–46. [CrossRef] [PubMed]
7. Liu, W.-Q.; Feng, Y.; Wang, Y.; Zou, Q.-H.; Chen, F.; Guo, J.-T.; Peng, Y.-H.; Jin, Y.; Li, Y.-G.; Hu, S.-N. Salmonella paratyphi C: Genetic divergence from Salmonella choleraesuis and pathogenic convergence with Salmonella typhi. *PLoS ONE* **2009**, *4*. [CrossRef]
8. Achtman, M.; Wain, J.; Weill, F.-X.; Nair, S.; Zhou, Z.; Sangal, V.; Krauland, M.G.; Hale, J.L.; Harbottle, H.; Uesbeck, A. Multilocus sequence typing as a replacement for serotyping in Salmonella enterica. *PLoS Pathog.* **2012**, *8*, e1002776. [CrossRef]
9. Didelot, X.; Achtman, M.; Parkhill, J.; Thomson, N.R.; Falush, D. A bimodal pattern of relatedness between the Salmonella Paratyphi A and Typhi genomes: Convergence or divergence by homologous recombination? *Genome Res.* **2007**, *17*, 61–68. [CrossRef]
10. Holt, K.E.; Thomson, N.R.; Wain, J.; Langridge, G.C.; Hasan, R.; Bhutta, Z.A.; Quail, M.A.; Norbertczak, H.; Walker, D.; Simmonds, M. Pseudogene accumulation in the evolutionary histories of Salmonella enterica serovars Paratyphi A and Typhi. *BMC Genom.* **2009**, *10*, 36. [CrossRef]
11. Key, F.M.; Posth, C.; Esquivel-Gomez, L.R.; Hübler, R.; Spyrou, M.A.; Neumann, G.U.; Furtwängler, A.; Sabin, S.; Burri, M.; Wissgott, A. Emergence of human-adapted Salmonella enterica is linked to the Neolithization process. *Nat. Ecol. Evol.* **2020**, *4*, 324–333. [CrossRef]
12. Maskey, A.P.; Day, J.N.; Tuan, P.Q.; Thwaites, G.E.; Campbell, J.I.; Zimmerman, M.; Farrar, J.J.; Basnyat, B. Salmonella enterica serovar Paratyphi A and S. enterica serovar Typhi cause indistinguishable clinical syndromes in Kathmandu, Nepal. *Clin. Infect. Dis.* **2006**, *42*, 1247–1253. [CrossRef] [PubMed]
13. Giglioli, G. Paratyphoid C an endemic disease of British Guiana: a clinical and pathological outline. B. paratyphosum C as a pyogenic organism. *Proc. R. Soc. Med.* **1929**, *23*, 165–167. [CrossRef] [PubMed]
14. Tenbroeck, C.; Li, C.; Yü, H. Studies on paratyphoid C bacilli isolated in China. *J. Exp. Med.* **1931**, *53*, 307–315. [CrossRef] [PubMed]
15. Giglioli, G. Paratyphoid C, an endemic disease in British Guiana. *Epidemiol. Infect.* **1929**, *29*, 273–281. [CrossRef] [PubMed]
16. Giglioli, G. Post-mortem and histo-pathological notes on twenty fatal cases of bact. Paratyphosum C infection in British Guiana. *West Indian Med. J.* **1958**, *7*, 29–38.
17. Jacobs, M.; Koornhof, H.; Crisp, S.; Palmhert, H.; Fitzstephens, A. Enteric fever caused by Salmonella paratyphi C in South and South West Africa. *S. Afr. Med. J.* **1978**, *54*, 434–438.
18. Chiu, C.-H.; Su, L.-H.; Chu, C. Salmonella enterica serotype Choleraesuis: Epidemiology, pathogenesis, clinical disease, and treatment. *Clin. Microbiol. Rev.* **2004**, *17*, 311–322. [CrossRef]
19. Langridge, G.C.; Fookes, M.; Connor, T.R.; Feltwell, T.; Feasey, N.; Parsons, B.N.; Seth-Smith, H.M.; Barquist, L.; Stedman, A.; Humphrey, T. Patterns of genome evolution that have accompanied host adaptation in Salmonella. *Proc. Natl. Acad. Sci. USA* **2015**, *112*, 863–868. [CrossRef]

20. Harris, S.R.; Feil, E.J.; Holden, M.T.; Quail, M.A.; Nickerson, E.K.; Chantratita, N.; Gardete, S.; Tavares, A.; Day, N.; Lindsay, J.A. Evolution of MRSA during hospital transmission and intercontinental spread. *Science* **2010**, *327*, 469–474. [CrossRef]
21. Zhou, Z.; Alikhan, N.-F.; Mohamed, K.; Fan, Y.; Achtman, M.; Brown, D.; Chattaway, M.; Dallman, T.; Delahay, R.; Kornschober, C. The EnteroBase user's guide, with case studies on Salmonella transmissions, Yersinia pestis phylogeny, and Escherichia core genomic diversity. *Genome Res.* **2020**, *30*, 138–152. [CrossRef]
22. Holt, K.E.; Parkhill, J.; Mazzoni, C.J.; Roumagnac, P.; Weill, F.-X.; Goodhead, I.; Rance, R.; Baker, S.; Maskell, D.J.; Wain, J. High-throughput sequencing provides insights into genome variation and evolution in Salmonella Typhi. *Nat. Genet.* **2008**, *40*, 987. [CrossRef] [PubMed]
23. Zerbino, D.R.; Birney, E. Velvet: Algorithms for de novo short read assembly using de Bruijn graphs. *Genome Res.* **2008**, *18*, 821–829. [CrossRef] [PubMed]
24. Staden, R.; Judge, D.P.; Bonfield, J.K. Managing sequencing projects in the GAP4 environment. In *Introduction to Bioinformatics*; Springer: Berlin/Heidelberg, Germany, 2003; pp. 327–344.
25. Assefa, S.; Keane, T.M.; Otto, T.D.; Newbold, C.; Berriman, M. ABACAS: Algorithm-based automatic contiguation of assembled sequences. *Bioinformatics* **2009**, *25*, 1968–1969. [CrossRef] [PubMed]
26. Otto, T.D.; Sanders, M.; Berriman, M.; Newbold, C. Iterative Correction of Reference Nucleotides (iCORN) using second generation sequencing technology. *Bioinformatics* **2010**, *26*, 1704–1707. [CrossRef] [PubMed]
27. Otto, T.D.; Dillon, G.P.; Degrave, W.S.; Berriman, M. RATT: Rapid annotation transfer tool. *Nucleic Acids Res.* **2011**, *39*, e57. [CrossRef] [PubMed]
28. Bolger, A.M.; Lohse, M.; Usadel, B. Trimmomatic: A flexible trimmer for Illumina sequence data. *Bioinformatics* **2014**, *30*, 2114–2120. [CrossRef]
29. Carver, T.J.; Rutherford, K.M.; Berriman, M.; Rajandream, M.-A.; Barrell, B.G.; Parkhill, J. ACT: The Artemis comparison tool. *Bioinformatics* **2005**, *21*, 3422–3423. [CrossRef]
30. Chen, F.; Mackey, A.J.; Stoeckert, C.J., Jr.; Roos, D.S. OrthoMCL-DB: Querying a comprehensive multi-species collection of ortholog groups. *Nucleic Acids Res.* **2006**, *34*, D363–D368. [CrossRef]
31. Kingsley, R.A.; Langridge, G.; Smith, S.E.; Makendi, C.; Fookes, M.; Wileman, T.M.; El Ghany, M.A.; Keith Turner, A.; Dyson, Z.A.; Sridhar, S. Functional analysis of Salmonella Typhi adaptation to survival in water. *Environ. Microbiol.* **2018**, *20*, 4079–4090. [CrossRef]
32. Conway, J.R.; Lex, A.; Gehlenborg, N. UpSetR: An R package for the visualization of intersecting sets and their properties. *Bioinformatics* **2017**, *33*, 2938–2940. [CrossRef]
33. Nuccio, S.-P.; Bäumler, A.J. Comparative analysis of Salmonella genomes identifies a metabolic network for escalating growth in the inflamed gut. *MBio* **2014**, *5*, e00929-14. [CrossRef] [PubMed]
34. Feng, Y.; Chien, K.-Y.; Chen, H.-L.; Chiu, C.-H. Pseudogene recoding revealed from proteomic analysis of Salmonella serovars. *J. Proteome Res.* **2012**, *11*, 171–1719. [CrossRef] [PubMed]
35. Wheeler, N.E.; Gardner, P.P.; Barquist, L. Machine learning identifies signatures of host adaptation in the bacterial pathogen Salmonella enterica. *PLoS Genet.* **2018**, *14*, e1007333. [CrossRef] [PubMed]
36. Zhou, Z.; Lundstrøm, I.; Tran-Dien, A.; Duchêne, S.; Alikhan, N.-F.; Sergeant, M.J.; Langridge, G.; Fotakis, A.K.; Nair, S.; Stenøien, H.K.; et al. Pan-genome analysis of ancient and modern Salmonella enterica demonstrates genomic stability of the invasive para C lineage for millennia. *Curr. Biol.* **2018**, *28*, 2420–2428.e2410. [CrossRef]
37. Vågene, Å.J.; Herbig, A.; Campana, M.G.; García, N.M.R.; Warinner, C.; Sabin, S.; Spyrou, M.A.; Valtueña, A.A.; Huson, D.; Tuross, N.; et al. Salmonella enterica genomes from victims of a major sixteenth century epidemic in Mexico. *Nat. Ecol. Evol.* **2018**, *2*, 520–528. [CrossRef]
38. Lou, L.; Zhang, P.; Piao, R.; Wang, Y. Salmonella pathogenicity island 1 (SPI-1) and its complex regulatory network. *Front. Cell Infect. Mi* **2019**, *9*, 270. [CrossRef]
39. Mohammed, M.; Cormican, M. Whole genome sequencing provides insights into the genetic determinants of invasiveness in Salmonella Dublin. *Epidemiol. Infect.* **2016**, *144*, 2430–2439. [CrossRef]
40. Winter, S.E.; Thiennimitr, P.; Winter, M.G.; Butler, B.P.; Huseby, D.L.; Crawford, R.W.; Russell, J.M.; Bevins, C.L.; Adams, L.G.; Tsolis, R.M. Gut inflammation provides a respiratory electron acceptor for Salmonella. *Nature* **2010**, *467*, 426–429. [CrossRef]

9

New Roles for Two-Component System Response Regulators of *Salmonella enterica* Serovar Typhi during Host Cell Interactions

Claudie Murret-Labarthe, Maud Kerhoas, Karine Dufresne and France Daigle *

Département de microbiologie, infectiologie, immunologie, Université de Montréal, Montréal, QC H3T 1J4, Canada; c.m.labarthe@gmail.com (C.M.-L.); maud1693@hotmail.com (M.K.); karine.dufresne@umontreal.ca (K.D.)

* Correspondence: france.daigle@umontreal.ca

Abstract: In order to survive external stresses, bacteria need to adapt quickly to changes in their environment. One adaptive mechanism is to coordinate and alter their gene expression by using two-component systems (TCS). TCS are composed of a sensor kinase that activates a transcriptional response regulator by phosphorylation. TCS are involved in motility, virulence, nutrient acquisition, and envelope stress in many bacteria. The pathogenic bacteria *Salmonella enterica* serovar Typhi (*S.* Typhi) possess 30 TCSs, is specific to humans, and causes typhoid fever. Here, we have individually deleted each of the 30 response regulators. We have determined their role during interaction with host cells (epithelial cells and macrophages). Deletion of most of the systems (24 out of 30) resulted in a significant change during infection. We have identified 32 new phenotypes associated with TCS of *S.* Typhi. Some previously known phenotypes associated with TCSs in *Salmonella* were also confirmed. We have also uncovered phenotypic divergence between *Salmonella* serovars, as distinct phenotypes between *S.* Typhi and *S.* Typhimurium were identified for *cpxR*. This finding highlights the importance of specifically studying *S.* Typhi to understand its pathogenesis mechanisms and to develop strategies to potentially reduce typhoid infections.

Keywords: *Salmonella* Typhi; two-component system; *cpxR*

1. Introduction

Bacteria possess a variety of systems that enable them to respond to diverse signals received from the external environment. These signals are mainly detected by two-component systems (TCS) composed of a histidine sensor kinase (SK) and a response regulator (RR). Physical or chemical signals, such as changes in extracellular ion concentrations, pH, oxygen, osmolarity, quorum sensing, and the presence of antibiotics are some of the signals detected by TCS. TCS are involved in adaptation to several conditions, notably stress conditions, host–pathogen interactions, symbiotic interactions, and intracellular signaling [1,2].

The SK partner of the TCS is located in the inner membrane and generally comprises two domains, a receiver and a transmitter domain that contains a kinase activity with a conserved histidine residue. Typically, the RR proteins are located in the cytoplasm and also comprise two domains, a receiver domain in the N-terminal section of the protein containing a conserved aspartate residue and a response domain in the C-terminal of the protein. When a signal is detected by the SK, this results in autophoshorylation of the conserved histidine residue, an ATP-dependent process. The SK then activates the RR through transfer of its phosphorylated group to the conserved RR aspartate residue.

Once activated, the RR initiates the adaptive transcriptional response, through activation or repression of genes that will adjust the bacterial lifestyle to the conditions encountered [3].

Salmonella enterica serovar Typhi (*S.* Typhi) is a human-specific bacterial pathogen and the etiologic agent of the typhoid fever. This disease is common in Africa and Southeast Asia and causes between 11.9 and 26.9 million cases and 128,000 to 216,500 deaths per year [4]. Infection with this pathogen occurs through the ingestion of contaminated food or water. Once ingested, *Salmonella* must first resist stomach acidity [5,6], then reach the small intestine, cross the mucosal barrier of the intestine, and gain access to intestinal epithelial cells. Bacteria can then invade epithelial cells using the type-three secretion system (T3SS) located on *Salmonella* pathogenicity island 1 (SPI-1) [7,8]. *S.* Typhi does not elicit a strong intestinal immune response or inflammation, mainly by producing the Vi capsule [9]. It crosses the intestinal barrier, infects macrophages, and survives within vacuoles by using a second T3SS located on SPI-2 [10,11]. *S.* Typhi then causes a systemic infection by disseminating to deeper tissues including spleen, liver, bone marrow, and gallbladder [12].

Currently, most of our knowledge concerning TCS was obtained from studies done in *Escherichia coli* or *Salmonella enterica* serovar Typhimurium. Thus far, only six TCS have been characterized in *S.* Typhi. Both the EnvZ-OmpR system and the Rcs system activate the expression of the Vi capsule [13,14]. The Rcs system also represses invasion proteins and flagellin [14–17]. The PhoPQ system regulates the *S.* Typhi-specific CdtB, ClyA, and TaiA toxins [18–20], is expressed in typhoid patients [21], and a *phoPQ* deletion was used in a live attenuated *S.* Typhi vaccine [22]. The SsrAB system had no role in survival in macrophages in *S.* Typhi [23]. The CpxAR system is involved in adhesion and invasion of human intestinal epithelial cells and is activated by osmolarity [24]. The QseCB system is activated by several signals, including neurotransmitters (epinephrine and norepinephrine) [25,26], and invasion of epithelial cells increased in a *qseB* mutant of *S.* Typhi [27]. UhpBA regulates glucose-6-phosphate transport [28]. A comparative study of the transcriptional profile performed in *S.* Typhi indicates that UhpA was involved in the sulfur assimilation pathway [29]. Other TCS have not been studied in *S.* Typhi and some TCS have not been investigated in *S.* Typhimurium (CitAB, CreCB, DpiBA, TctED, and TorSR).

As some TCS play a role in *S.* Typhi infection, it is likely that other TCS may have a significant role in different stages of disease by this pathogen. To study the TCS of *S.* Typhi, we have deleted each of the genes encoding RR proteins, since it has been shown that some SK can also activate non-specific RR and complement defects of the specific corresponding SK mutant [30]. Non-polar deletions of genes encoding each RR protein were created by allelic exchange and we evaluated the ability of each mutant to adhere, invade, and replicate in human epithelial cells and to be phagocytosed and survive in human macrophages. This study represents a comprehensive characterization of all *S.* Typhi TCS and identifies a potential role for each of these systems in *S.* Typhi pathogenesis.

2. Materials and Methods

2.1. Bacterial Strains and Growth Conditions

S. Typhi strain ISP1820 was used throughout this study as the main wild-type strain [31]. Strains and plasmids used in this study are listed in Supplementary Tables S1 and S2, respectively. Bacteria were routinely grown overnight in Luria-Bertani (LB) broth, with agitation at 37 °C, unless indicated otherwise. Antibiotic or supplements were added at the following concentration: 34 μg/mL chloramphenicol and 50 μg/mL diaminopimelic acid, when required. Bacterial transformation was performed using the calcium/manganese-based method, as previously described [32].

2.2. Chromosomal Deletion of TCS Regulatory Genes

Thirty TCS were identified in the sequenced genome of *S.* Typhi strain CT18 [33] by searching for DNA binding protein and regulator. The non-polar deletion of all the response regulator (RR) encoding genes were obtained by allelic exchange, as described previously [34], using the overlap-extension

PCR method [35]. Deletions were confirmed by PCR. The primers used for mutagenesis are listed in Supplementary Table S3.

2.3. Interaction with Cultured Human Epithelial Intestinal Cells

The INT-407 (ATCC CCL-6) cells were cultivated in Eagle minimal essential medium (EMEM) (Wisent, St-Bruno, QC, Canada) supplemented with 10% heat-inactivated fetal bovine serum (FBS) (Wisent) and 25 mM HEPES (Wisent, St-Bruno, QC, Canada). The gentamicin protection assay described previously was adapted to 96-well plates and performed at a multiplicity of infection (MOI) of 20 [34]. Bacteria were grown overnight in static condition (low aeration) in LB-NaCl (300 mM) to induce SPI-1 and were added in triplicate. After 90 min, infected cells were washed with phosphate-buffer saline (PBS) and fresh medium supplemented with 50 μg/mL gentamicin was added to kill the extracellular bacteria. Cells were lysed with PBS and 0.1% sodium deoxycholate (PBS-DOC) at 90 min (adhesion), 180 min (invasion), and 18 h (survival) post-infection. Serial dilutions were performed for enumeration of viable colony counts by colony-forming units (CFU/mL). The assay was performed at least three times in triplicate.

2.4. Infection of Cultured Macrophages

The THP-1 (ATCC TIB-202) cells were cultivated in RPMI 1640 (Wisent, St-Bruno, QC, Canada) supplemented with 10% heat-inactivated FBS (Wisent), 1 mM sodium pyruvate (Wisent), and 1% MEM non-essential amino acids (Wisent, St-Bruno, QC, Canada). The human monocytes cells were differentiated into macrophages by addition of 10^{-7} M phorbol 12-myristate 13 acetate (Sigma) for 48 h before the infection. Similarly, the RAW264.7 (ATCC TIB-71) murine macrophages were cultivated in Dulbecco's Modified Eagle's Medium (DMEM; Wisent, St-Bruno, QC, Canada). The method was adapted to 96-well plates and performed at a MOI of 10 [36]. To obtain a similar number of intracellular bacteria, a MOI of 10 was used for macrophages to compensate for the phagocytic activity. Briefly, following an overnight growth in LB broth, the strains were added in triplicate. After 30 min, infected cells were washed with PBS, treated with gentamicin (50 ug/mL), and lysed with PBS-DOC 0.1% at 30 min (phagocytosis), and 18 h (survival) post-infection, then, serial dilutions were performed for enumeration of viable colony counts (CFU/mL). Each deletion was tested at least three times in triplicate.

2.5. Motility Assays

Motility assays were performed in a tube, containing the «Motility Test Medium» (BBL, BD, Mississauga, ON, Canada), in which a solution of 1% of triphenyltetrazolium chloride was added. These agar tubes were inoculated by stabbing the agar with an overnight culture of bacteria. The tubes were then incubated at 37 °C for approximately 18 h, to evaluate the motility of the mutants. For each deletion, this assay was performed at least three times. Motility assays on plates were performed as described previously [37].

3. Results

3.1. Deletion and Characterization of RR Mutants

We have identified 30 RR genes in the genome of *S.* Typhi and an overview of their putative functions is summarized in Table 1. These TCS were all detected in the genome of the closely related serovar Typhimurium. However, these two serovars have a different host range, and cause distinct disease, suggesting that potential differences between these serovars may involve differences in gene regulation. All RR were deleted individually. Deletion of an internal fragment of each RR was achieved by allelic exchange in *S.* Typhi strain ISP1820. Each marker-less deletion was in frame, to avoid any polar effect. Mutants were characterized for their growth, susceptibility to aminoglycoside, and motility. All mutants had a similar growth curve in LB compared to the wild-type parent strain (data not shown). The *arcA* mutant produced smaller colonies on LB agar. The mutants were all sensitive to gentamicin and most mutants were motile as the wild-type (except for *cheY*, as expected, and *ompR*, which demonstrated a reduced swimming area, 85% of the wild-type, in motility medium).

Table 1. Two-component systems of *Salmonella* Typhi and their putative function.

SK	RR	Function
ArcB (STY3507)	ArcA (STY4947)	Global aerobic respiration control; oxidative stress [38,39]; SPI-1 activation [40]; motility [41]; defective in invasion and survival [42]
BaeS (STY2343)	BaeR (STY2155)	Envelope stress: (antimicrobial resistance (AMR) and metal resistance) [43,44]
CitA (STY0062)	CitB (STY0061)	Anaerobic citrate fermentation [a] [45]
CheA (STY2130)	CheY (STY2125)	Chemotaxis; required for virulence in mice [46], and in invasion [47]
CopS (STY1127)	CopR (STY1128)	Uncharacterized [a]
CpxA (STY3813)	CpxR (STY3812)	Membrane stress (AMR and metal resistance) [48–52]; SPI-1 repression [53,54] and SPI-2 regulation [55]; virulence [53,55,56]
CreC (STY4936)	CreB (STY4935)	Carbon source metabolism [a] [57]
DcuS (STY4502)	DcuR (STY4501)	C4-dicarboxylates catabolism [a] [57–59]
DpiB (STY0674)	DpiA (STY0675)	SOS response [a] [60]
GlnL (STY3875)	GlnG (STY3876)	Nitrogen response [61,62]
HydH (STY3712)	HydG (STY3211)	Zinc transport [a] [63]
KdpD (STY0744)	KdpE (STY0743)	Potassium transport [64], *C. elegans* colonization [65]
NarX (STY1286)	NarL (STY1285)	Nitrate responsive [66,67]
NarQ (STY2718)	NarP (STY2472)	Nitrate respiration [66] [a]; Involved in virulence [68]
EnvZ (STY4295)	OmpR (STY4294)	Envelope stress response. Osmolarity and acid resistance [69,70]; virulence [71], SPI-1 and SPI-2 control [72–75], Vi capsule activation [13,14]; adhesion and invasion [76]
PgtB (STY2634)	PgtA (STY2633)	Phosphoglycerate transport [77]
PhoR (STY0433)	PhoB (STY0432)	Inorganic phosphate assimilation [78]; SPI-1 regulation [79]
PhoQ (STY1270)	PhoP (STY1271)	Global virulence regulator [80]; Magnesium transport [81]; AMR [82–84]; invasion [85]; survival in macrophages [80]
PmrB (STY4490)	PmrA (STY4491)	LPS modification, AMR resistance, virulence [27,86]; SPI-2 repression [87]
QseC (STY3355)	QseB (STY3354)	Motility, invasion [27], macrophage survival [25], virulence [25,88,89]
QseE (STY2811)	QseF (STY2809)	Invasion and intramacrophage replication [25]; virulence [25]
RcsC (STY2496)	RcsB (STY2495)	Cell envelope stress response, Vi capsule activation [16]; virulence [90]; AMR [91]; LPS modifications; oxidative and acidic stress [92]; invasion [17]
RstB (STY1651)	RstA (STY1647)	Motility [93]; iron acquisition [94,95]
BarA (STY3096)	SirA (STY2155)	Virulence [96], SPI-1 [97], SPI-2 [97], motility [98], Vi capsule [99]; invasion [100]
SsrA (STY1728)	SsrB (STY1729)	SPI-2 regulator [11,101], oxidative stress [102]; SPI-1 repression [103]
TctE (STY2903)	TctD (STY2904)	Tricarboxylate transport [104]
TorS (STY3951)	*TorR* (STY3954)	Trimethylamine-N-oxide respiration (anaerobic) [a] [105]
TtrS (STY1735)	TtrR (STY1733)	Tetrathionate respiration [106]
UhpB (STY3993)	UhpA (STY3992)	Hexose phosphate transport [28], sulfur assimilation [29]
YehU (STY2389)	YehT (STY2388)	Poorly characterized, regulation of the carbon starvation protein (CstA) [107]

[a] Role in Escherichia coli.

3.2. Adhesion, Invasion, and Replication in Epithelial Cells

Passage through the intestinal epithelial cell barrier is a key step in the pathogenesis of *S.* Typhi. We used infection of epithelial cells to evaluate adhesion, invasion, and replication effects of the TCS mutant of *S.* Typhi in these cell type. The wild-type *S.* Typhi ISP1820 strain was used as the reference control and its isogenic *invA* (SPI-1)/*ssrB* (SPI-2) mutant (here referred as ΔSPIs) were used as a low virulence control, as this strain exhibits impaired host cell entry.

The adhesion level for the different TCS mutants ranged from 45 to 144% of the wild-type (Figure 1A). There were 5 mutants that showed a significant change in adherence compared to the wild-type strain. Three mutants (*cheY*, *ompR* and *pgtA*) were less adherent and 2 mutants (*narP* and *rcsB*) were more adherent. The *ompR* was the least adherent, whereas the *rcsB* mutant had the highest level of cell adherence.

For the cell invasion phenotype, differences in invasion varied from 7 to 370% of the wild-type, and several mutants (16/30) showed a significant difference in cell invasion compared to the wild-type strain. Seven mutants showed increased invasion (*cheY*, *citB*, *narP*, *pgtA*, *pmrA*, *qseB* and *rcsB*) and 9 showed decreased invasion (*arcA*, *baeR*, *cpxR*, *ompR*, *phoP*, *qseF*, *sirA*, *tctD* and *torR*) (Figure 1B). The negative control (ΔSPIs) showed only 1.3% invasion compared to the wild-type, as expected. The TCS mutant demonstrating the most decreased invasion was *sirA* and the mutant with the highest increased invasion was *rcsB*.

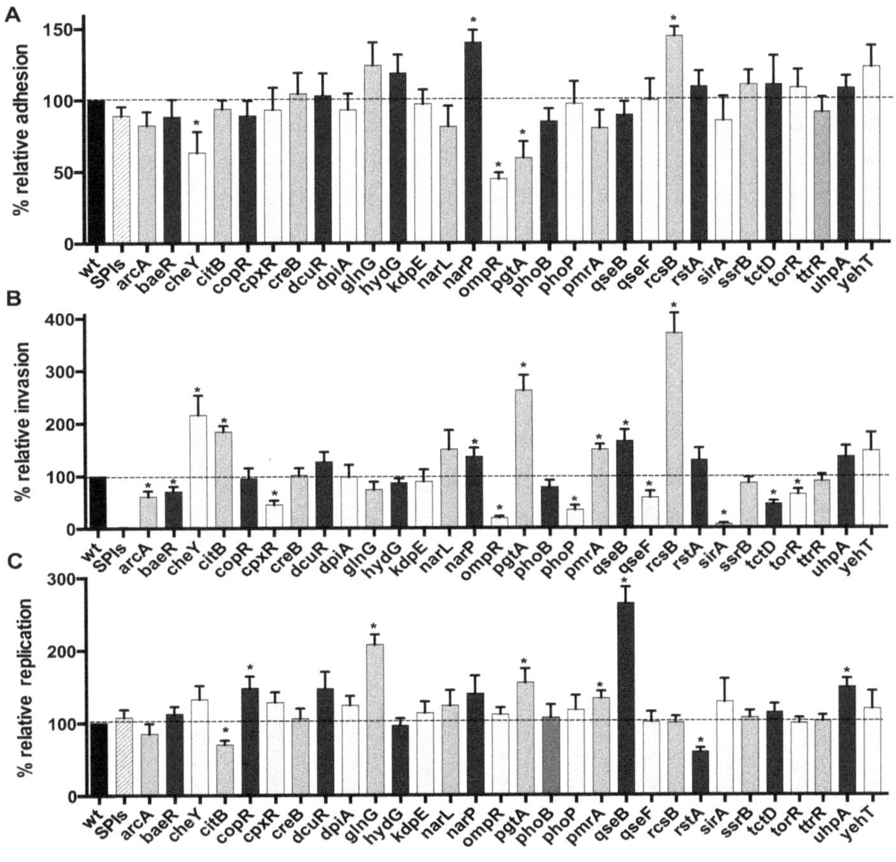

Figure 1. Effect of loss of TCS response regulators on interaction with human epithelial cells. INT-407 epithelial cells were infected with *S.* Typhi wild-type strain and the isogenic RR mutants, and the level of bacteria associated with cells was determined upon adherence (90 min) (**A**), invasion (180 min) (**B**), or after 18 h (**C**). All assays were conducted in triplicate and repeated independently at least three times. The results are expressed as the mean ± SEM of the replicate experiments. Significant differences (* $p < 0.0001$) in the levels recovered as compared to the wild-type were determined by the Student's unpaired *t*-test. The dashed line corresponds to the wild-type level.

For intracellular replication, the range was from 70 to 264% of the wild-type. There were 8 mutants demonstrating significantly different levels of replication, 6 that were higher (*copR*, *glnG*, *pgtA*, *pmrA*, *qseB*, and *uhpA*) and 2 that were lower (*citB* and *rstA*) than the wild-type control (Figure 1C). The *rstA* mutant had the greatest decrease, whereas the *qseB* mutant had the highest level of replication in epithelial cells. Interestingly, several mutants that were defective in invasion were able to replicate similarly to the wild-type.

3.3. Uptake and Survival in Macrophages

Some TCSs are important for survival of *Salmonella* inside macrophages, and survival within these cells represents a crucial step in the pathogenesis and virulence of *S.* Typhi to disseminate systemically. Thus, we investigated the role of each TCS in uptake and survival in macrophages. The wild-type *S.* Typhi ISP1820 strain was used as the reference control and the *phoP24* isogenic mutant (PhoP constitutive) [108], known to be defective in virulence and macrophages survival [109], was used as a low virulence control. This control was chosen as the isogenic *invA* (SPI-1)/*ssrB* (SPI-2) mutant (ΔSPIs) to survive as the wild-type strain in macrophage [23]. The level of internalization by macrophage varied from between 76 to 404% of the wild-type (Figure 2A). There were 10 mutants with a significant difference in uptake by macrophage compared to the wild-type strain. Seven of the mutants showed increased uptake (*arcA*, *kdpE*, *narL*, *narP*, *ompR*, *pgtA*, and *rcsB*) and three mutants (*cpxR*, *dcuR*, and *glnG*) showed decreased macrophage uptake. The *glnG* mutant demonstrated the lowest level of uptake and the *rcsB* mutant showed the highest level of uptake by macrophage.

The level of survival in macrophages ranged from 29 to 249% of the wild-type (Figure 2B). There were 16 mutants with a significant difference in survival compared to the wild-type strain, 6 showed an increased survival (*copR*, *pmrA*, *rcsB*, *sirA*, *tctD*, and *torR*) and 10 demonstrated a decreased survival (*arcA*, *baeR*, *cheY*, *citB*, *cpxR*, *dpiA*, *kdpE*, *narP*, *ompR*, and *phoP*). The *phoP* mutant demonstrated the lowest survival and the *rcsB* mutant had the highest level of survival in macrophage.

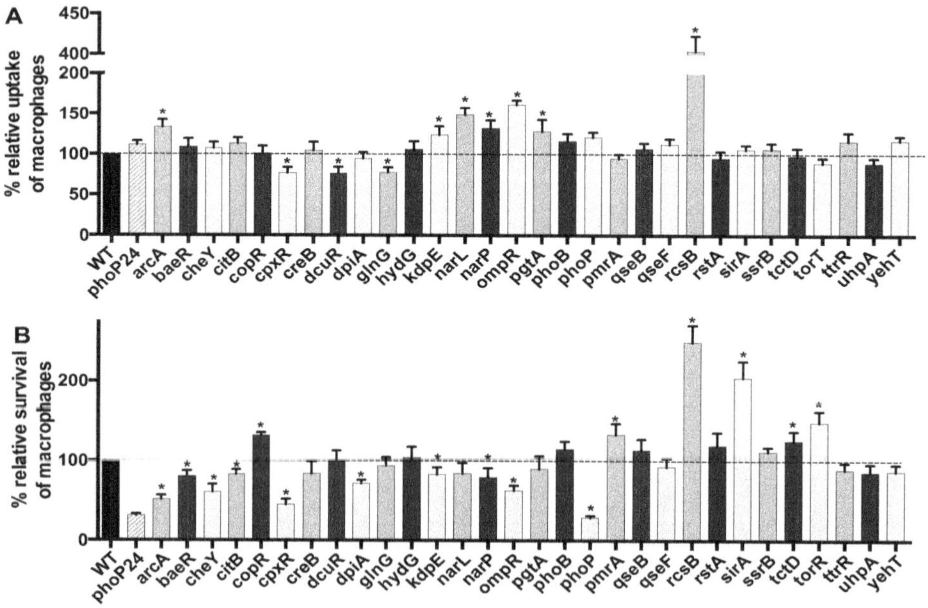

Figure 2. Effect of loss of TCS response regulators during interaction with human macrophages. THP-1 cells were differentiated into macrophages and infected with *S.* Typhi wild-type strain and the isogenic RR mutants. The level of bacterial uptake (phagocytosis) (**A**) and the level of survival after 18 h infection (**B**) were determined. All assays were conducted in duplicate and repeated independently at least three times. The results are expressed as the mean ± SEM of replicate experiments. Significant differences (* $p < 0.0001$) as compared to wild-type were determined by the Student's unpaired *t*-test. The dashed line corresponds to the wild-type level.

3.4. Complementation

In order to confirm that the phenotypic difference was associated with the RR mutation, we selected 4 mutants that were strongly under- or over-represented compared to the wild-type strain in invasion or survival level in macrophages. The *cpxR*, *ompR*, *rcsB*, and *sirA* mutants were complemented with a wild-type copy of the gene on a low-copy vector. Interactions with epithelial cells and macrophages were evaluated. The wild-type levels association with cells were restored in the complemented strains (Figure 3).

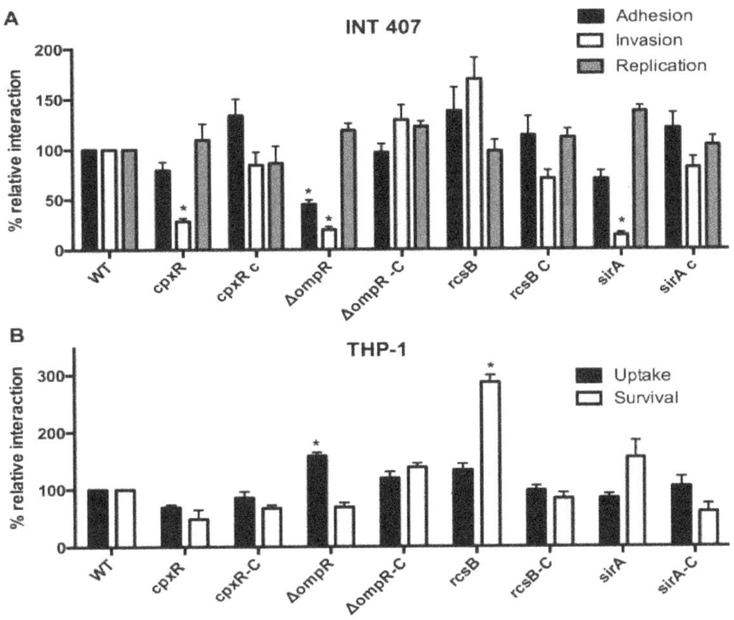

Figure 3. Complementation. Epithelial INT-407 cells (**A**) and THP-1 macrophages (**B**) were infected with *S.* Typhi wild-type strain, the *cpxR*, *ompR*, *rcsB*, and *sirA* mutants and complemented mutants with a wild-type copy on a low-copy vector. All assays were conducted in triplicate and repeated independently at least three times. The results are expressed as the mean ± SEM of the replicate experiments. Significant differences (* $p < 0.0001$) in the level between the wild-type and the mutant were determined by the Student's unpaired *t*-test. The dashed line corresponds to the wild-type level.

3.5. Impact of the Vi Antigen

It was previously demonstrated that RscB and OmpR regulate the Vi capsule [14–17,19,20]. As these TCS showed strong phenotypes, often opposite, except for phagocytosis, we investigated the role of the Vi antigen during host cell interaction. We have constructed a *tviB* mutant as well as a double *tviB-ompR* and a double *tviB-rcsB* mutant and evaluated these strains with epithelial cells and macrophages (Figure 4). The lower level of adhesion to epithelial cells observed for the *ompR* mutant was specific to *ompR* as the *tviB* mutant was not significantly different than the wild-type, whereas the double *tviB-ompR* was similar to the *ompR* mutant. Similarly, the high level of invasion of epithelial cells observed for the *rcsB* mutant was specific to the *rcsB* mutation as the mutant and the double mutant *tviB-rcsB* were both significantly different than the wild-type but not the *tviB* mutant. The loss of the Vi antigen did not increase the phagocytosis and survival level in macrophages, suggesting that the phenotypes observed were specific to the *ompR* and the *rcsB* mutation. We have confirmed by immuno-staining that the *ompR*, *rcsB*, and *tviB* mutants did not express the Vi antigen compared to the wild-type strain and other mutants (Figure 4C).

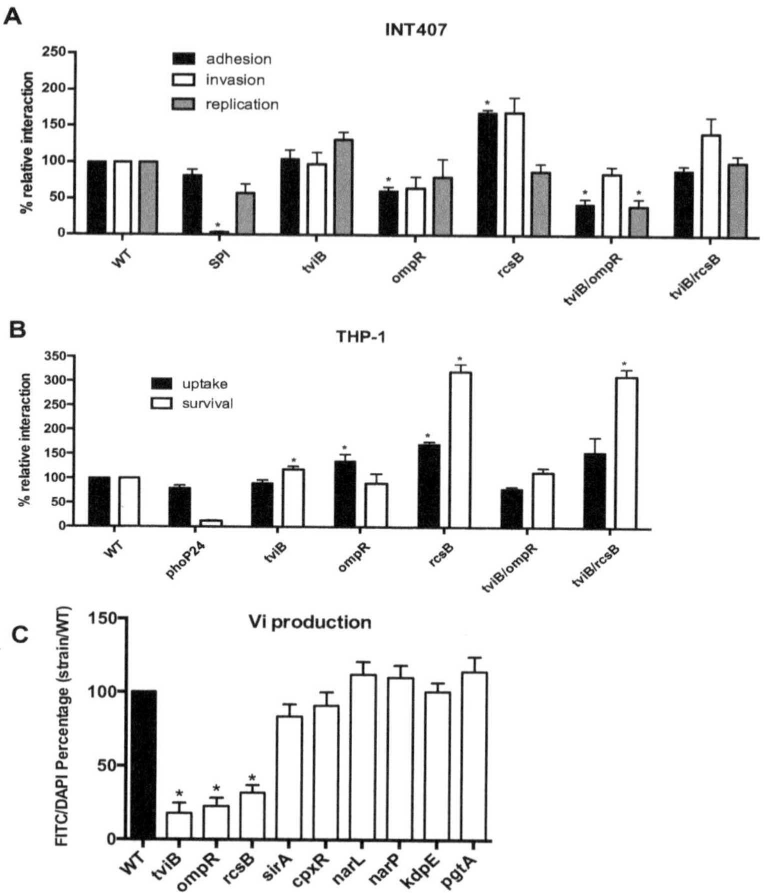

Figure 4. Role of Vi capsule. Epithelial INT-407 cells (**A**) and THP-1 macrophages (**B**) were infected with *S.* Typhi wild-type strain, the *tviB, ompR, rcsB* and *the double mutant tviB-ompR* and *tviB-rcsB* mutants. (**C**) Production of the Vi antigen by immuno-staining. All assays were conducted in triplicate and repeated independently at least three times. The results are expressed as the mean ± SEM of the replicate experiments. Significant differences (* $p < 0.0001$) in the level between the wild-type and the mutant were determined by the Student's unpaired *t*-test.

3.6. Strain Specificity

As all mutants were tested in *S.* Typhi strain ISP1820, we also investigated if the *ompR* phenotype was conserved in another *S.* Typhi strain. We generated an *ompR* deletion in *S.* Typhi Ty2, and this mutant also showed decreased infection of epithelial cells or macrophages (Figure 5).

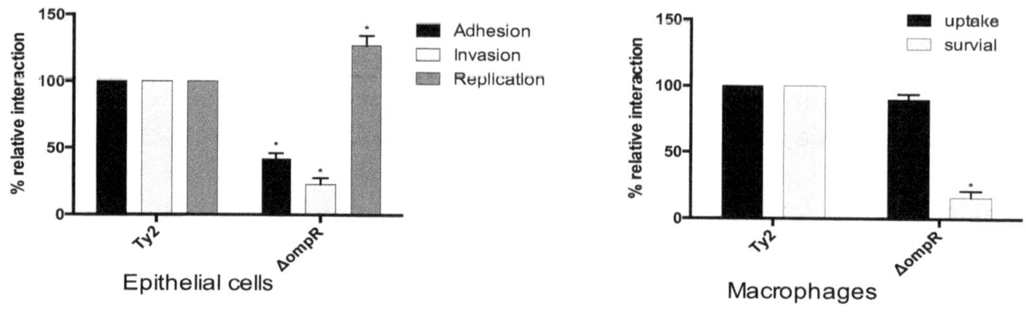

Figure 5. Role of *ompR* mutant in *S.* Typhi strain Ty2. Epithelial INT-407 cells and THP-1 macrophages were infected with *S.* Typhi Ty2 strain and its isogenic *ompR* mutant. All assays were conducted in triplicate and repeated independently at least three times. The results are expressed as the mean ± SEM of the replicate experiments. Significant differences (* $p < 0.05$) compared to the wild-type were determined by the Student's unpaired *t*-test.

Then, as the *cpxR* mutant was found to be significantly less invasive than the wild-type strain in *S.* Typhi, but was able to invade and replicate in epithelial cells at levels comparable to the wild-type strain in *S.* Typhimurium [53,76], we constructed this mutant in *S.* Typhimurium SL1344 and investigated its interaction with cells (Figure 6). During interaction with epithelial cells, the *cpxR* mutant of *S.* Typhimurium was similar to the wild-type strain, suggesting that the effect is strain-specific to *S.* Typhi. There was also no difference between the wild-type and the SL1344 *cpxR* mutant when tested in the murine macrophages RAW264.7.

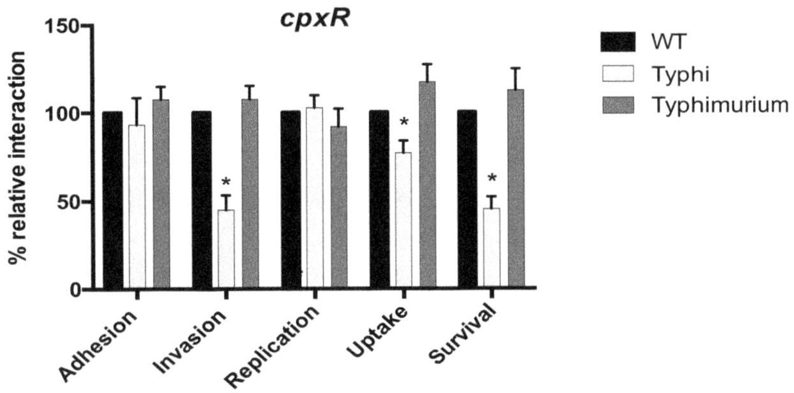

Figure 6. Comparison of the *cpxR* mutant of *S.* Typhi and *S.* Typhimurium. Epithelial INT-407 cells and THP-1 macrophages were infected with *S.* Typhi ISP1820 strain and *S.* Typhimurium SL1344 and their isogenic *cpxR* mutant. Both WT strains are settled at 100 percent. All assays were conducted in triplicate and repeated independently at least three times. The results are expressed as the mean ± SEM of the replicate experiments. Significant differences (* $p < 0.0001$) compared to the wild-type were determined by the Student's unpaired *t*-test.

4. Discussion

TCS are usually the first to detect a perturbation in the intracellular or extracellular environment and will react quickly to modify bacterial gene expression. They are involved in sensing a variety of signals (pH, ions, nutrients, stress, etc.). Therefore, TCS are critical for bacterial adaptation and survival. Here, we have identified 30 TCS in the genome of *S.* Typhi and summarized their putative function and role in *Salmonella* (Table 1). We have deleted each of the TCS regulator encoding genes from *S.* Typhi and tested interactions with human epithelial cells (adhesion, invasion, and replication) and macrophages (uptake and survival), which constitute two important niches of *S.* Typhi infection. Moreover, these mutants represent important tools to advance our knowledge of *S.* Typhi pathogenesis by investigating their roles during interactions with cells or under different environmental conditions.

All the TCS mutants grew similarly to the wild-type strain in liquid culture. Most of the TCS mutants (24/30) showed a significant difference compared to the wild-type strain during at least one step of infection (adhesion, invasion, replication, uptake, or survival) (Table 2). There were 9 phenotypes previously associated with 8 TCS in *S.* Typhimurium that were confirmed in *S.* Typhi (*arcA*, *cheY*, *phoP*, *qseB*, *qseF*, *rcsB*, *sirA*, and *yehT*) (Table 2). Interestingly, several of the TCS previously associated with *S.* Typhimurium virulence in mice (*cheY*, *cpxR*, *narP*, *ompR*, *phoP*, *qseB*, *qseF*, *rcsB*, *sirA*, and *ssrB*) display a phenotype during host cell interaction with *S.* Typhi, except for *cpxR* and *ssrB*, see below (Table 2). An important aspect of this study was the identification of 32 new phenotypes associated with *S.* Typhi TCS mutants (Table 2). Interestingly, the *cpxR* mutant had phenotypes distinct from *S.* Typhimurium found in the literature (Table 2). The *S.* Typhimurium *cpxR* mutant was not affected for invasion or intracellular replication in epithelial cells (HEp2 and Caco-2) or survival in RAW264.7 macrophages [53], while the *S.* Typhi *cpxR* mutant was defective in invasion of INT407 cells and survival in THP-1 macrophages (Table 2). Thus, we have deleted *cpxR* in *S.* Typhimurium SL1344 and evaluated its level of adhesion, invasion, and replication in epithelial cells and in macrophages

(Figure 6). No significant difference between the wild-type was observed, confirming a difference in the role of CpxR between *S.* Typhi and *S.* Typhimurium.

Table 2. Phenotype of regulator mutant during interaction with host.

RR	Epithelial Cells (INT407) Adhesion	Epithelial Cells (INT407) Invasion	Epithelial Cells (INT407) Rep	Macrophages (THP1) Uptake	Macrophages (THP1) Survial
ArcA		C (blue)		N (red)	C (blue)
BaeR		N (blue)			N (blue)
CitB		N (red)	N (red)		N (blue)
CheY	N (blue)	C (red)			N (blue)
CopR			N (red)		N (red)
CpxR		* (blue)		N (blue)	* (blue)
CreB					
DcuR					
DpiA					N (blue)
GlnG			N (red)	N (blue)	
HydG					
KdpE				N (blue)	N (red)
NarL				N (red)	
NarP	N (red)	N (red)		N (red)	N (blue)
OmpR	* (blue)	* (blue)		N (red)	* (blue)
PgtA	N (blue)	N (red)	N (red)	N (red)	
PhoB					
PhoP		C (blue)			C (blue)
PmrA		N (red)	N (red)		N (red)
QseB		C (red)	N (red)		
QseF		C (blue)			
RcsB	N (red)	C (red)		N (red)	N (red)
RstA			N (blue)		
SirA		C (blue)			N (red)
SsrB					
TctD		N (blue)			N (red)
TorR		N (blue)			N (red)
TtrR					
UhpA			N (red)		
YehT		C (grey)			

Blue = significantly lower; Grey = no difference, Red = significantly higher than the wild-type. C = confirmed phenotype; N = new phenotype; * = divergent phenotype.

Six RR mutants, *creB*, *hydG*, *phoB*, *ssrB*, *ttrR* and *yehT* were similar to the wild-type strain in all conditions tested. The mutation of 4 TCS (*creB*, *hydG*, *phoB*, *ssrB*) in *S.* Dublin also resulted in a phenotype similar to the wild-type strain during infection of epithelial cells [110]. The deletion of the Ttr system of *S.* Dublin caused a higher level of invasion, but in *S.* Typhi, the *ttrS* sensor is a pseudogene (see below), which may explain why no phenotypes were observed. It may be surprising that the SsrAB system, which is the principal regulator of SPI-2, demonstrated no defect, but we have previously demonstrated that the entire SPI-2 deletion was not essential for *S.* Typhi survival in macrophages [23], and SPI-2 was not required for *S.* Typhi infection in a humanized mice model [111], highlighting one of the major differences with *S.* Typhimurium.

S. Typhi has evolved as a human-restricted pathogen without any known environmental niche. This specialization is associated with genome degradation, as up to 5% of its genome includes predicted open reading frames that have become pseudogenes. There are two TCS that are pseudogenes in *S.* Typhi: TorR and the sensor TtrS. The TtrSR system is involved in tetrathionate respiration in the inflamed gut, which provides a competitive advantage against the intestinal microbiota [112]. However, the production of the Vi capsule by *S.* Typhi prevents intestinal inflammation [9], suggesting that *S.* Typhi does not need the TtrRS system and the *ttrR* mutant did not show any phenotype in the tested conditions here. The TorSR system is not characterized in *Salmonella*. In *E. coli*, TorR activates the transcription of *torCAD* [113], which encodes proteins required for anaerobic respiration [114–116].

Here, even in the absence of a functional sensor, the *torR* mutant was defective in invasion and had a higher level of survival in macrophages.

Epithelial cell invasion was the infection step in epithelial cells where TCS mutants differed significantly when compared to the wild-type, as 16 mutants demonstrated changes in invasion (7 increased invasion and 9 decreased invasion). As expected, the *sirA* (*Salmonella* invasion regulator) deletion resulted in decreased invasion, consistent with the role of SirA in inducing SPI-1 [97,117]. The complementation of this mutant restored the wild-type level (Figure 3). By contrast, only 5 mutants were affected in their adhesion level and 8 in intracellular replication, compared to the wild-type. Interestingly, none of the TCS mutants had the same phenotypic pattern (Table 1), except for the 6 aforementioned mutants that did not differ from the wild-type. This emphasizes the diversity of TCS used to respond to environmental changes as well as the specificity of each system, as each TCS is unique.

The *rcsB* mutant showed increases in cell interactions for almost all tested conditions, except for intracellular replication in epithelial cells. RcsB belongs to the Rcs phosphorelay, a complex TCS with three members, RcsC, RcsD, and RcsB, and several accessory proteins involved in the stress envelope response. RcsB was shown to repress important virulence factors, including fimbriae, SPI-1, and also activation expression of the Vi capsule [16,90]. Thus, some virulence genes are expressed in the *rcsB* mutant, which lead to increased adhesion and invasion and the Vi capsule is repressed, which increased phagocytosis by these cells [118].

The *ompR* mutant showed the lowest level of adhesion and one of the lowest levels of invasion (Figure 1). These defects were restored by the addition of a wild-type copy of *ompR* (Figure 3). The motility of the *ompR* mutant was also reduced to 85% of the wild-type. An *ompR* mutant was attenuated in *S.* Typhimurium [71] and OmpR was associated with the activation of SPI-2 [73–75] and motility genes [119]. This regulation pattern is exactly the opposite of the Rcs system, which may explain why these mutants have strong and opposite phenotypes. These phenotypes are specific to each mutation and did not involve the Vi capsule.

5. Conclusions

Virulence genes expression needed to be tightly regulated in order for *S.* Typhi to adapt and survive within the host. TCS participate in the regulation of several virulence factors and we have shown that several TCS contribute to adhesion, invasion, replication, uptake, and survival of *S.* Typhi. Distinct phenotypes of the CpxR mutant of *S.* Typhi compared to *S.* Typhimurium may reveal fundamental regulatory differences associated with *S.* Typhi niche specialization. Further characterization of the regulons associated with TCS involved in virulence and identification of the signals required for their activation will be important to understand *S.* Typhi pathogenesis. This will help to identify and develop strategies to prevent and or to reduce typhoid infections.

Author Contributions: Conceptualization, C.M.-L. and F.D.; methodology, C.M.-L., M.K. and K.D.; validation, C.M.-L., M.K., K.D. and F.D.; formal analysis, C.M.-L., F.D.; resources, F.D.; writing—original draft preparation, C.M.-L.; writing—review and editing, C.M.-L., M.K., K.D. and F.D.; supervision, F.D.; funding acquisition, F.D. All authors have read and agreed to the published version of the manuscript.

References

1. Beier, D.; Gross, R. Regulation of bacterial virulence by two-component systems. *Curr. Opin. Microbiol.* **2006**, *9*, 143–152. [CrossRef] [PubMed]

2. Stock, A.M.; Robinson, V.L.; Goudreau, P.N. Two-component signal transduction. *Annu. Rev. Biochem.* **2000**, *69*, 183–215. [CrossRef] [PubMed]
3. Parkinson, J.S.; Kofoid, E.C. Communication modules in bacterial signaling proteins. *Annu. Rev. Genet.* **1992**, *26*, 71–112. [CrossRef] [PubMed]
4. Gibani, M.M.; Britto, C.; Pollard, A.J. Typhoid and paratyphoid fever: A call to action. *Curr. Opin. Infect. Dis.* **2018**, *31*, 440–448. [CrossRef]
5. Audia, J.P.; Webb, C.C.; Foster, J.W. Breaking through the acid barrier: An orchestrated response to proton stress by enteric bacteria. *Int. J. Med. Microbiol.* **2001**, *291*, 97–106. [CrossRef]
6. Tiwari, R.P.; Sachdeva, N.; Hoondal, G.S.; Grewal, J.S. Adaptive acid tolerance response in *Salmonella enterica* serovar Typhimurium and *Salmonella enterica* serovar Typhi. *J. Basic Microbiol.* **2004**, *44*, 137–146. [CrossRef]
7. Lostroh, C.P.; Lee, C.A. The Salmonella pathogenicity island-1 type III secretion system. *Microbes Infect.* **2001**, *3*, 1281–1291. [CrossRef]
8. Lara-Tejero, M.; Galan, J.E. The Injectisome, a Complex Nanomachine for Protein Injection into Mammalian Cells. *EcoSal Plus* **2019**, *8*. [CrossRef]
9. Raffatellu, M.; Chessa, D.; Wilson, R.P.; Dusold, R.; Rubino, S.; Baumler, A.J. The Vi capsular antigen of *Salmonella enterica* serotype Typhi reduces Toll-like receptor-dependent interleukin-8 expression in the intestinal mucosa. *Infect. Immun.* **2005**, *73*, 3367–3374. [CrossRef]
10. Waterman, S.R.; Holden, D.W. Functions and effectors of the Salmonella pathogenicity island 2 type III secretion system. *Cell. Microbiol.* **2003**, *5*, 501–511. [CrossRef]
11. Hensel, M.; Shea, J.E.; Waterman, S.R.; Mundy, R.; Nikolaus, T.; Banks, G.; Vazquez-Torres, A.; Gleeson, C.; Fang, F.C.; Holden, D.W. Genes encoding putative effector proteins of the type III secretion system of *Salmonella* pathogenicity island 2 are required for bacterial virulence and proliferation in macrophages. *Mol. Microbiol.* **1998**, *30*, 163–174. [CrossRef] [PubMed]
12. Parry, C.M.; Hien, T.T.; Dougan, G.; White, N.J.; Farrar, J.J. Typhoid fever. *N. Engl. J. Med.* **2002**, *347*, 1770–1782. [CrossRef] [PubMed]
13. Pickard, D.; Li, J.; Roberts, M.; Maskell, D.; Hone, D.; Levine, M.; Dougan, G.; Chatfield, S. Characterization of defined ompR mutants of Salmonella typhi: ompR is involved in the regulation of Vi polysaccharide expression. *Infect. Immun.* **1994**, *62*, 3984–3993. [CrossRef] [PubMed]
14. Santander, J.; Roland, K.L.; Curtiss, R., 3rd. Regulation of Vi capsular polysaccharide synthesis in *Salmonella enterica* serotype Typhi. *J. Infect. Dev. Ctries* **2008**, *2*, 412–420.
15. Virlogeux, I.; Waxin, H.; Ecobichon, C.; Lee, J.O.; Popoff, M.Y. Characterization of the rcsA and rcsB genes from Salmonella typhi: rcsB through tviA is involved in regulation of Vi antigen synthesis. *J. Bacteriol.* **1996**, *178*, 1691–1698. [CrossRef] [PubMed]
16. Winter, S.E.; Winter, M.G.; Thiennimitr, P.; Gerriets, V.A.; Nuccio, S.P.; Russmann, H.; Baumler, A.J. The TviA auxiliary protein renders the *Salmonella enterica* serotype Typhi RcsB regulon responsive to changes in osmolarity. *Mol. Microbiol.* **2009**, *74*, 175–193. [CrossRef]
17. Arricau, N.; Hermant, D.; Waxin, H.; Ecobichon, C.; Duffey, P.S.; Popoff, M.Y. The RcsB-RcsC regulatory system of *Salmonella typhi* differentially modulates the expression of invasion proteins, flagellin and Vi antigen in response to osmolarity. *Mol. Microbiol.* **1998**, *29*, 835–850. [CrossRef]
18. Fowler, C.C.; Galan, J.E. Decoding a *Salmonella* Typhi Regulatory Network that Controls Typhoid Toxin Expression within Human Cells. *Cell Host Microbe* **2018**, *23*, 65–76, e66. [CrossRef]
19. Faucher, S.P.; Forest, C.; Beland, M.; Daigle, F. A novel PhoP-regulated locus encoding the cytolysin ClyA and the secreted invasin TaiA of *Salmonella enterica* serovar Typhi is involved in virulence. *Microbiology* **2009**, *155*, 477–488. [CrossRef]
20. Charles, R.C.; Harris, J.B.; Chase, M.R.; Lebrun, L.M.; Sheikh, A.; LaRocque, R.C.; Logvinenko, T.; Rollins, S.M.; Tarique, A.; Hohmann, E.L.; et al. Comparative proteomic analysis of the PhoP regulon in *Salmonella enterica* serovar Typhi versus Typhimurium. *PLoS ONE* **2009**, *4*, e6994. [CrossRef]
21. Sheikh, A.; Charles, R.C.; Sharmeen, N.; Rollins, S.M.; Harris, J.B.; Bhuiyan, M.S.; Arifuzzaman, M.; Khanam, F.; Bukka, A.; Kalsy, A.; et al. In vivo expression of *Salmonella enterica* serotype Typhi genes in the blood of patients with typhoid fever in Bangladesh. *PLoS Negl. Trop. Dis.* **2011**, *5*, e1419. [CrossRef] [PubMed]

22. Hohmann, E.L.; Oletta, C.A.; Killeen, K.P.; Miller, S.I. phoP/phoQ-deleted Salmonella typhi (Ty800) is a safe and immunogenic single-dose typhoid fever vaccine in volunteers. *J. Infect. Dis.* **1996**, *173*, 1408–1414. [CrossRef] [PubMed]
23. Forest, C.G.; Ferraro, E.; Sabbagh, S.C.; Daigle, F. Intracellular survival of Salmonella enterica serovar Typhi in human macrophages is independent of Salmonella pathogenicity island (SPI)-2. *Microbiology* **2010**, *156*, 3689–3698. [CrossRef] [PubMed]
24. Leclerc, G.J.; Tartera, C.; Metcalf, E.S. Environmental regulation of *Salmonella typhi* invasion-defective mutants. *Infect. Immun.* **1998**, *66*, 682–691. [CrossRef]
25. Moreira, C.G.; Sperandio, V. Interplay between the QseC and QseE bacterial adrenergic sensor kinases in *Salmonella enterica* serovar Typhimurium pathogenesis. *Infect. Immun.* **2012**, *80*, 4344–4353. [CrossRef]
26. Bearson, B.L.; Bearson, S.M. The role of the QseC quorum-sensing sensor kinase in colonization and norepinephrine-enhanced motility of *Salmonella enterica* serovar Typhimurium. *Microb. Pathog.* **2008**, *44*, 271–278. [CrossRef]
27. Ji, Y.; Li, W.; Zhang, Y.; Chen, L.; Zhang, Y.; Zheng, X.; Huang, X.; Ni, B. QseB mediates biofilm formation and invasion in *Salmonella enterica* serovar Typhi. *Microb. Pathog.* **2017**, *104*, 6–11. [CrossRef]
28. Island, M.D.; Wei, B.Y.; Kadner, R.J. Structure and function of the uhp genes for the sugar phosphate transport system in *Escherichia coli* and *Salmonella typhimurium*. *J. Bacteriol.* **1992**, *174*, 2754–2762. [CrossRef]
29. Sheng, X.; Huang, X.; Li, J.; Xie, X.; Xu, S.; Zhang, H.; Xu, H. Regulation of sulfur assimilation pathways in *Salmonella enterica* serovar Typhi upon up-shift high osmotic treatment: The role of UhpA revealed through transcriptome profiling. *Curr. Microbiol.* **2009**, *59*, 628–635. [CrossRef]
30. Wanner, B.L. Is cross regulation by phosphorylation of two-component response regulator proteins important in bacteria? *J. Bacteriol.* **1992**, *174*, 2053–2058. [CrossRef]
31. Hone, D.M.; Harris, A.M.; Chatfield, S.; Dougan, G.; Levine, M.M. Construction of genetically defined double aro mutants of *Salmonella typhi*. *Vaccine* **1991**, *9*, 810–816. [CrossRef]
32. O'Callaghan, D.; Charbit, A. High efficiency transformation of *Salmonella typhimurium* and *Salmonella typhi* by electroporation. *Mol. Gen. Genet.* **1990**, *223*, 156–158. [CrossRef] [PubMed]
33. Parkhill, J.; Dougan, G.; James, K.D.; Thomson, N.R.; Pickard, D.; Wain, J.; Churcher, C.; Mungall, K.L.; Bentley, S.D.; Holden, M.T.; et al. Complete genome sequence of a multiple drug resistant *Salmonella enterica* serovar Typhi CT18. *Nature* **2001**, *413*, 848–852. [CrossRef] [PubMed]
34. Forest, C.; Faucher, S.; Poirier, K.; Houle, S.; Dozois, C.; Daigle, F. Contribution of the *stg* fimbrial operon of *Salmonella enterica* serovar Typhi during interaction with human cells. *Infect. Immun.* **2007**, *75*, 5264–5271. [CrossRef]
35. Ho, S.N.; Hunt, H.D.; Horton, R.M.; Pullen, J.K.; Pease, L.R. Site-directed mutagenesis by overlap extension using the polymerase chain reaction. *Gene* **1989**, *77*, 51–59. [CrossRef]
36. Daigle, F.; Graham, J.; Curtiss, R., 3rd. Identification of *Salmonella typhi* genes expressed within macrophages by selective capture of transcribed sequences (SCOTS). *Mol. Microbiol.* **2001**, *41*, 1211–1222. [CrossRef]
37. Sabbagh, S.C.; Lepage, C.; McClelland, M.; Daigle, F. Selection of *Salmonella enterica* serovar Typhi genes involved during interaction with human macrophages by screening of a transposon mutant library. *PLoS ONE* **2012**, *7*, e36643. [CrossRef]
38. Lu, S.; Killoran, P.B.; Fang, F.C.; Riley, L.W. The global regulator ArcA controls resistance to reactive nitrogen and oxygen intermediates in *Salmonella enterica* serovar Enteritidis. *Infect. Immun.* **2002**, *70*, 451–461. [CrossRef]
39. Morales, E.H.; Calderon, I.L.; Collao, B.; Gil, F.; Porwollik, S.; McClelland, M.; Saavedra, C.P. Hypochlorous acid and hydrogen peroxide-induced negative regulation of *Salmonella enterica* serovar Typhimurium ompW by the response regulator ArcA. *BMC Microbiol.* **2012**, *12*, 63. [CrossRef]
40. Lim, S.; Yoon, H.; Kim, M.; Han, A.; Choi, J.; Choi, J.; Ryu, S. Hfq and ArcA are involved in the stationary phase-dependent activation of *Salmonella* pathogenicity island 1 (SPI1) under shaking culture conditions. *J. Microbiol. Biotechnol.* **2013**, *23*, 1664–1672. [CrossRef]
41. Evans, M.R.; Fink, R.C.; Vazquez-Torres, A.; Porwollik, S.; Jones-Carson, J.; McClelland, M.; Hassan, H.M. Analysis of the ArcA regulon in anaerobically grown *Salmonella enterica* sv. Typhimurium. *BMC Microbiol.* **2011**, *11*, 58. [CrossRef]

42. Pardo-Este, C.; Hidalgo, A.A.; Aguirre, C.; Briones, A.C.; Cabezas, C.E.; Castro-Severyn, J.; Fuentes, J.A.; Opazo, C.M.; Riedel, C.A.; Otero, C.; et al. The ArcAB two-component regulatory system promotes resistance to reactive oxygen species and systemic infection by *Salmonella* Typhimurium. *PLoS ONE* **2018**, *13*, e0203497. [CrossRef] [PubMed]
43. Guerrero, P.; Collao, B.; Morales, E.H.; Calderon, I.L.; Ipinza, F.; Parra, S.; Saavedra, C.P.; Gil, F. Characterization of the BaeSR two-component system from *Salmonella* Typhimurium and its role in ciprofloxacin-induced *mdtA* expression. *Arch. Microbiol.* **2012**, *194*, 453–460. [CrossRef] [PubMed]
44. Appia-Ayme, C.; Patrick, E.; Sullivan, M.J.; Alston, M.J.; Field, S.J.; AbuOun, M.; Anjum, M.F.; Rowley, G. Novel inducers of the envelope stress response BaeSR in *Salmonella* Typhimurium: BaeR is critically required for tungstate waste disposal. *PLoS ONE* **2011**, *6*, e23713. [CrossRef] [PubMed]
45. Bott, M. Anaerobic citrate metabolism and its regulation in enterobacteria. *Arch. Microbiol.* **1997**, *167*, 78–88. [CrossRef]
46. Stecher, B.; Hapfelmeier, S.; Muller, C.; Kremer, M.; Stallmach, T.; Hardt, W.D. Flagella and chemotaxis are required for efficient induction of Salmonella enterica serovar Typhimurium colitis in streptomycin-pretreated mice. *Infect. Immun.* **2004**, *72*, 4138–4150. [CrossRef]
47. Lee, C.A.; Jones, B.D.; Falkow, S. Identification of a Salmonella typhimurium invasion locus by selection for hyperinvasive mutants. *Proc. Natl. Acad. Sci. USA* **1992**, *89*, 1847–1851. [CrossRef]
48. Pezza, A.; Pontel, L.B.; Lopez, C.; Soncini, F.C. Compartment and signal-specific codependence in the transcriptional control of *Salmonella* periplasmic copper homeostasis. *Proc. Natl. Acad. Sci. USA* **2016**, *113*, 11573–11578. [CrossRef]
49. Kato, A.; Higashino, N.; Utsumi, R. Fe(3+)-dependent epistasis between the CpxR-activated loci and the PmrA-activated LPS modification loci in *Salmonella enterica*. *J. Gen. Appl. Microbiol.* **2017**, *62*, 286–296. [CrossRef]
50. Cerminati, S.; Giri, G.F.; Mendoza, J.I.; Soncini, F.C.; Checa, S.K. The CpxR/CpxA system contributes to *Salmonella* gold-resistance by controlling the GolS-dependent *gesABC* transcription. *Environ. Microbiol.* **2017**, *19*, 4035–4044. [CrossRef]
51. Weatherspoon-Griffin, N.; Zhao, G.; Kong, W.; Kong, Y.; Andrews-Polymenis, H.; McClelland, M.; Shi, Y. The CpxR/CpxA two-component system up-regulates two Tat-dependent peptidoglycan amidases to confer bacterial resistance to antimicrobial peptide. *J. Biol. Chem.* **2011**, *286*, 5529–5539. [CrossRef] [PubMed]
52. Lopez, C.; Checa, S.K.; Soncini, F.C. CpxR/CpxA Controls scsABCD Transcription To Counteract Copper and Oxidative Stress in *Salmonella enterica* Serovar Typhimurium. *J. Bacteriol.* **2018**, *200*. [CrossRef] [PubMed]
53. Humphreys, S.; Rowley, G.; Stevenson, A.; Anjum, M.F.; Woodward, M.J.; Gilbert, S.; Kormanec, J.; Roberts, M. Role of the two-component regulator CpxAR in the virulence of *Salmonella enterica* serotype Typhimurium. *Infect. Immun.* **2004**, *72*, 4654–4661. [CrossRef] [PubMed]
54. De la Cruz, M.A.; Perez-Morales, D.; Palacios, I.J.; Fernandez-Mora, M.; Calva, E.; Bustamante, V.H. The two-component system CpxR/A represses the expression of *Salmonella* virulence genes by affecting the stability of the transcriptional regulator HilD. *Front. Microbiol.* **2015**, *6*, 807. [CrossRef] [PubMed]
55. Subramaniam, S.; Muller, V.S.; Hering, N.A.; Mollenkopf, H.; Becker, D.; Heroven, A.K.; Dersch, P.; Pohlmann, A.; Tedin, K.; Porwollik, S.; et al. Contribution of the Cpx envelope stress system to metabolism and virulence regulation in *Salmonella enterica* serovar Typhimurium. *PLoS ONE* **2019**, *14*, e0211584. [CrossRef]
56. Fujimoto, M.; Goto, R.; Haneda, T.; Okada, N.; Miki, T. *Salmonella enterica* Serovar Typhimurium CpxRA Two-Component System Contributes to Gut Colonization in *Salmonella*-Induced Colitis. *Infect. Immun.* **2018**, *86*. [CrossRef] [PubMed]
57. Avison, M.B.; Horton, R.E.; Walsh, T.R.; Bennett, P.M. *Escherichia coli* CreBC is a global regulator of gene expression that responds to growth in minimal media. *J. Biol. Chem.* **2001**, *276*, 26955–26961. [CrossRef] [PubMed]
58. Scheu, P.D.; Kim, O.B.; Griesinger, C.; Unden, G. Sensing by the membrane-bound sensor kinase DcuS: Exogenous versus endogenous sensing of C(4)-dicarboxylates in bacteria. *Future Microbiol.* **2010**, *5*, 1383–1402. [CrossRef]
59. Golby, P.; Davies, S.; Kelly, D.J.; Guest, J.R.; Andrews, S.C. Identification and characterization of a two-component sensor-kinase and response-regulator system (DcuS-DcuR) controlling gene expression in response to C4-dicarboxylates in *Escherichia coli*. *J. Bacteriol.* **1999**, *181*, 1238–1248. [CrossRef]

60. Miller, C.; Thomsen, L.E.; Gaggero, C.; Mosseri, R.; Ingmer, H.; Cohen, S.N. SOS response induction by beta-lactams and bacterial defense against antibiotic lethality. *Science* **2004**, *305*, 1629–1631. [CrossRef]
61. Ferro-Luzzi Ames, G.; Nikaido, K. Nitrogen regulation in *Salmonella typhimurium*. Identification of an *ntrC* protein-binding site and definition of a consensus binding sequence. *EMBO J.* **1985**, *4*, 539–547. [CrossRef] [PubMed]
62. Klose, K.E.; Mekalanos, J.J. Simultaneous prevention of glutamine synthesis and high-affinity transport attenuates *Salmonella typhimurium* virulence. *Infect. Immun.* **1997**, *65*, 587–596. [CrossRef] [PubMed]
63. Leonhartsberger, S.; Huber, A.; Lottspeich, F.; Bock, A. The *hydH/G* Genes from *Escherichia coli* code for a zinc and lead responsive two-component regulatory system. *J. Mol. Biol.* **2001**, *307*, 93–105. [CrossRef] [PubMed]
64. Rhoads, D.B.; Waters, F.B.; Epstein, W. Cation transport in *Escherichia coli*. VIII. Potassium transport mutants. *J. Gen. Physiol.* **1976**, *67*, 325–341. [CrossRef]
65. Alegado, R.A.; Chin, C.Y.; Monack, D.M.; Tan, M.W. The two-component sensor kinase KdpD is required for *Salmonella* typhimurium colonization of *Caenorhabditis elegans* and survival in macrophages. *Cell. Microbiol.* **2011**, *13*, 1618–1637. [CrossRef]
66. Noriega, C.E.; Lin, H.Y.; Chen, L.L.; Williams, S.B.; Stewart, V. Asymmetric cross-regulation between the nitrate-responsive NarX-NarL and NarQ-NarP two-component regulatory systems from *Escherichia coli* K-12. *Mol. Microbiol.* **2010**, *75*, 394–412. [CrossRef]
67. Rabin, R.S.; Stewart, V. Dual response regulators (NarL and NarP) interact with dual sensors (NarX and NarQ) to control nitrate- and nitrite-regulated gene expression in *Escherichia coli* K-12. *J. Bacteriol.* **1993**, *175*, 3259–3268. [CrossRef]
68. Lopez, C.A.; Rivera-Chavez, F.; Byndloss, M.X.; Baumler, A.J. The Periplasmic Nitrate Reductase NapABC Supports Luminal Growth of *Salmonella enterica* Serovar Typhimurium during Colitis. *Infect. Immun.* **2015**, *83*, 3470–3478. [CrossRef]
69. Bang, I.S.; Kim, B.H.; Foster, J.W.; Park, Y.K. OmpR regulates the stationary-phase acid tolerance response of Salmonella enterica serovar typhimurium. *J. Bacteriol.* **2000**, *182*, 2245–2252. [CrossRef]
70. Chakraborty, S.; Kenney, L.J. A New Role of OmpR in Acid and Osmotic Stress in *Salmonella* and *E. coli*. *Front. Microbiol.* **2018**, *9*, 2656. [CrossRef]
71. Dorman, C.J.; Chatfield, S.; Higgins, C.F.; Hayward, C.; Dougan, G. Characterization of porin and *ompR* mutants of a virulent strain of *Salmonella typhimurium*: *ompR* mutants are attenuated in vivo. *Infect. Immun.* **1989**, *57*, 2136–2140. [CrossRef] [PubMed]
72. Cameron, A.D.; Dorman, C.J. A fundamental regulatory mechanism operating through OmpR and DNA topology controls expression of *Salmonella* pathogenicity islands SPI-1 and SPI-2. *PLoS Genet.* **2012**, *8*, e1002615. [CrossRef] [PubMed]
73. Lee, A.K.; Detweiler, C.S.; Falkow, S. OmpR regulates the two-component system SsrA-ssrB in Salmonella pathogenicity island 2. *J. Bacteriol.* **2000**, *182*, 771–781. [CrossRef] [PubMed]
74. Garmendia, J.; Beuzon, C.R.; Ruiz-Albert, J.; Holden, D.W. The roles of SsrA-SsrB and OmpR-EnvZ in the regulation of genes encoding the Salmonella typhimurium SPI-2 type III secretion system. *Microbiology* **2003**, *149*, 2385–2396. [CrossRef] [PubMed]
75. Feng, X.; Oropeza, R.; Kenney, L.J. Dual regulation by phospho-OmpR of *ssrA/B* gene expression in *Salmonella* pathogenicity island 2. *Mol. Microbiol.* **2003**, *48*, 1131–1143. [CrossRef]
76. Mills, S.D.; Ruschkowski, S.R.; Stein, M.A.; Finlay, B.B. Trafficking of porin-deficient *Salmonella typhimurium* mutants inside HeLa cells: *ompR* and *envZ* mutants are defective for the formation of Salmonella-induced filaments. *Infect. Immun.* **1998**, *66*, 1806–1811. [CrossRef]
77. Yang, Y.L.; Goldrick, D.; Hong, J.S. Identification of the products and nucleotide sequences of two regulatory genes involved in the exogenous induction of phosphoglycerate transport in Salmonella typhimurium. *J. Bacteriol.* **1988**, *170*, 4299–4303. [CrossRef]
78. Pontes, M.H.; Groisman, E.A. Protein synthesis controls phosphate homeostasis. *Genes Dev.* **2018**, *32*, 79–92. [CrossRef]
79. Lucas, R.L.; Lee, C.A. Roles of hilC and hilD in regulation of hilA expression in Salmonella enterica serovar Typhimurium. *J. Bacteriol.* **2001**, *183*, 2733–2745. [CrossRef]
80. Miller, S.I.; Kukral, A.M.; Mekalanos, J.J. A two-component regulatory system (phoP phoQ) controls *Salmonella typhimurium* virulence. *Proc. Natl. Acad. Sci. USA* **1989**, *86*, 5054–5058. [CrossRef]

81. Choi, E.; Groisman, E.A.; Shin, D. Activated by different signals, the PhoP/PhoQ two-component system differentially regulates metal uptake. *J. Bacteriol.* **2009**, *191*, 7174–7181. [CrossRef] [PubMed]
82. Shi, Y.; Cromie, M.J.; Hsu, F.F.; Turk, J.; Groisman, E.A. PhoP-regulated *Salmonella* resistance to the antimicrobial peptides magainin 2 and polymyxin B. *Mol. Microbiol.* **2004**, *53*, 229–241. [CrossRef] [PubMed]
83. Navarre, W.W.; Halsey, T.A.; Walthers, D.; Frye, J.; McClelland, M.; Potter, J.L.; Kenney, L.J.; Gunn, J.S.; Fang, F.C.; Libby, S.J. Co-regulation of *Salmonella enterica* genes required for virulence and resistance to antimicrobial peptides by SlyA and PhoP/PhoQ. *Mol. Microbiol.* **2005**, *56*, 492–508. [CrossRef] [PubMed]
84. van Velkinburgh, J.C.; Gunn, J.S. PhoP-PhoQ-regulated loci are required for enhanced bile resistance in Salmonella spp. *Infect. Immun.* **1999**, *67*, 1614–1622. [CrossRef] [PubMed]
85. Palmer, A.D.; Kim, K.; Slauch, J.M. PhoP-Mediated Repression of the SPI1 Type 3 Secretion System in *Salmonella enterica* Serovar Typhimurium. *J. Bacteriol.* **2019**, *201*. [CrossRef]
86. Gunn, J.S.; Ryan, S.S.; Van Velkinburgh, J.C.; Ernst, R.K.; Miller, S.I. Genetic and functional analysis of a PmrA-PmrB-regulated locus necessary for lipopolysaccharide modification, antimicrobial peptide resistance, and oral virulence of *Salmonella enterica* serovar *typhimurium*. *Infect. Immun.* **2000**, *68*, 6139–6146. [CrossRef]
87. Choi, J.; Groisman, E.A. The lipopolysaccharide modification regulator PmrA limits Salmonella virulence by repressing the type three-secretion system Spi/Ssa. *Proc. Natl. Acad. Sci. USA* **2013**, *110*, 9499–9504. [CrossRef]
88. Moreira, C.G.; Weinshenker, D.; Sperandio, V. QseC mediates *Salmonella enterica* serovar typhimurium virulence in vitro and in vivo. *Infect. Immun.* **2010**, *78*, 914–926. [CrossRef]
89. Merighi, M.; Septer, A.N.; Carroll-Portillo, A.; Bhatiya, A.; Porwollik, S.; McClelland, M.; Gunn, J.S. Genome-wide analysis of the PreA/PreB (QseB/QseC) regulon of *Salmonella enterica* serovar Typhimurium. *BMC Microbiol.* **2009**, *9*, 42. [CrossRef]
90. Mouslim, C.; Delgado, M.; Groisman, E.A. Activation of the RcsC/YojN/RcsB phosphorelay system attenuates *Salmonella* virulence. *Mol. Microbiol.* **2004**, *54*, 386–395. [CrossRef]
91. Farris, C.; Sanowar, S.; Bader, M.W.; Pfuetzner, R.; Miller, S.I. Antimicrobial peptides activate the Rcs regulon through the outer membrane lipoprotein RcsF. *J. Bacteriol.* **2010**, *192*, 4894–4903. [CrossRef] [PubMed]
92. Farizano, J.V.; Torres, M.A.; Pescaretti Mde, L.; Delgado, M.A. The RcsCDB regulatory system plays a crucial role in the protection of *Salmonella enterica* serovar Typhimurium against oxidative stress. *Microbiology* **2014**, *160*, 2190–2199. [CrossRef] [PubMed]
93. Cabeza, M.L.; Aguirre, A.; Soncini, F.C.; Vescovi, E.G. Induction of RpoS degradation by the two-component system regulator RstA in *Salmonella enterica*. *J. Bacteriol.* **2007**, *189*, 7335–7342. [CrossRef] [PubMed]
94. Jeon, J.; Kim, H.; Yun, J.; Ryu, S.; Groisman, E.A.; Shin, D. RstA-promoted expression of the ferrous iron transporter FeoB under iron-replete conditions enhances Fur activity in *Salmonella enterica*. *J. Bacteriol.* **2008**, *190*, 7326–7334. [CrossRef]
95. Tran, T.K.; Han, Q.Q.; Shi, Y.; Guo, L. A comparative proteomic analysis of *Salmonella typhimurium* under the regulation of the RstA/RstB and PhoP/PhoQ systems. *Biochim. Biophys. Acta* **2016**, *1864*, 1686–1695. [CrossRef]
96. Ahmer, B.M.; van Reeuwijk, J.; Watson, P.R.; Wallis, T.S.; Heffron, F. *Salmonella* SirA is a global regulator of genes mediating enteropathogenesis. *Mol. Microbiol.* **1999**, *31*, 971–982. [CrossRef]
97. Martinez, L.C.; Yakhnin, H.; Camacho, M.I.; Georgellis, D.; Babitzke, P.; Puente, J.L.; Bustamante, V.H. Integration of a complex regulatory cascade involving the SirA/BarA and Csr global regulatory systems that controls expression of the *Salmonella* SPI-1 and SPI-2 virulence regulons through HilD. *Mol. Microbiol.* **2011**, *80*, 1637–1656. [CrossRef]
98. Teplitski, M.; Goodier, R.I.; Ahmer, B.M. Pathways leading from BarA/SirA to motility and virulence gene expression in *Salmonella*. *J. Bacteriol.* **2003**, *185*, 7257–7265. [CrossRef]
99. Pickard, D.; Kingsley, R.A.; Hale, C.; Turner, K.; Sivaraman, K.; Wetter, M.; Langridge, G.; Dougan, G. A genomewide mutagenesis screen identifies multiple genes contributing to Vi capsular expression in Salmonella enterica serovar Typhi. *J. Bacteriol.* **2013**, *195*, 1320–1326. [CrossRef]
100. Johnston, C.; Pegues, D.A.; Hueck, C.J.; Lee, A.; Miller, S.I. Transcriptional activation of *Salmonella typhimurium* invasion genes by a member of the phosphorylated response-regulator superfamily. *Mol. Microbiol.* **1996**, *22*, 715–727. [CrossRef]
101. Ochman, H.; Soncini, F.C.; Solomon, F.; Groisman, E.A. Identification of a pathogenicity island required for *Salmonella* survival in host cells. *Proc. Natl. Acad. Sci. USA* **1996**, *93*, 7800–7804. [CrossRef] [PubMed]

102. Brown, N.F.; Rogers, L.D.; Sanderson, K.L.; Gouw, J.W.; Hartland, E.L.; Foster, L.J. A horizontally acquired transcription factor coordinates *Salmonella* adaptations to host microenvironments. *MBio* **2014**, *5*, e01727-14. [CrossRef]
103. Perez-Morales, D.; Banda, M.M.; Chau, N.Y.E.; Salgado, H.; Martinez-Flores, I.; Ibarra, J.A.; Ilyas, B.; Coombes, B.K.; Bustamante, V.H. The transcriptional regulator SsrB is involved in a molecular switch controlling virulence lifestyles of *Salmonella*. *PLoS Pathog.* **2017**, *13*, e1006497. [CrossRef] [PubMed]
104. Widenhorn, K.A.; Somers, J.M.; Kay, W.W. Expression of the divergent tricarboxylate transport operon *(tctI)* of *Salmonella typhimurium*. *J. Bacteriol.* **1988**, *170*, 3223–3227. [CrossRef] [PubMed]
105. Baraquet, C.; Theraulaz, L.; Guiral, M.; Lafitte, D.; Mejean, V.; Jourlin-Castelli, C. TorT, a member of a new periplasmic binding protein family, triggers induction of the Tor respiratory system upon trimethylamine N-oxide electron-acceptor binding in *Escherichia coli*. *J. Biol. Chem.* **2006**, *281*, 38189–38199. [CrossRef] [PubMed]
106. Hensel, M.; Hinsley, A.P.; Nikolaus, T.; Sawers, G.; Berks, B.C. The genetic basis of tetrathionate respiration in *Salmonella typhimurium*. *Mol. Microbiol.* **1999**, *32*, 275–287. [CrossRef]
107. Wong, V.K.; Pickard, D.J.; Barquist, L.; Sivaraman, K.; Page, A.J.; Hart, P.J.; Arends, M.J.; Holt, K.E.; Kane, L.; Mottram, L.F.; et al. Characterization of the *yehUT* two-component regulatory system of *Salmonella enterica* Serovar Typhi and Typhimurium. *PLoS ONE* **2013**, *8*, e84567. [CrossRef]
108. Kier, L.D.; Weppelman, R.M.; Ames, B.N. Regulation of nonspecific acid phosphatase in *Salmonella*: phoN and phoP genes. *J. Bacteriol.* **1979**, *138*, 155–161. [CrossRef]
109. Miller, S.I.; Mekalanos, J.J. Constitutive expression of the phoP regulon attenuates *Salmonella* virulence and survival within macrophages. *J. Bacteriol.* **1990**, *172*, 2485–2490. [CrossRef]
110. Pullinger, G.D.; van Diemen, P.M.; Dziva, F.; Stevens, M.P. Role of two-component sensory systems of *Salmonella enterica* serovar Dublin in the pathogenesis of systemic salmonellosis in cattle. *Microbiology* **2010**, *156*, 3108–3122. [CrossRef]
111. Karlinsey, J.E.; Stepien, T.A.; Mayho, M.; Singletary, L.A.; Bingham-Ramos, L.K.; Brehm, M.A.; Greiner, D.L.; Shultz, L.D.; Gallagher, L.A.; Bawn, M.; et al. Genome-wide Analysis of *Salmonella enterica* serovar Typhi in Humanized Mice Reveals Key Virulence Features. *Cell Host Microbe* **2019**, *26*, 426–434 e426. [CrossRef] [PubMed]
112. Winter, S.E.; Thiennimitr, P.; Winter, M.G.; Butler, B.P.; Huseby, D.L.; Crawford, R.W.; Russell, J.M.; Bevins, C.L.; Adams, L.G.; Tsolis, R.M.; et al. Gut inflammation provides a respiratory electron acceptor for Salmonella. *Nature* **2010**, *467*, 426–429. [CrossRef]
113. Jourlin, C.; Ansaldi, M.; Mejean, V. Transphosphorylation of the TorR response regulator requires the three phosphorylation sites of the TorS unorthodox sensor in *Escherichia coli*. *J. Mol. Biol.* **1997**, *267*, 770–777. [CrossRef] [PubMed]
114. Mejean, V.; Iobbi-Nivol, C.; Lepelletier, M.; Giordano, G.; Chippaux, M.; Pascal, M.C. TMAO anaerobic respiration in *Escherichia coli: Involvement* of the tor operon. *Mol. Microbiol.* **1994**, *11*, 1169–1179. [CrossRef] [PubMed]
115. Gon, S.; Giudici-Orticoni, M.T.; Mejean, V.; Iobbi-Nivol, C. Electron transfer and binding of the c-type cytochrome TorC to the trimethylamine N-oxide reductase in *Escherichia coli*. *J. Biol. Chem.* **2001**, *276*, 11545–11551. [CrossRef]
116. McCrindle, S.L.; Kappler, U.; McEwan, A.G. Microbial dimethylsulfoxide and trimethylamine-N-oxide respiration. *Adv. Microb. Physiol.* **2005**, *50*, 147–198. [CrossRef]
117. Teplitski, M.; Goodier, R.I.; Ahmer, B.M. Catabolite repression of the SirA regulatory cascade in *Salmonella enterica*. *Int. J. Med. Microbiol.* **2006**, *296*, 449–466. [CrossRef]
118. Kossack, R.E.; Guerrant, R.L.; Densen, P.; Schadelin, J.; Mandell, G.L. Diminished neutrophil oxidative metabolism after phagocytosis of virulent *Salmonella typhi*. *Infect. Immun.* **1981**, *31*, 674–678. [CrossRef]
119. Perkins, T.T.; Kingsley, R.A.; Fookes, M.C.; Gardner, P.P.; James, K.D.; Yu, L.; Assefa, S.A.; He, M.; Croucher, N.J.; Pickard, D.J.; et al. A strand-specific RNA-Seq analysis of the transcriptome of the typhoid bacillus Salmonella typhi. *PLoS Genet.* **2009**, *5*, e1000569. [CrossRef]

10

The *Salmonella enterica* Plasmidome as a Reservoir of Antibiotic Resistance

Jean-Guillaume Emond-Rheault [1], Jérémie Hamel [1], Julie Jeukens [1], Luca Freschi [1], Irena Kukavica-Ibrulj [1], Brian Boyle [1], Sandeep Tamber [2], Danielle Malo [3,4], Eelco Franz [5], Elton Burnett [6], France Daigle [7,8], Gitanjali Arya [9], Kenneth Sanderson [10], Martin Wiedmann [11], Robin M. Slawson [12], Joel T. Weadge [12], Roger Stephan [13], Sadjia Bekal [14], Samantha Gruenheid [15], Lawrence D. Goodridge [16,*] and Roger C. Levesque [1,*]

[1] Institut de Biologie Intégrative et des Systèmes (IBIS), Université Laval, Québec, QC G1V 0A6, Canada; jean-guillaume.emond-rheault.1@ulaval.ca (J.-G.E.-R.); jeremie.hamel.1@ulaval.ca (J.H.); julie.jeukens.1@ulaval.ca (J.J.); l.freschi@gmail.com (L.F.); kukavica@fmed.ulaval.ca (I.K.-I.); brian.boyle@ibis.ulaval.ca (B.B.)

[2] Health Canada, Bureau of Microbial Hazards, Ottawa, ON K1A 0K9, Canada; sandeep.tamber@canada.ca

[3] McGill Research Center on Complex Traits, McGill University, Montréal, QC H3G 0B1, Canada; danielle.malo@mcgill.ca

[4] Departments of Medicine and Human Genetics, McGill University, Montréal, QC H3G 0B1, Canada

[5] Centre for Infectious Disease Control (CIb), National Institute for Public Health and the Environment (RIVM), 3720 BA Bilthoven, The Netherlands; eelco.franz@rivm.nl

[6] Institute of Parasitology, McGill University, Montréal, QC H9X 3L9, Canada; elton.burnett@mail.mcgill.ca

[7] Département de Microbiologie, Infectiologie et Immunologie, Université de Montréal, Montréal, QC H3T 1J4, Canada; france.daigle@umontreal.ca

[8] Swine and poultry Infectious Diseases Research Center (CRIPA-FRQNT), Montréal, QC H3C 3J7, Canada

[9] National Microbiology Laboratory, Public Health Agency of Canada, Guelph, ON N1G 3W4, Canada; gitanjali.arya@phac-aspc.gc.ca

[10] Department of Biological Sciences, University of Calgary, Calgary, AB T2N 1N4, Canada; kesander@ucalgary.ca

[11] Department of Food Science, Cornell University, Ithaca, NY 14853-7201, USA; mw16@cornell.edu

[12] Department of Biology, Wilfrid Laurier University, Waterloo, ON N2L 3C5, Canada; rslawson@wlu.ca (R.M.S.); jweadge@wlu.ca (J.T.W.)

[13] Institute for Food Safety and hygiene, University of Zürich, CH-8057 Zürich, Switzerland; stephanr@fsafety.uzh.ch

[14] Laboratoire de santé publique du Québec, Sainte-Anne-de-Bellevue, QC H9X 3R5, Canada; sadjia.bekal@inspq.qc.ca

[15] Department of Microbiology & Immunology, McGill University, Montréal, QC H3G 0B1, Canada; samantha.gruenheid@mcgill.ca

[16] Food Science Department, University of Guelph, Guelph, ON N1G 2W1, Canada

* Correspondence: goodridl@uoguelph.ca (L.D.G.); rclevesq@ibis.ulaval.ca (R.C.L.)

Abstract: The emergence of multidrug-resistant bacterial strains worldwide has become a serious problem for public health over recent decades. The increase in antimicrobial resistance has been expanding via plasmids as mobile genetic elements encoding antimicrobial resistance (AMR) genes that are transferred vertically and horizontally. This study focuses on *Salmonella enterica*, one of the leading foodborne pathogens in industrialized countries. S. enterica is known to carry several plasmids involved not only in virulence but also in AMR. In the current paper, we present an integrated strategy to detect plasmid scaffolds in whole genome sequencing (WGS) assemblies. We developed a two-step procedure to predict plasmids based on i) the presence of essential elements for plasmid replication and mobility, as well as ii) sequence similarity to a reference plasmid. Next, to confirm the accuracy of the prediction in 1750 *S. enterica* short-read sequencing data, we combined Oxford Nanopore MinION long-read sequencing with Illumina MiSeq short-read sequencing in hybrid assemblies for 84 isolates to evaluate the proportion of plasmid that has been detected. At least one scaffold with an origin of replication (ORI) was predicted in 61.3% of the *Salmonella* isolates tested. The results indicated that IncFII and IncI1 ORIs were distributed in many *S. enterica* serotypes and were the most prevalent AMR genes carrier, whereas IncHI2A/IncHI2 and IncA/C2 were more serotype restricted but bore several AMR genes. Comparison between hybrid and short-read assemblies revealed that 81.1% of plasmids were found in the short-read sequencing using our pipeline. Through this process, we established that plasmids are prevalent in *S. enterica* and we also substantially expand the AMR genes in the resistome of this species.

Keywords: plasmid; *Salmonella enterica*; antimicrobial resistance; long-read sequencing; hybrid assembly

---

1. Introduction

Non-typhoidal *Salmonella enterica* is responsible for 88,000 cases of gastroenteritis in Canada each year. The symptoms of gastroenteritis can be mild to severe depending on the health conditions of individuals. Generally, the patient may recover without antibiotic treatment. However, antibiotic intervention may be necessary for children, the elderly, and immunosuppressed patients.

The *Salmonella* genus belongs to the *Enterobacteriaceae* family and includes two species, *bongori* and *enterica*. According to the Kauffman–White scheme, more than 2500 serotypes have been characterized [1]. As reported by the US Centers for Disease Control and Prevention (CDC), although all *S. enterica* serotypes can cause disease in humans, less than 100 serotypes account for much of the infections.

In 2014, a global report by the World Health Organization (WHO) on the surveillance of antimicrobial resistance (AMR) revealed that increasing resistance across many different infections has become a serious concern for public health worldwide [2]. AMR can be acquired by either spontaneous mutations or by horizontal gene transfer (HGT), in which plasmids are known to play a key role [3]. Plasmids are mobile genetic elements (MGE) encoding for their self-replication and transfer. The genes responsible for plasmid maintenance and transmission form a "backbone" that is a core set of genes encoding for essential plasmid functions [4]. Plasmids also provide non-essential cellular functions, such as virulence factors, AMRs, metabolic pathways, and unknown functions that are defined by genes encoding hypothetical and unknown proteins, which all confer competitive advantages to the bacterial host in specific situations. Once an AMR gene becomes stable on a plasmid through environmental pressures, it can quickly spread across species and ecosystems that can lead to its transfer from the surrounding environment to human pathogens [5,6].

Plasmids are amenable to detailed analysis using data from whole genome sequencing (WGS), using complementary software including mlplasmid, PlasmidFinder, cBar, plasmidSPAdes, Recycler, and PLACNET [7–12]. A recent comparison between five bioinformatics software showed that plasmidSPAdes was capable of fully or partially predicting 84% of plasmids used as references [12]. However, as plasmidSPAdes separates plasmids from chromosomes based on read coverage, plasmid contigs with a similar coverage to the chromosomal contigs are often mislabelled [8].

Plasmids are widespread in *S. enterica,* where they are known to carry nonessential genes involved in AMR and virulence [13,14]. Given that the spreading of AMR genes through microorganisms is a major issue for public health worldwide, the prediction of plasmid-carrying AMR genes will give insight into their dissemination across bacterial strains. In the current study, we expanded our knowledge of AMR genes carried by the plasmidome of 1750 *S. enterica* genomes. These genomes sequenced by Illumina MiSeq as part of a *Salmonella* Syst-OMICS project were analyzed by Plasmid-Gather, a pipeline designed to predict plasmid scaffolds based on the presence of essential genes for plasmid replication, mobility, and sequence similarity to a reference plasmid.

2. Materials and Methods

2.1. Bacterial Isolates and Growth Conditions

The *Salmonella enterica* isolates used in this study are described in Supplementary Table S1. The isolates were grown for 16–18 h at 37 °C on brain heart infusion agar (BHIA; Difco). The isolates were then transferred into Luria–Bertani (LB) broth with either 15% (*v/v*) glycerol or 8% (*v/v*) DMSO and stored at -80 °C until needed.

2.2. DNA Preparation and Sequencing

Genomic DNA was extracted from 1 mL of 4 mL LB broth cultures incubated for 16–18 h at 37 °C in agitation at 200 rpm, using the E–Z 96 Tissue DNA Kit (Omega Bio-tek, Norcross, GA, USA). Approximately 500 ng of genomic DNA was mechanically fragmented for 40 s with a Covaris M220 (Covaris, Woburn, MA, USA) using the default settings. Libraries were synthesized using the NEBNext Ultra II DNA library prep kit for Illumina (New England Biolabs, Ipswich, MA, USA) according to the manufacturer's instructions and sequenced to obtain 30Xs coverage in an Illumina MiSeq 300 bp paired-end run at the Plateforme d'Analyses Génomiques of the Institut de Biologie Intégrative et des Systèmes (Université Laval, Québec, QC, Canada).

2.3. Library Preparation and Oxford Nanopore MinION Sequencing

Genomic DNA was extracted from 16-18 h LB broth cultures at 37 °C using the DNeasy Blood and Tissue Kit (QIAGEN, Toronto, ON, Canada). The manufacturer's protocol has been adapted to maximize the read length (performed without any rapid pipetting, vortexing, and only homogenization by inversion). We used 1.2 µg of a genomic DNA for library preparation with the SQK-LSK109 Kit and followed the manufacturer's recommendations. Native barcoding expansion PCR-free EXP-NBD104 (1–12) and EXP-NBD114 (13–24) kits were used according to the manufacturers' protocol. Twenty-four libraries were pooled and sequenced with a R9.4.1 flow cell (FLO-MIN106D) on a MinION device. On average, one sequencing run gave between 20 to 28 Gb of raw data per run.

2.4. Bio-informatic Analysis and Databases

The origins of replication (ORIs) database (PlasmidFinder-DB) was downloaded from the PlasmidFinder web server [7] (accessed 23/10/2018 10:10). A homemade database (MOBs-DB) of proteins involved in plasmids conjugation, mobilization, or transfer was constructed with annotated proteins encoded by plasmids described in the UniProtKB database [15] (accessed 29/08/2017 20:48). The resulting plasmid mobility proteins were clustered by CD-HIT [16] using 60% and 85% amino acids identity as a cut-off and minimal alignment coverage for the longer and shorter sequences, respectively. By this process, the mobility proteins database contained 361 reference proteins. A plasmids database (Plasmids-DB), containing 13,924 plasmids on 23 October 2018, was downloaded from the National Center for Biotechnology Information (NCBI) (ftp://ftp.ncbi.nlm.nih.gov/genomes/refseq/plasmids/, accessed 23/10/2018 10:15). To ensure that the sequences in the Plasmids-DB were of plasmid origin and not mislabeled chromosomal DNA, we examined all the plasmids with more than 550 kb of DNA. We identified 2 sequences belonging to *Salmonella* plasmids with large sizes (NZ_CP022019.1 = 4,627 kb and NZ_LN868944.1 = 728 kb). NZ_CP022019.1 is most likely a complete chromosome mislabeled as a plasmid because it has the same size as a typical *Salmonella* chromosome. A search of the NCBI non-redundant nucleotide collection database (nr/nt) using the basic local alignement search tool (BLAST) revealed that NZ_LN868944.1 aligned completely with the *Salmonella* chromosomes; these 2 sequences were removed from the Plasmids-DB.

2.5. *Plasmid-Gather Pipeline*

With the aim of detecting plasmids that can carry AMR or virulence genes, we developed an approach that combines 2 types of databases, thereby enhancing the discovery rate of contigs as plasmid fragments. The Plasmid-Gather pipeline is summarized in Figure 1. Briefly, reads were trimmed using Trimmomatic (v. 0.36) [17] and assembled by SPAdes (v. 3.10.1) [18]. We chose SPAdes as an assembler instead of plasmidSPAdes (an algorithm based on Bruijn graph to assemble plasmids), because the latter assembles only reads with coverage different from the chromosome, and therefore low copy plasmids with similar coverage to the chromosome are missed. SPAdes was used to obtain the whole genome assembly, and the plasmids were recovered based on two databases. BLAST (v. 2.6.0) [19] was performed on the resulting scaffolds against the PlasmidFinder-DB (see the above section on databases) to predict the ORI. Since it was expected that some plasmids assembled in several scaffolds were caused by repeated elements [20,21], we added a BLAST (v. 2.6.0) [19] search against a MOBs-DB (see the above section on databases) instead of using exclusively the PlasmidFinder-DB to maximize the discovery of contigs as plasmid fragments. To remove the possible chromosome contigs from the resulting scaffolds predicted by the pipeline, scaffolds with more than 300 kb were not taken in account. Another threshold to exclude sequences less than or equal to 1 kb was also included. To investigate whether the scaffolds corresponded to a known plasmid, the resulting scaffolds were aligned using BLAST (v. 2.6.0) [19] against the NCBI Plasmid database (≥ 95% sequence identity). The percentage of GC content was calculated using the infoseq application from the EMBOSS package (v. 6.5.7) [22].

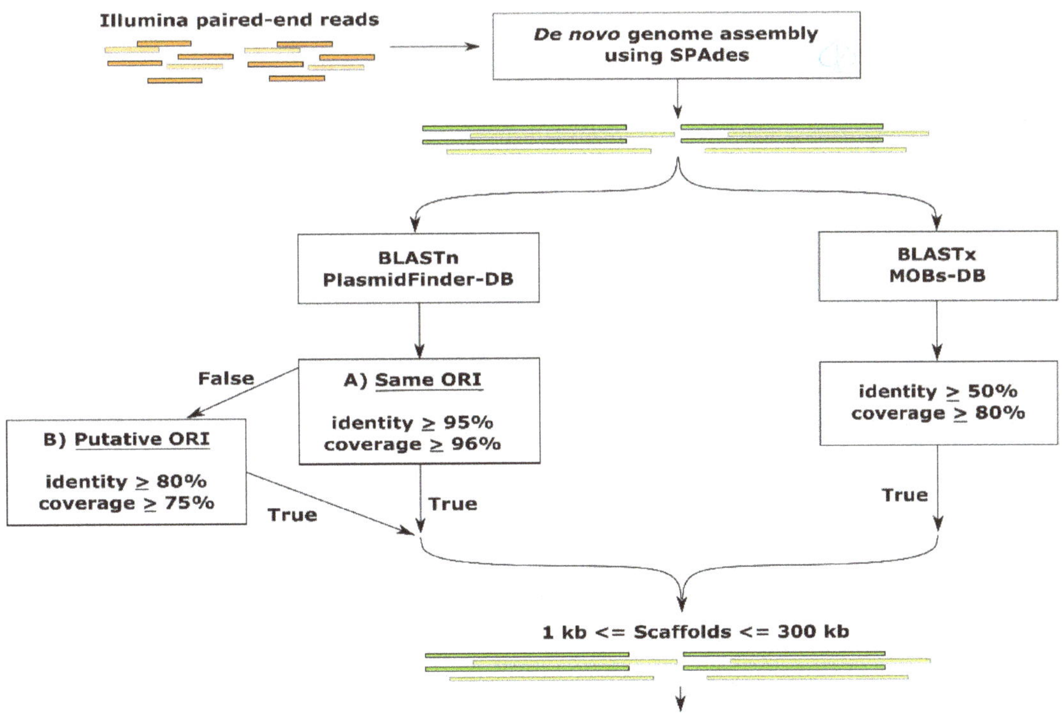

Figure 1. Plasmid-Gather workflow. First, MiSeq Illumina paired-end reads were trimmed using Trimmomatic (version 0.36) [17] and assembled by SPAdes (version 3.10.1) [18]. BLAST analysis (version 2.6.0) [19] against the origin of replications (ORIs) (PlasmidFinder-DB) and mobility proteins databases (MOBs-DB) were performed to predict which scaffolds carried one of these elements. The significant matches against the PlasmidFinder-DB were separated into two groups depending on the threshold: A) the highly similar ORIs with the database or B) the ORIs related to ORIs in the PlasmidFinder-DB. By the latter threshold, we wanted potentially to expand the discovery of plasmid scaffolds. Only scaffolds encoding an ORI and/or a plasmid mobility protein between 1 and 300 kb in size were kept for future analysis.

2.6. Antibiotic Resistance Gene Analysis

AMR genes were predicted using Resistance Gene Identifier (RGI) (v. 4.2.2) based on the BLAST search against the Comprehensive Antibiotic Resistance Database (CARD) [23]. The presence of AMR genes was determined based on the curated e-value cut-offs.

2.7. SISTR

The *Salmonella* serotypes were predicted from the genome assemblies using the *Salmonella In Silico* Typing Resource (SISTR) (v. 1.0.2) [24].

2.8. Plasmid Fragments Recovery (Post-Recovery)

To increase the discovery rate in the Illumina MiSeq assembly of contigs as DNA plasmid fragments, we added an additional step in the Plasmid-Gather pipeline illustrated in Figure 1 to recover plasmid fragments without ORI or mobility proteins. For each scaffold with an ORI identified by Plasmid-Gather, we identified the plasmid with the highest bit score using BLAST against the NCBI Plasmid database (≥ 95% sequence identity, ≥ 15% query coverage per subject, and ≤ 550 kb of subject length). This plasmid, which varied with the plasmid scaffold containing an ORI(s) (query sequence), was used as a reference plasmid to align the Illumina MiSeq assembly. To be considered as a plasmid fragment, the scaffolds must share a ≥ 95% sequence identity and a ≥ 25% query coverage per subject with the reference.

3. Results

3.1. Construction of a Bioinformatics Pipeline for Plasmid Identification

In the framework of the Syst-OMICs genome project, 1750 *S. enterica* isolates (Supplementary Table S1) representing 153 serotypes analyzed by WGS (Supplementary Table S2) and available in the SalFoS database (https://salfos.ibis.ulaval.ca/) [25], were analyzed using the Plasmid-Gather pipeline depicted in Figure 1. Plasmid-Gather was developed to identify plasmid-related scaffolds in WGS data for *S. enterica* isolates by combining a systematic integrated strategy.

Plasmid-Gather identified 2211 scaffolds matching our criteria (i.e., scaffolds between 1 and 300 kb in size encoding either a plasmid mobility protein and/or an ORI) (Supplementary Table S3). There were three scaffolds > 300 kb (750, 515, and 421 kb) that were predicted to be plasmids based upon protein homology with sequences contained in the MOBs-DB (none encoded an ORI). A BLAST of these scaffolds against the NCBI Nucleotide collection (nr/nt) database revealed that they aligned with *Salmonella* chromosomes, but at 94%, 84%, and 94% of query cover, respectively. The genomic regions encoding the mobility proteins predicted by Plasmid-Gather were missed in these three alignments. A BLAST against the NCBI Nucleotide collection (nr/nt) database of these genomic regions where mobility proteins were identified revealed they corresponded to partial plasmid sequences. By evaluating this information, these three scaffolds could presumably be chromosomal DNA contigs carrying an integrated plasmid or an integrated conjugative element (ICE).

Scaffolds identified by Plasmid-Gather were labelled as "plasmid scaffolds". Of these 2211 plasmid scaffolds, our pipeline predicted at least one ORI for 1910 of them. The GC-content, ORI type(s), and presence of the mobility protein are described in Supplementary Table S3. To provide an overview of the plasmid scaffolds that have already been characterized, the percentage coverage of the best alignments using BLAST (identity ≥ 95%) against the NCBI Plasmid database are presented in Supplementary Table S3.

We predicted from 1 to 10 plasmid scaffolds in 1097 *S. enterica* isolates. Of these 1097 isolates, one or several ORIs have been predicted in 1073 isolates. Some plasmids belonging to the *Enterobacteriaceae* were characterized and confirmed to contain more than one ORI [26]. We assume that possessing multiple ORIs would presumably allow plasmids the ability to replicate when transferred into another species or serotype and broaden the range of hosts. Overall, we predicted 2350 ORIs, of which 851 were termed as putative ORIs (Supplementary Table S4). Although the ORI termed as "putative ORI" contains the name of its closest BLAST match (e.g., putative-*IncFII*), putative ORIs were considered as a different type of ORI. Further analysis will be needed to consider a putative ORI as part of the same incompatibility group (Inc) to its closest BLAST match. A collection of 12 plasmid scaffolds carried three ORIs (10 IncFIB/IncFII/IncX1, 1 IncFIB/IncFII/IncI1, and 1 IncFIA/IncHI1A/IncHI1B), 416 had two ORIs (251 IncFIB/IncFII and 16 other combinations), and 1471 had one ORI. The three most frequent ORIs identified in *Salmonella* isolates, excluding the 851 putative ORIs, were the transferable IncFII ($n_{isolate} = 533$), IncFIB ($n_{isolate} = 371$), and IncI ($n_{isolate} = 142$) (Table 1). All three Inc group plasmids have been shown to carry virulence-associated and AMR genes within *Enterobacteriaceae* [14,27–30]. The majority of the IncFII and IncFIB ORIs were identified from *S.* Enteritidis and *S.* Typhimurium (Table 1) (at 33% and 28% for IncFII and at 47% and 39% for IncFIB, respectively). Moreover, IncFII was co-carried with IncFIB in 97% of the isolates (359/371). Even putative ORIs were excluded in Table 1; the three most widespread ORIs between *Salmonella* serotypes were IncFII ($n_{serotype} = 50$), IncI1 ($n_{serotype} = 43$), and ColpVC ($n_{serotype} = 37$). In contrast, the two ORIs, IncX1 ($n_{serotype} = 10$) and IncA/C2 ($n_{serotype} = 12$), were limited to few serotypes (Table 1).

Table 1. Nine most frequent ORIs found across the most frequent *S. enterica* serotypes.

Serotype	Number of Isolates (Given by SISTR V. 1.0.2)	Nine Most Frequent ORIs (if $n_{replicon} \geq 20$)								
		IncFII	IncFIB	IncI1	IncX1	ColpVC	IncA/C2	Col156	IncHI2A	IncHI2
Typhimurium	201	147	145	28	3	7	11	6	-	-
Enteritidis	200	179	178	9	24	3	-	1	-	-
Newport	80	14	-	2	3	-	25	-	1	1
Heidelberg	51	-	-	13	35	19	1	2	4	4
Oranienburg	49	30	-	-	-	1	-	-	-	-
Thompson	44	2	-	-	-	3	-	-	-	-
Muenchen	43	4	2	3	-	-	-	-	-	-
Infantis	38	-	-	5	-	-	1	-	-	-
Anatum	38	13	-	5	-	1	3	-	1	1
Senftenberg	36	-	1	-	-	-	-	-	-	-
Braenderup	34	3	3	-	-	1	-	-	-	-
Javiana	28	2	-	2	-	-	-	-	-	-
Saintpaul	26	4	1	3	-	2	-	1	2	2
Agona	26	1	-	7	-	1	1	-	1	1
I_4 [5]; 12:i:-	25	17	17	6	-	1	1	-	1	1
Montevideo	24	1	-	1	1	-	-	-	-	-
Paratyphi_B_var._Java_monophasic	23	16	-	1	-	1	-	-	-	-
Give	23	-	-	1	-	1	-	1	-	-
Gaminara	21	-	-	-	-	-	-	-	-	
Paratyphi_B_var._Java	20	1	-	3	-	1	-	-	-	-
Paratyphi_B	20	-	-	2	-	-	-	-	-	-
Kentucky	20	9	9	11	13	1	-	1	3	3
Typhi	17	-	1	-	-	-	-	-	-	-
Hartford	17	17	-	-	-	1	-	-	-	-
Tennessee	16	-	-	1	-	-	1	1	1	1
Mississippi	16	1	-	1	-	-	-	-	-	-
Mbandaka	16	-	1	-	-	1	-	-	1	1
Rubislaw	15	2	-	-	2	5	-	3	-	-
Manhattan	15	-	-	2	-	1	-	-	-	-
Dublin	15	15	-	-	15	-	5	-	-	-
Total of isolates	1197	478	358	106	96	51	49	16	15	15
Total of isolates in other serotypes	553	55	13	36	2	37	4	13	9	9
Total of isolates in all serotypes	1750	533	371	142	98	88	53	29	24	24
Count of serotypes	153	50	18	43	10	37	12	16	17	17

3.2. Antibiotic Resistance Genes of the S. enterica Plasmidome

To evaluate the diversity of plasmid-encoded AMR genes that can potentially complicate disease treatments and potentially be transferred to other bacteria, we next predicted AMR genes carried by the *S. enterica* plasmidome using the Resistance Gene Identifier (RGI v. 4.2.2) [23]. The RGI predicted 863 AMR genes across 375 plasmid scaffolds in 327 *S. enterica* genomes (Supplementary Table S5). Plasmid scaffolds encoded 55 different AMR genes, and 96 unique resistomes encoded by plasmid scaffolds were found across the 327 genomes (Figure 2).

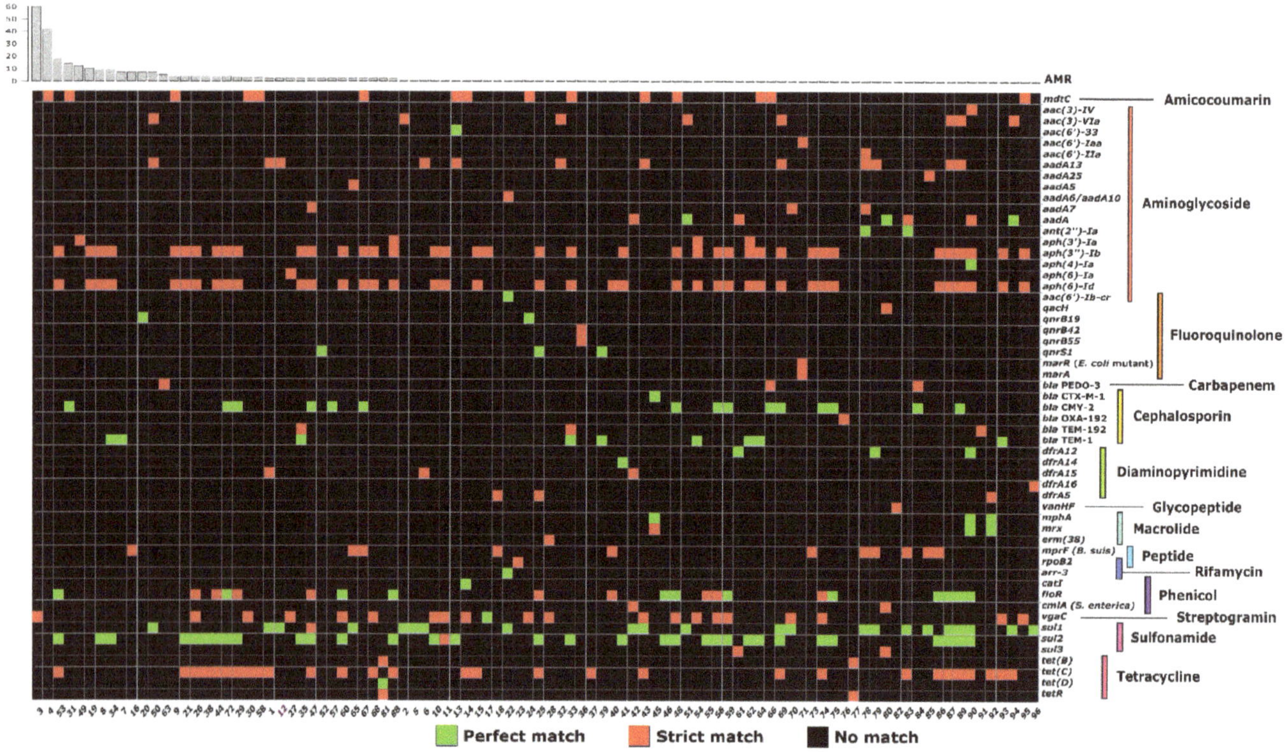

Figure 2. Antimicrobial resistance (AMR) genes of the *S. enterica* plasmidome predicted using the Resistance Gene Identifier (RGI) (v. 4.2.2), based on the Comprehensive Antibiotic Resistance Database (CARD) [23]. The bar plot above shows the frequency of unique resistomes. Numbers below the heatmap indicate the antimicrobial resistance profile (AMRp) (Supplementary Table S5). The AMRps were assigned to the resistome of each isolate plasmidome. The antibiotic family or function are shown on the right.

The plasmid scaffolds with the highest number of AMR genes were a single without ORI (absent) (n_{AMR} = 9), three containing IncA/C2 (n_{AMR} = 8), and one with IncL/M (n_{AMR} = 7). We found that the three most frequent ORIs carrying the AMR gene(s) were IncI1 (n_{ORI} = 98), followed by IncFII (n_{ORI} = 50) and IncX1 (n_{ORI} = 25). IncI1 has previously been the most common ORI type identified in multi-drugs resistance isolates [31]. However, in our studies plasmid scaffolds without an ORI are the second most common AMR gene carriers (86 scaffolds into 76 isolates). These are likely DNA fragments of larger plasmids of which the ORI assembled on another scaffold. Plasmids can be assembled in several scaffolds because of repeated elements. Further analysis using PCR or DNA long-read sequencing will be required to order scaffolds for assembly.

AMR genes were also identified for the 1750 *S. enterica* genomes in which plasmid scaffolds were removed and both resistomes were compared (Supplementary Table S6). The prevalence of AMR genes available from the CARD website (v. 4.2.2) among *Salmonella* genomes from the NCBI Chromosome and NCBI Plasmid databases were included in Supplementary Table S6 for comparative purposes. An analysis of 1750 *Salmonella* chromosomes showed an average of 39 AMR genes by genome (from 30 to 56 AMR genes/ genome), which represented 207 different AMR genes. Thirty-four AMR genes were predicted in nearly all chromosomes (from 95 to 100% of chromosomes) (26 out of these 34 resistance mechanisms belong to an antibiotic efflux pump complex) (Supplementary Table S6). These genes may likely correspond to the core resistome of *S. enterica*. Moreover, the prevalence of 25 of these AMR genes in the NCBI Plasmid and Chromosome databases found in the CARD database were consistent with our prediction (Supplementary Table S6). Overall, 17 AMR genes that were infrequently predicted in chromosomes are normally limited to the NCBI Plasmid database according to CARD (0% in NCBI Chromosome database) (Supplementary Table S6), which suggests that some plasmid scaffolds may remain unidentified among chromosome scaffolds.

3.3. *Increasing Recovery of Plasmid Scaffolds Using a Reference*

To investigate whether plasmid scaffolds remained within the *S. enterica* chromosome scaffolds, the four chromosomal scaffolds carrying *aac(3)-VIa*, a resistance gene limited to the NCBI Plasmid database, were aligned against the NCBI Plasmid database, and their best match was used as reference to map the Illumina MiSeq assemblies (Figure 3).

In three of the four cases, the best match from the NCBI Plasmid database was the multidrug-resistant plasmid IncA/C pSN254, while the fourth was identified as IncHI2 pAPEC-01-R [32,33]. To confirm the ORI type of the plasmids from Plasmids-DB, we aligned all the plasmids of the NCBI Plasmid database using BLAST against the PlasmidFinder-DB [7]. The plasmid pSN254, as well as many *Salmonella* plasmids first published as IncA/C (pAM04528, peH4H, pAR060302, p1643_10, p33676, pCVM2245, pCVM22462, pCVM22513, pCVM21538, pCVMN1543, and pCVM21550), perfectly matched with IncA/C2; meanwhile, pRA1 and pRAx matched with IncA/C [34–38]. As mentioned by Carattoli et al. (2006), IncA/C and IncA/C2 exhibit 26 nucleotide substitutions [39]. As demonstrated in Figure 3, at least two scaffolds that aligned with the reference plasmid had already been detected in the WGS using our pipeline; one encoded the TraI mobility protein, whereas the second carried the ORI(s) (IncA/C2 or IncHI2/IncHI2A). Furthermore, as depicted in Figure 3, several new plasmid scaffolds were recovered using the closest homologous plasmid from NCBI as the reference plasmid. Figure 3 also shows the complexity of plasmid reconstruction, which is probably due to the high plasticity of some plasmids, as observed for IncHI2 and IncA/C [31,40,41].

To improve the detection of plasmid fragments, we added a last step that used a reference plasmid to the Plasmid-Gather pipeline, which is illustrated in Figure 1. However, instead of using the scaffold encoding the AMR gene to select the closest reference plasmid, we picked the reference based on the best match with the scaffold bearing the ORI. We recovered 1172 scaffolds for the *S. enterica* plasmidome, giving a total of 3383 scaffolds. By taking this data into account, the scaffolds were re-assorted into two groups as plasmid and chromosome scaffolds.

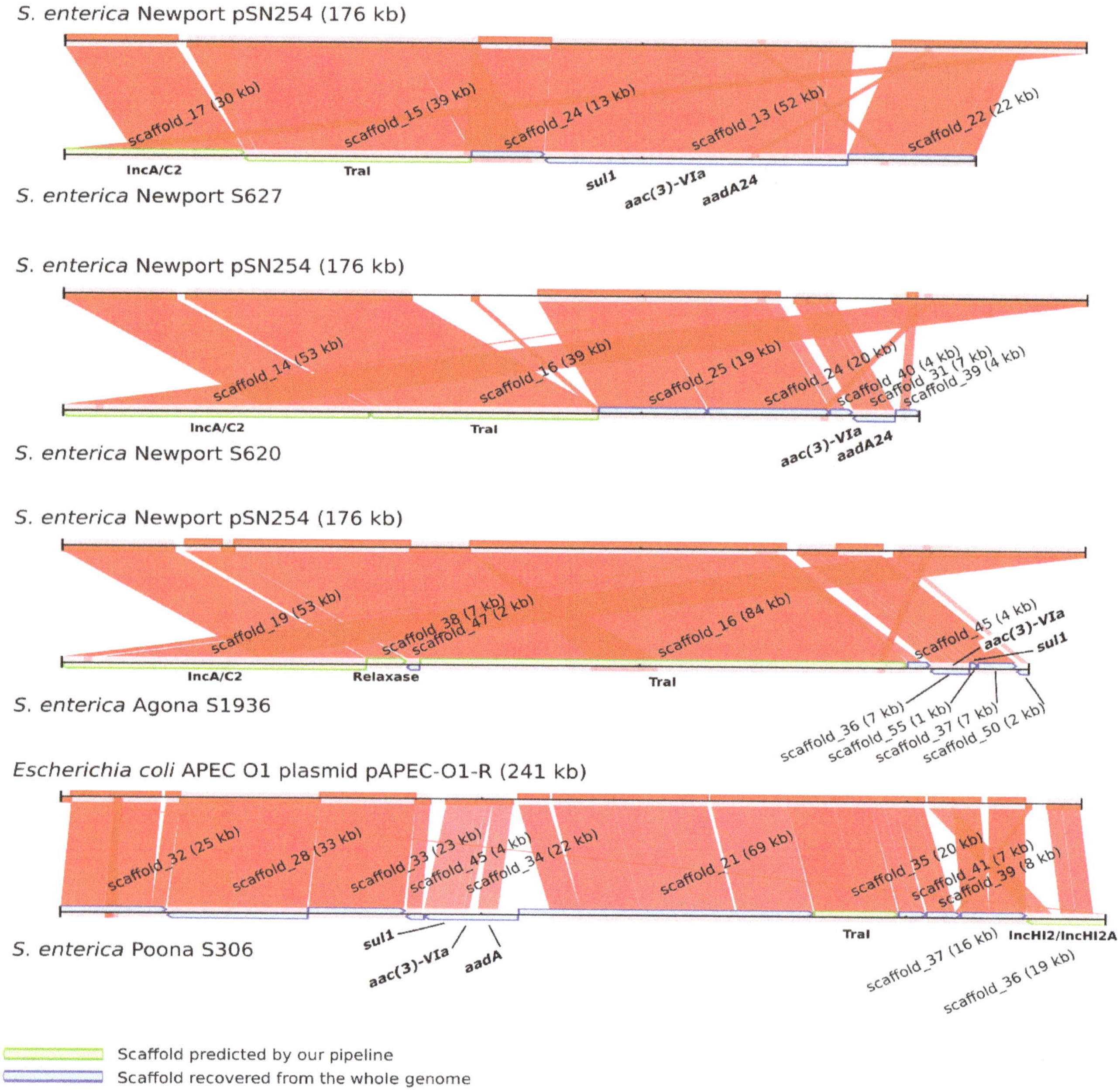

Figure 3. Recovery of plasmid fragments in whole genome sequencing (WGS) data based on comparisons with reference plasmids. The reference plasmids above each alignment were selected based on the best match against the National Center for Biotechnology Information (NCBI) Plasmid database with the scaffold encoding *aac(3)-VIa* gene usually found in plasmid sequences. The WGS data were mapped using CONTIGuator v. 2.7 against the reference plasmids. Several scaffolds without ORI or mobility protein have been identified as plasmid scaffolds in the four *Salmonella* genomes using a reference plasmid.

3.4. The Resistome of S. enterica Plasmids and Chromosomes

We predicted AMR genes using RGI v. 4.2.2 [23], but in the *S. enterica* plasmid and chromosome scaffolds that were separated using the strategy that we called post-recovery. The AMR genes predicted in either the post-recovery plasmid or chromosome scaffolds of *S. enterica* showed a better AMR gene specificity carried by each. RGI predicts in plasmids a total of 1174 AMR genes (311 new AMR comparing with the previous prediction). Several predicted AMR genes, which are frequently found in the NCBI Plasmid database when compared to the NCBI Chromosome database, showed similar distributions with CARD (Supplementary Table S7). For instance, before the recovery of plasmid scaffolds, 36 and 37 $bla_{\text{CMY-2}}$ genes were predicted in plasmids and chromosomes, respectively (Supplementary Table S6). After the post-recovery strategy based on a reference plasmid, 69 (6.26%) and 4 (0.23%) $bla_{\text{CMY-2}}$ were identified within plasmids and chromosomes (Supplementary Table S7). The prevalence of the $bla_{\text{CMY-2}}$ gene in the *S. enterica* genomes from the NCBI Plasmid and NBCI Chromosome databases are 6.62% and 0.73%, respectively, which is consistent with what we obtained post-recovery (Supplementary Table S7). A similar trend was observed for the *sul1*, $bla_{\text{TEM-1}}$, *tet(B)*, *tet(C)*, *tet(D)*, *tetR*, and *aph(3')-Ia* AMR genes.

To determine whether there is an enrichment of certain AMR genes between the plasmids and chromosomes of *S. enterica*, we calculated *p* values using Fisher's exact test (Supplementary Table S7). We noted that 52 and 13 AMR genes were significantly enriched ($p < 0.001$) in chromosomes and plasmids, respectively (Supplementary Table S8 and Table 2).

Table 2. Additional antimicrobial genes found in the *S. enterica* plasmidome.

AMR Genes with a p-Value ≤ 0.001	Prevalence (%)	Resistance Mechanism	Drug Class	Confers Resistance to
aac(3)-Via	1.4	antibiotic inactivation	aminoglycoside antibiotic	gentamicin B and C
aph(3")-Ib (strA)	10.5	antibiotic inactivation	aminoglycoside antibiotic	streptomycin
aph(6)-Id (strB)	10.4	antibiotic inactivation	aminoglycoside antibiotic	streptomycin
aadA8	0.8	antibiotic inactivation	aminoglycoside antibiotic	streptomycin and spectinomycin
aadA13	2.5	antibiotic inactivation	aminoglycoside antibiotic	streptomycin and spectinomycin
$bla_{CMY\text{-}2}$	6.3	antibiotic inactivation	cephamycin and cephalosporin	cefoxitin, cephamycin and ceftazidime
$bla_{TEM\text{-}1}$	4.3	antibiotic inactivation	penem, cephalosporin, monobactam, penam	amoxicillin, ampicillin and cefalotin
floR	4.7	antibiotic efflux	phenicol antibiotic	chloramphenicol and florfenicol
sul2	8.5	antibiotic target replacement	sulfonamide antibiotic, sulfone antibiotic	sulfadiazine, sulfadimidine, sulfadoxine, sulfamethoxazole, sulfisoxazole, sulfacetamide, mafenide, sulfasalazine and sulfamethizole
tet(C)	7.9	antibiotic efflux	tetracycline antibiotic	tetracycline
tet(D)	2.2	antibiotic efflux	tetracycline antibiotic	tetracycline
mprF (Brucella suis)	2.1	antibiotic target alteration	peptide antibiotic	defensin
qnrB19	0.7	antibiotic target protection	fluoroquinolone antibiotic	-

3.5. Analysis of Plasmid Content Using Long-Read DNA Sequencing

As depicted in Supplementary Table S9, 84 *Salmonella* isolates were selected from distant branches of a phylogenetic tree representing 2544 *S. enterica* genomes to get the inter alia maximum genome and plasmid diversity contained in the *S. enterica* species (Figure 4). Additionally, expanding the WGS using the Oxford Nanopore giving DNA long-reads and combining this data with Illumina MiSeq short-reads in the hybrid genome assembly of the complete chromosome and plasmid contents allowed us to evaluate our prediction in the short-reads data using Plasmid-Gather.

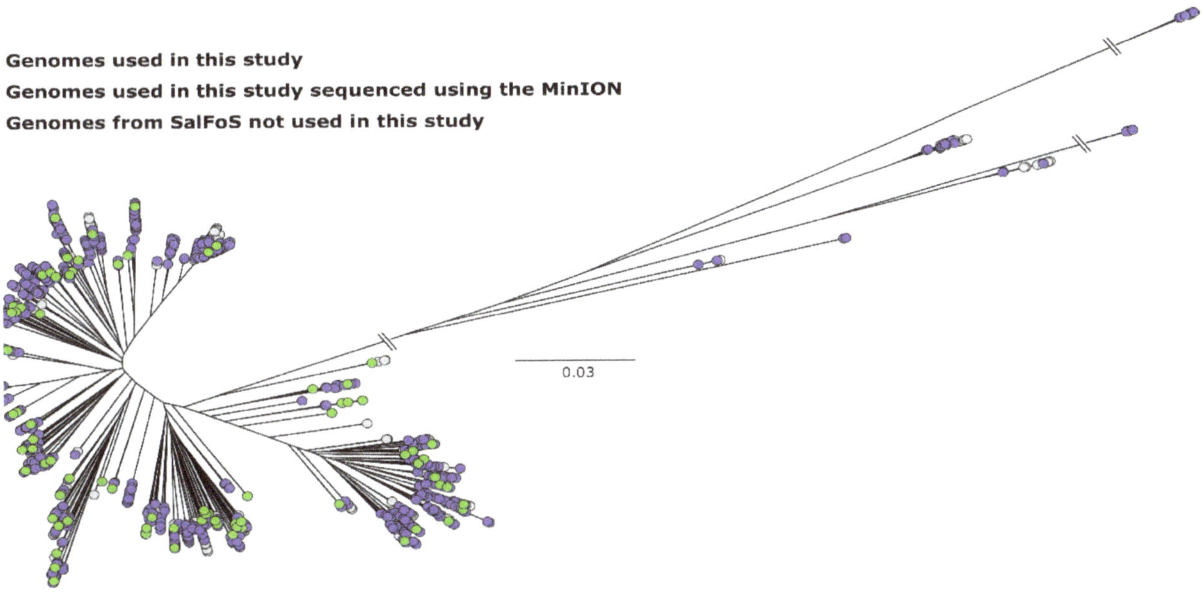

Figure 4. Unrooted maximum likelihood tree of 2544 *S. enterica* genomes based on 173,657 single nucleotide polymorphisms (SNPs). Genomes were assembled using SPAdes. Isolates used are labelled in green and blue. Green nodes were isolates sequenced using Oxford Nanopore.

The combined hybrid assemblies gave the complete bacterial chromosome in all the 84 isolates selected. Hybrid assemblies of the complete chromosomes also indicated 73 scaffolds, of which 64 were predicted as plasmids (87.7%) using the ORIs (PlasmidFinder-DB) and the mobility proteins (MOBs-DB) databases that predicted plasmids in the short-read assemblies (Supplementary Table S9). Mobility proteins or ORI sequences were not identified in the *Salmonella* chromosomes, demonstrating a high specificity of the two databases for extrachromosomal elements. The percentage of each plasmid assembled using hybrid assemblies covered by those predicted in the MiSeq data has been calculated, and the sum showed that 81.1% of plasmids were found in the short-read assemblies. Nine extrachromosomal elements, of which eight are small elements (less than 7 kb), could not be identified as plasmids in both assemblies, although the online BLAST searches on NCBI indicated that they matched with the plasmid sequences.

The AMR genes were predicted using RGI v. 4.2.2 in the 73 extrachromosomal elements only [23] (Supplementary Table S9). This analysis gave two major observations: 1) the most frequent ORI carrying AMR genes was IncI1 (4/5), and 2) the plasmid with the greatest number of AMR genes was an IncA/C2 ($n_{AMR} = 12$; *aac(3)-VIa, aph(3")-Ib, aph(6)-Id,* $bla_{CMY\text{-}35}$, $bla_{CMY\text{-}44}$, $bla_{CMY\text{-}80}$, $bla_{CMY\text{-}90}$, *aadA13, floR, sul1, sul2* and *tet(C)*) (Supplementary Table S9). Both observations were consistent with our prediction in the MiSeq data described above.

4. Discussion

By combining a collection of public and SalFoS data, we identified a high proportion of plasmid contigs in Illumina MiSeq WGS assemblies using two databases containing essential conserved plasmid elements (PlasmidFinder-DB and MOBs-DB) combined with known reference plasmids. One of the added values will be to increase the plasmid sequences identified. The databases can be regularly updated to include new ORIs and mobility genes for future analyses.

By using Plasmid-Gather and the combined strategies described here, IncFII and IncFIB were the most frequent ORIs predicted in *S. enterica*; this was presumably caused by the over-representation of the *S.* Enteritidis and *S.* Typhimurium isolates in the dataset (Table 1). These two serotypes accounted for more than 23% of all the isolates and carried together 61% and 87%, respectively, of all th eIncFII and IncFIB (Table 1). The distribution of ORIs among the *S. enterica* serotypes showed that IncFII, IncI1, and ColpVC were found in a broad range of serotypes, whereas IncA/C2 and IncX1 are restricted to a dozen serotypes (Table 1). Interestingly, Lindsey et al. (2009) demonstrated by a cluster-based analysis using the pulsed field gel electrophoresis (PFGE) of 216 multidrug resistance *S. enterica* that IncI1 is not clonally distributed, whereas IncA/C is commonly observed in the same serotypes. Hence, IncI1 is presumably much more mobile than IncA/C [42]. IncI1 incompatibility was often associated with multi-drug resistance and with the widespread distribution of Beta-lactam resistance genes [28,29,41,43]. Likewise, we observed that plasmids with IncI1 are among the most important carriers of AMR genes (Supplementary Table S5 and Supplementary Table S9). Hence, one may assume that the mobility of IncI1 also leads to the spread of AMR genes in many *S. enterica* serotypes, whereas IncA/C2 seems more serotype restricted, but were associated with several AMR genes.

Large plasmids, representing different Inc ORIs, are known to integrate and carry transposons or integrons conferring AMR [3,14]. Several multi-resistance plasmids have been identified in *Salmonella*. Among them is the Inc group A/C (IncA/C and A/C2), consisting of 150 kb plasmids [31,33,38,42,44]. In our study, 49 of the 53 IncA/C2 plasmid scaffolds had less than 54 kb. This may be due to the limitations of plasmid assembly, as demonstrated in Figure 3. Three of the four IncA/C2 assembled with expected sizes encoding seven AMR genes each (*aph(3″)-Ib*, *aph(6)-Ib*, $bla_{CMY\text{-}2}$, *sul1*, *sul2*, *aad* or *aad7*, and *florR* or *aac(3)-IV*) (Supplementary Table S5). In addition, the IncA/C2 plasmid reconstructed by hybrid assembly from the S624 isolate possessed 12 AMR genes, a greater number than the other plasmids carrying AMR genes obtained using hybrid assemblies (Supplementary Table S9). Furthermore, in the Illumina MiSeq data we noted that nearly all the *S. enterica* isolates with IncA/C2 (52/53) had one or more AMR encoded by scaffolds in their plasmidome. Isolates with IncA/C2 plasmids carried on average five AMR genes (up to 11 for the S628 isolate); IncA/C2 is the only ORI predicted in 23/53 genomes. Multidrug resistance isolates have been linked previously to IncA/C [42].

Regarding the 52 AMR genes significantly enriched amongst *S. enterica* chromosomes, 34 were part of what we call "the core resistome"—i.e., AMR genes found in more than 95% of *S. enterica* genomes (described in Supplementary Table S8). The predominant AMR mechanism in the so-called core resistome is antibiotic efflux (26/34). Efflux transporters exist as either single- (e.g., Tet) or multi-component pumps (e.g., MdsABC complex) [45]. Multidrug efflux pumps are common resistance mechanisms among Gram-negative bacteria [45]. However, due to various efflux pumps that can compensate with wide substrate specificity, it remains a challenge to identify which drug efflux pump confers AMR. For other less frequent AMR genes found in *S. enterica*, *aac(6′)-Ia,a* and *aac(6′)-Iy* sharing a 99% amino acid identity were found in different serotypes (e.g., Typhimurium, Braenderup, and I 4 [5];12;i;- for *aac(6′)-Iaa*; Enteritidis, Newport, and Heidelberg for *aac(6′)-Iy*). Together, these 2 *N*-acetyltranferases (AAC) were encoded within 1738 chromosomes (99.3%), as shown in Supplementary Table S8. The gene *fosA7*, conferring resistance to fosfomycin, was predicted in 100% of the *S.* Heidelberg (51/51) isolates. In alignment with these results, fosfomycin resistance has previously been found in *S.* Heidelberg isolated from broiler chickens [46]. Similarly, *fosA7* was observed predominantly in almost all the isolates from the same serotype: in 96% of *S.* Agona (25/26), in 100% of the *S.* Telelkebir (8/8), in

67% of the *S.* Derby (8/12), and in 70% of the *S.* Alachua (7/10). The remaining *fosA7* genes ($n = 23$) were distributed among 14 under-represented serotypes.

Although considered as chromosome encoded, some efflux pumps have been identified on plasmids, such as the *tetA* gene encoding tetracycline resistance [47]. As shown in Table 2, 3 of the 13 AMR genes enriched in the *Salmonella* plasmidome encoded efflux pumps, 2 conferred resistance to tetracycline (*tet(C)* and *tet(D)*) and the last one was the resistance to chloramphenicol/florfenicol (*floR*). Tetracycline has been overused in human and veterinary medicines as growth promoters in animals [48,49]. The *tet(C)* and *tet(D)* AMR genes were often reported on MGEs, such as genomic islands (GEIs), as part of conjugative elements and in plasmids [50–54]. We observed a low abundance of *tet(C)* and *tet(D)* in isolates carrying plasmid scaffolds (7.9% and 2.2%, respectively) (Table 2). Previous studies have shown the rare occurrence of these AMR genes in *Salmonella enterica* strains [55,56]. The serotypes of *S. enterica* from SalFoS harboring *tet* genes were mostly *S.* Newport (29.9%, $n = 26$) and *S.* Typhimurium (23%, $n = 20$) for *tet(C)* and *S.* Kentucky (41.7%, $n = 10$) for *tet(D)*. The *floR* gene is the only significant plasmid gene conferring resistance to chloramphenicol (Table 2). We also noticed that 92.3% of the plasmidomes coding for *floR* also carried an IncA/C2, thereby leading to the conclusion that this ORI is likely to be strongly associated with its dissemination. The connection between *floR* and IncA/C2 can also be seen in hybrid assemblies, because *floR* was only predicted once in an IncA/C2 plasmid (Supplementary Table S9). The *floR* gene was already highlighted as the most common in *Salmonella* chloramphenicol-resistant strains [56,57].

In examining the AMR genes detected in plasmids (Table 2), the most common resistance encoded was resistance to streptomycin (*strA* and *strB* resistance genes). In addition to being used for human medicine, streptomycin is used as a feed supplements for pigs and as a pesticide for agriculture [48,58]. Likely because it is extensively used in agriculture, resistance to streptomycin was frequently found in environmental and pathogenic isolates [59,60]. Moreover, aminoglycoside antibiotic was the most prevalent drug class identified.

In this study, we were also interested in AMR genes that may complicate the treatment of salmonellosis and cause possible public health issues by the HGT of AMR genes. In 2014, of all antimicrobials prescribed in human medicine used for treating bacterial infections, the beta-lactam amoxicillin represented the largest proportion used (26%), followed by azithromycin (9%) and ciprofloxacin (8%) [61]. In the same year, 5% of the non-typhoidal *Salmonella* isolates were resistant to amoxicillin, while no resistance to azithromycin or ciprofloxacin was observed; these last two antimicrobials were largely prescribed to treat severe and invasive salmonellosis [61]. Three AMR genes identified in the *S. enterica* plasmidome confer resistance to either amoxicillin ($bla_{\text{TEM-1}}$ ($n = 47$)), azithromycin (*mphA* ($n = 4$)) or ciprofloxacin (*aac(6′)-Ib-cr* ($n = 1$)) (Supplementary Table S7); the last two antibiotics are used to treat severe and invasive *Salmonella* infections [62–64]. Fortunately, these three AMR genes are infrequent in the *S. enterica* plasmidome, except for $bla_{\text{TEM-1}}$, and are not co-carried by the same isolate. However, once an AMR gene is plasmid-stable, AMR resistance can quickly spread through bacterial communities, and so this is something that may need future monitoring. In contrast, there is no clear pattern among *S. enterica* isolates harboring $bla_{\text{TEM-1}}$; these strains were isolated from 1981 to 2011 in five countries from eight species representing 15 *Salmonella* serotypes. Furthermore, nine different ORIs were found to be associated with scaffolds carrying $bla_{\text{TEM-1}}$.

5. Conclusions

Dealing with the increasing multi-resistance of *S. enterica* isolates remains a major worldwide challenge. Over the last decade, mobile genetic elements including plasmids have contributed to the spread of AMR genes vertically and horizontally between serotypes. *S. enterica*, one of the leading foodborne pathogens in industrialized countries, is known to carry plasmids encoding AMR and virulence. We present an integrated strategy to identify plasmid scaffolds using WGS. We combined two databases containing essential elements for plasmid DNA replication (PlasmidFinder-DB) and for plasmid mobility (MOBs-DB). In the current study, we highlight the great diversity of plasmids present in *S. enterica* as reflected on the basis of ORIs diversity. Plasmids were identified in 1750 *S. enterica* genomes, representing 153 serotypes, and 61.3% of the genomes from 1073 of 1750 WGS data had at least one plasmid carrying an ORI, thereby confirming plasmid prevalence in *S. enterica*. Whereas the databases from NCBI, EMBL, and DDBJ are overflowing with WGS data, this is not significantly informative without metadata and the availability of isolates for future functional studies. The SalFoS *Salmonella* database was constructed for the public distribution of isolates for functional studies and serves as a convenient resource to accomplish the expansion of the metadata.

Author Contributions: J.-G.E.-R., J.H., J.J., L.F., I.K.-I., B.B. participated in the technology development, database construction, and experiments. S.T., D.M., E.F., E.B., F.D., G.A., K.S., M.W., R.M.S., J.T.W., R.S., S.B., S.G., L.D.G. furnished isolates and metadata. R.C.L., J.-G.E.-R., L.D.G., D.M., F.D. wrote and revised the manuscript. All authors have read and agreed to the published version of the manuscript.

Acknowledgments: We express our gratitude to the team of the IBIS Genomics analysis platform for excellent work and collaborations (http://www.ibis.ulaval.ca/en/services-2/genomic-analysis-platform/). We also would like to thank Alexander Gill from Health Canada, Bureau of Microbial Hazards, Ottawa, ON, for the *S. enterica* isolates provided for the study.

References

1. Grimont, P.A.; Weill, F.-X. *Antigenic Formulae of the Salmonella Servovars*, 9th ed.; Institut Pasteur: Paris, France, 2007; Volume 13.
2. *World Health Organization Antimicrobial Resistance: Global Report on Surveillance*; World Heath Organization: Geneva, Switzerland, 2014.
3. Rozwandowicz, M.; Brouwer, M.S.M.; Fischer, J.; Wagenaar, J.A.; González-Zorn, B.; Guerra, B.; Mevius, D.J.; Hordijk, J. Plasmids carrying antimicrobial resistance genes in Enterobacteriaceae. *J. Antimicrob. Chemother.* **2018**, *73*, 1121–1137. [CrossRef] [PubMed]
4. Thomas, C.M. Paradigms of plasmid organization. *Mol. Microb.* **2000**, *37*, 485–491. [CrossRef] [PubMed]
5. Morosini, M.I.; Blázquez, J.; Negri, M.-C.; Cantón, R.; Loza, E.; Baquero, F. Characterization of a Nosocomial Outbreak Involving an Epidemic Plasmid Encoding for TEM-27 in Salmonella enterica Subspecies enterica Serotype Othmarschen. *J. Infect. Dis.* **1996**, *17*, 1015–1020. [CrossRef] [PubMed]
6. Cantón, R.; Gonzalez-Alba, J.M.; Galán, J.C. CTX-M Enzymes: Origin and Diffusion. *Front. Microbiol.* **2012**, *3*, 110. [CrossRef]
7. Carattoli, A.; Zankari, E.; Garcia-Fernandez, A.; Larsen, M.V.; Lund, O.; Villa, L.; Aarestrup, F.M.; Hasman, H. In SilicoDetection and Typing of Plasmids using PlasmidFinder and Plasmid Multilocus Sequence Typing. *Antimicrob. Agents Chemother.* **2014**, *58*, 3895–3903. [CrossRef]
8. Antipov, D.; Hartwick, N.; Shen, M.; Rayko, M.; Lapidus, A.; Pevzner, P.A. plasmidSPAdes: Assembling Plasmids from Whole Genome Sequencing Data. *Bioinformatics* **2016**, *32*, 3380–3387. [CrossRef]
9. Rozov, R.; Kav, A.B.; Bogumil, D.; Shterzer, N.; Halperin, E.; Mizrahi, I.; Shamir, R. Recycler: An algorithm for detecting plasmids from de novo assembly graphs. *Bioinformatics* **2017**, *33*, 475–482. [CrossRef]
10. Lanza, V.F.; De Toro, M.; Garcillán-Barcia, M.P.; Mora, A.; Blanco, J.; Coque, T.M.; De La Cruz, F. Plasmid Flux in Escherichia coli ST131 Sublineages, Analyzed by Plasmid Constellation Network (PLACNET), a New Method for Plasmid Reconstruction from Whole Genome Sequences. *PLoS Genet.* **2014**, *10*, e1004766. [CrossRef]
11. Zhou, F.; Xu, Y. cBar: A computer program to distinguish plasmid-derived from chromosome-derived sequence fragments in metagenomics data. *Bioinformatics* **2010**, *26*, 2051–2052. [CrossRef]
12. Arredondo-Alonso, S.; Willems, R.J.; Van Schaik, W.; Schürch, A.C. On the (im)possibility of reconstructing plasmids from whole-genome short-read sequencing data. *Microb. Genom.* **2017**, *3*. [CrossRef]

13. Guiney, D.G.; Fierer, J.M. The Role of the spv Genes in Salmonella Pathogenesis. *Front. Microbiol.* **2011**, *2*, 1–10. [CrossRef]
14. Carattoli, A. Resistance Plasmid Families in Enterobacteriaceae. *Antimicrob. Agents Chemother.* **2009**, *53*, 2227–2238. [CrossRef]
15. The UniProt Consortium UniProt: The universal protein knowledgebase. *Nucleic Acids Res.* **2018**, *46*, 2699. [CrossRef]
16. Fu, L.; Niu, B.; Zhu, Z.; Wu, S.; Li, W. CD-HIT: Accelerated for clustering the next-generation sequencing data. *Bioinformatics* **2012**, *28*, 3150–3152. [CrossRef]
17. Bolger, A.M.; Lohse, M.; Usadel, B. Trimmomatic: A flexible trimmer for Illumina sequence data. *Bioinformatics* **2014**, *30*, 2114–2120. [CrossRef]
18. Bankevich, A.; Nurk, S.; Antipov, D.; Gurevich, A.A.; Dvorkin, M.; Kulikov, A.S.; Lesin, V.M.; Nikolenko, S.I.; Pham, S.; Prjibelski, A.D.; et al. SPAdes: A New Genome Assembly Algorithm and Its Applications to Single-Cell Sequencing. *J. Comput. Biol.* **2012**, *19*, 455–477. [CrossRef]
19. Altschul, S.F.; Gish, W.; Miller, W.; Myers, E.W.; Lipman, D.J. Basic local alignment search tool. *J. Mol. Biol.* **1990**, *215*, 403–410. [CrossRef]
20. Treangen, T.J.; Salzberg, S.L. Repetitive DNA and next-generation sequencing: Computational challenges and solutions. *Nat. Rev. Genet.* **2011**, *13*, 36–46. [CrossRef]
21. Utturkar, S.M.; Klingeman, D.M.; Hurt, R.A.J.; Brown, S.D. A Case Study into Microbial Genome Assembly Gap Sequences and Finishing Strategies. *Front. Microbiol.* **2017**, *8*, 1–11. [CrossRef] [PubMed]
22. Rice, P.; Longden, I.; Bleasby, A. EMBOSS: The European Molecular Biology Open Software Suite. *Trends Genet.* **2000**, *16*, 276–277. [CrossRef]
23. McArthur, A.G.; Waglechner, N.; Nizam, F.; Yan, A.; Azad, M.A.; Baylay, A.J.; Bhullar, K.; Canova, M.J.; De Pascale, G.; Ejim, L.; et al. The Comprehensive Antibiotic Resistance Database. *Antimicrob. Agents Chemother.* **2013**, *57*, 3348–3357. [CrossRef] [PubMed]
24. Yoshida, C.E.; Kruczkiewicz, P.; Laing, C.R.; Lingohr, E.J.; Gannon, V.P.J.; Nash, J.H.E.; Taboada, E.N. The Salmonella In Silico Typing Resource (SISTR): An Open Web-Accessible Tool for Rapidly Typing and Subtyping Draft Salmonella Genome Assemblies. *PLoS ONE* **2016**, *11*, e0147101. [CrossRef] [PubMed]
25. Emond-Rheault, J.-G.; Jeukens, J.; Freschi, L.; Kukavica-Ibrulj, I.; Boyle, B.; Dupont, M.-J.; Colavecchio, A.; Barrere, V.; Cadieux, B.; Arya, G.; et al. A Syst-OMICS Approach to Ensuring Food Safety and Reducing the Economic Burden of Salmonellosis. *Front. Microbiol.* **2017**, *8*, 8. [CrossRef] [PubMed]
26. Villa, L.; Garcia-Fernandez, A.; Fortini, D.; Carattoli, A. Replicon sequence typing of IncF plasmids carrying virulence and resistance determinants. *J. Antimicrob. Chemother.* **2010**, *65*, 2518–2529. [CrossRef]
27. Rychlik, I.; Gregorova, D.; Hradecka, H. Distribution and function of plasmids in Salmonella enterica. *Veter. Microbiol.* **2006**, *112*, 1–10. [CrossRef]
28. Martín, I.F.; AbuOun, M.; Reichel, R.; La Ragione, R.; Woodward, M.J. Sequence analysis of a CTX-M-1 IncI1 plasmid found in Salmonella 4,5,12:i:—, Escherichia coli and Klebsiella pneumoniae on a UK pig farm. *J. Antimicrob. Chemother.* **2014**, *69*, 2098–2101. [CrossRef] [PubMed]
29. García-Ferná Ndez, A.; Chiaretto, G.; Bertini, A.; Villa, L.; Fortini, D.; Ricci, A.; Carattoli, A. Multilocus sequence typing of IncI1 plasmids carrying extended-spectrum b-lactamases in Escherichia coli and Salmonella of human and animal origin. *J. Antimicrob. Chemother.* **2008**, *61*, 1229–1233. [CrossRef]
30. Kaldhone, P.R.P.R.; Han, J.; Deck, J.; Khajanchi, B.K.; Nayak, R.; Foley, S.L.; Ricke, S.C. Evaluation of the Genetics and Functionality of Plasmids in Incompatibility Group I1-Positive Salmonella enterica. *Foodborne Pathog. Dis.* **2018**, *15*, 168–176. [CrossRef]
31. Han, J.; Pendleton, S.J.; Deck, J.; Singh, R.; Gilbert, J.; Johnson, T.J.; Sanad, Y.M.; Nayak, R.; Foley, S.L. Impact of co-carriage of IncA/C plasmids with additional plasmids on the transfer of antimicrobial resistance in Salmonella enterica isolates. *Int. J. Food Microbiol.* **2018**, *271*, 77–84. [CrossRef]
32. Johnson, T.; Wannemeuhler, Y.M.; Scaccianoce, J.A.; Johnson, S.J.; Nolan, L.K. Complete DNA Sequence, Comparative Genomics, and Prevalence of an IncHI2 Plasmid Occurring among Extraintestinal Pathogenic Escherichia coli Isolates. *Antimicrob. Agents Chemother.* **2006**, *50*, 3929–3933. [CrossRef]
33. Welch, T.J.; Fricke, W.F.; McDermott, P.F.; White, D.G.; Rosso, M.-L.; Rasko, D.A.; Mammel, M.K.; Eppinger, M.; Rosovitz, M.; Wagner, D.; et al. Multiple Antimicrobial Resistance in Plague: An Emerging Public Health Risk. *PLoS ONE* **2007**, *2*, e309. [CrossRef]

34. Cao, G.; Allard, M.W.; Hoffmann, M.; Monday, S.R.; Muruvanda, T.; Luo, Y.; Payne, J.; Rump, L.; Meng, K.; Zhao, S.; et al. Complete Sequences of Six IncA/C Plasmids of Multidrug-Resistant Salmonella enterica subsp. enterica Serotype Newport. *Genome Announc.* **2015**, *3*, e00027-15. [CrossRef]
35. Call, D.; Singer, R.S.; Meng, D.; Broschat, S.L.; Orfe, L.H.; Anderson, J.M.; Herndon, D.R.; Kappmeyer, L.; Daniels, J.B.; Besser, T.E. bla CMY-2-Positive IncA/C Plasmids from Escherichia coli and Salmonella enterica Are a Distinct Component of a Larger Lineage of Plasmids. *Antimicrob. Agents Chemother.* **2009**, *54*, 590–596. [CrossRef]
36. Wasyl, D.; Kern-Zdanowicz, I.; Domanska-Blicharz, K.; Zając, M.; Hoszowski, A. High-level fluoroquinolone resistant Salmonella enterica serovar Kentucky ST198 epidemic clone with IncA/C conjugative plasmid carrying blaCTX-M-25 gene. *Veter. Microbiol.* **2015**, *175*, 85–91. [CrossRef]
37. Silva, C.; Calva, E.; Calva, J.J.; Wiesner, M.; Fernández-Mora, M.; Puente, J.L.; Vinuesa, P. Complete Genome Sequence of a Human-Invasive Salmonella enterica Serovar Typhimurium Strain of the Emerging Sequence Type 213 Harboring a Multidrug Resistance IncA/C Plasmid and a blaCMY-2-Carrying IncF Plasmid. *Genome Announc.* **2015**, *3*, e01323-15. [CrossRef]
38. Fricke, W.F.; Welch, T.J.; McDermott, P.F.; Mammel, M.K.; Leclerc, J.E.; White, D.G.; Cebula, T.A.; Ravel, J. Comparative Genomics of the IncA/C Multidrug Resistance Plasmid Family. *J. Bacteriol.* **2009**, *191*, 4750–4757. [CrossRef] [PubMed]
39. Carattoli, A.; Miriagou, V.; Bertini, A.; Loli, A.; Colinon, C.; Villa, L.; Whichard, J.M.; Rossolini, G. Replicon Typing of Plasmids Encoding Resistance to Newer β-Lactams. *Emerg. Infect. Dis.* **2006**, *12*, 1145–1148. [CrossRef]
40. Fang, L.-X.; Li, X.-P.; Deng, G.-H.; Li, S.-M.; Yang, R.-S.; Wu, Z.-W.; Liao, X.-P.; Sun, J.; Liu, Y.-H. High Genetic Plasticity in Multidrug-Resistant Sequence Type 3-IncHI2 Plasmids Revealed by Sequence Comparison and Phylogenetic Analysis. *Antimicrob. Agents Chemother.* **2018**, *62*, e02068-17. [CrossRef]
41. Han, J.; Lynne, A.M.; David, D.E.; Tang, H.; Xu, J.; Nayak, R.; Kaldhone, P.; Logue, C.M.; Foley, S.L. DNA Sequence Analysis of Plasmids from Multidrug Resistant Salmonella enterica Serotype Heidelberg Isolates. *PLoS ONE* **2012**, *7*, e51160. [CrossRef] [PubMed]
42. Lindsey, R.L.; Fedorka-Cray, P.J.; Frye, J.G.; Meinersmann, R.J. Inc A/C Plasmids Are Prevalent in Multidrug-Resistant Salmonella enterica Isolates. *Appl. Environ. Microbiol.* **2009**, *75*, 1908–1915. [CrossRef]
43. Bleicher, A.; Schöfl, G.; Rodicio, M.D.R.; Saluz, H.P. The plasmidome of a Salmonella enterica serovar Derby isolated from pork meat. *Plasmid* **2013**, *69*, 202–210. [CrossRef]
44. Papagiannitsis, C.C.; Kutilova, I.; Medvecky, M.; Hrabák, J.; Dolejska, M. Characterization of the Complete Nucleotide Sequences of IncA/C2 Plasmids Carrying In809-Like Integrons from Enterobacteriaceae Isolates of Wildlife Origin. *Antimicrob. Agents Chemother.* **2017**, *61*, e01093-17. [CrossRef]
45. Li, X.-Z.; Plésiat, P.; Nikaido, H. The Challenge of Efflux-Mediated Antibiotic Resistance in Gram-Negative Bacteria. *Clin. Microbiol. Rev.* **2015**, *28*, 337–418. [CrossRef]
46. Rehman, M.A.; Yin, X.; Persaud-Lachhman, M.G.; Diarra, M.S. First Detection of a Fosfomycin Resistance Gene, fosA7, in Salmonella enterica Serovar Heidelberg Isolated from Broiler Chickens. *Antimicrob. Agents Chemother.* **2017**, *61*, e00410-17. [CrossRef]
47. Levy, S.B. Active efflux mechanisms for antimicrobial resistance. *Antimicrob. Agents Chemother.* **1992**, *36*, 695–703. [CrossRef]
48. Witte, W. Selective pressure by antibiotic use in livestock. *Int. J. Antimicrob. Agents* **2000**, *16*, 19–24. [CrossRef]
49. Chopra, I.; Roberts, M.C. Tetracycline Antibiotics: Mode of Action, Applications, Molecular Biology, and Epidemiology of Bacterial Resistance. *Microbiol. Mol. Boil. Rev.* **2001**, *65*, 232–260. [CrossRef] [PubMed]
50. Marti, H.; Kim, H.; Joseph, S.J.; Dojiri, S.; Read, T.D.; Dean, D. Tet(C) Gene Transfer between Chlamydia suis Strains Occurs by Homologous Recombination after Co-infection: Implications for Spread of Tetracycline-Resistance among Chlamydiaceae. *Front. Microbiol.* **2017**, *8*, 313. [CrossRef]
51. Dugan, J.; Rockey, D.D.; Jones, L.; Andersen, A.A. Tetracycline Resistance in Chlamydia suis Mediated by Genomic Islands Inserted into the Chlamydial inv-Like Gene. *Antimicrob. Agents Chemother.* **2004**, *48*, 3989–3995. [CrossRef]
52. Furushita, M.; Shiba, T.; Maeda, T.; Yahata, M.; Kaneoka, A.; Takahashi, Y.; Torii, K.; Hasegawa, T.; Ohta, M. Similarity of Tetracycline Resistance Genes Isolated from Fish Farm Bacteria to Those from Clinical Isolates. *Appl. Environ. Microbiol.* **2003**, *69*, 5336–5342. [CrossRef] [PubMed]

53. Mulvey, M.R.; Boyd, D.A.; Baker, L.; Mykytczuk, O.; Reis, E.M.F.; Asensi, M.D.; Rodrigues, D.P.; Ng, L. Characterization of a Salmonella enterica serovar Agona strain harbouring a class 1 integron containing novel OXA-type B-lactamase (blaoxa-53) and 6′-N-aminoglycoside acetyltransferase genes. *J. Antimicrob. Chemother.* **2004**, *54*, 354–359. [CrossRef] [PubMed]
54. L'Abée-Lund, T.M.; Sørum, H. A global non-conjugative Tet C plasmid, pRAS3, from Aeromonas salmonicida. *Plasmid* **2002**, *47*, 172–181. [CrossRef]
55. Frech, G.; Schwarz, S. Molecular analysis of tetracycline resistance in Salmonella enterica subsp. enterica serovars Typhimurium, Enteritidis, Dublin, Choleraesuis, Hadar and Saintpaul: Construction and application of specific gene probes. *J. Appl. Microbiol.* **2000**, *89*, 633–641. [CrossRef]
56. Miko, A.; Pries, K.; Schroeter, A.; Helmuth, R. Molecular mechanisms of resistance in multidrug-resistant serovars of Salmonella enterica isolated from foods in Germany. *J. Antimicrob. Chemother.* **2005**, *56*, 1025–1033. [CrossRef]
57. Thai, T.H.; Hirai, T.; Lan, N.T.; Shimada, A.; Ngoc, P.T.; Yamaguchi, R. Antimicrobial resistance of Salmonella serovars isolated from beef at retail markets in the north Vietnam. *J. Veter. Med. Sci.* **2012**, *74*, 1163–1169. [CrossRef] [PubMed]
58. Levy, S.B. Factors impacting on the problem of antibiotic resistance. *J. Antimicrob. Chemother.* **2002**, *49*, 25–30. [CrossRef]
59. Sundin, G.W.; Bender, C.L. Dissemination of the strA-strB streptomycin-resistance genes among commensal and pathogenic bacteria from humans, animals, and plants. *Mol. Ecol.* **1996**, *5*, 133–143. [CrossRef]
60. Van Overbeek, L.S.; Wellington, E.M.H.; Egan, S.; Smalla, K.; Heuer, H.; Collard, J.M.; Guillaume, G.; Karagouni, A.D.; Nikolakopoulou, T.L.; Van Elsas, J.D. Prevalence of streptomycin-resistance genes in bacterial populations in European habitats. *FEMS Microbiol. Ecol.* **2002**, *42*, 277–288. [CrossRef]
61. Public Health Agency of Canada. *Canadian Antimicrobial Resistance Surveillance System Report Ontario*; Public Health Agency of Canada: Ottawa, ON, Canada, 2016; ISBN 6139572991.
62. Gunell, M.; Kotilainen, P.; Jalava, J.; Huovinen, P.; Siitonen, A.; Hakanen, A. In Vitro Activity of Azithromycin against Nontyphoidal Salmonella enterica. *Antimicrob. Agents Chemother.* **2010**, *54*, 3498–3501. [CrossRef]
63. Mandalakas, A.M.; Menzies, D. Outpatient treatment of patients with enteric fever. *Lancet Infect. Dis.* **2011**, *11*, 419–421.
64. Guerrant, R.L.; Van Gilder, T.; Steiner, T.S.; Thielman, N.M.; Slutsker, L.; Tauxe, R.V.; Hennessy, T.; Griffin, P.M.; Dupont, H.; Sack, R.B.; et al. Practice Guidelines for the Management of Infectious Diarrhea. *Clin. Infect. Dis.* **2001**, *32*, 331–351. [CrossRef] [PubMed]

11

Iron-Uptake Systems of Chicken-Associated *Salmonella* Serovars and their Role in Colonizing the Avian Host

Dinesh H. Wellawa [1,2], Brenda Allan [1], Aaron P. White [1,2] and Wolfgang Köster [1,2,*]

1 Vaccine & Infectious Disease Organization-International Vaccine Centre, University of Saskatchewan, 120 Veterinary Rd., Saskatoon, SK S7N 5E3, Canada; dinesh.wellawa@usask.ca (D.H.W.); brenda.allan@usask.ca (B.A.); aaron.white@usask.ca (A.P.W.)
2 Department of Veterinary Microbiology, Western College of Veterinary Medicine, University of Saskatchewan, Saskatoon, SK S7N 5B4, Canada
* Correspondence: wolfgang.koester@usask.ca

Abstract: Iron is an essential micronutrient for most bacteria. *Salmonella enterica* strains, representing human and animal pathogens, have adopted several mechanisms to sequester iron from the environment depending on availability and source. Chickens act as a major reservoir for *Salmonella enterica* strains which can lead to outbreaks of human salmonellosis. In this review article we summarize the current understanding of the contribution of iron-uptake systems to the virulence of non-typhoidal *S. enterica* strains in colonizing chickens. We aim to address the gap in knowledge in this field, to help understand and define the interactions between *S. enterica* and these important hosts, in comparison to mammalian models.

Keywords: *Salmonella*; iron homeostasis and regulation; chicken; pathogenicity; iron transport

---

1. Introduction

The genus *Salmonella* is composed of two species, *Salmonella enterica* and *Salmonella bongori*. *Salmonella enterica* is subdivided into six subspecies; *enterica* (I), *arizonae* (IIIa), *diarizonae* (IIIb), *houtenae* (IV), *salamae* (II) and *indica* (VI), based on antigenic properties (somatic (O), flagellar (H1, H2) and capsule (K) antigens) and biochemical properties [1–3]. *Salmonella bongori* predominantly resides as commensal in ectotherms and except for a few incidences, mammalian infections are rare [4,5]. It is hypothesized that adaptation to different niches paved the pathway for speciation of *S. enterica* and *S. bongori* from a common ancestor by means of gene gain, gene loss and conjugation events [6–8]. *Salmonella enterica* contains >2600 serovars which can infect insects, wild birds, reptiles and mammals. A significant proportion of human salmonellosis (>99%) are caused by serovars under subspecies I (*enterica*) hence it is the most important category in terms of public health. Clinical manifestation of salmonellosis can vary among serovars. The gastroenteritis-causing strains are collectively known as non-typhoidal *Salmonella* (NTS) strains and this review mainly focuses on NTS. Gastroenteritis is associated with intestinal inflammation and diarrhea without fever in general. NTS strains have the capacity to infect broad livestock species, yet chickens (*Gallus gallus domesticus*) are known to be a major reservoir. This is supported by epidemiological data indicating that poultry represent a major epicenter for human salmonellosis (non-typhoidal) globally (Table 1) [9,10].

Table 1. Some of the global incidences of human salmonellosis linked to poultry.

Serotype	Source	Year(s)	Geographical Region	No of Cases [a]	References
Enteritidis	Chicken (shell eggs)	2010	USA	1939 [b]	CDC 2020 [d]
Enteritidis Virchow	Chicken	2010 (from 2007)	Brazil	>260	[11]
Enteritidis Virchow	Chicken	2010	Taiwan	>1000	[12]
Stanley	Turkey (meat)	2011–2013	EU	710	[13]
Heidelberg	Chicken (meat)	2011	USA	190	CDC 2020 [d]
Infantis Newport Lille	Chicks, ducklings (live)	2012	USA	195	CDC 2020 [d]
Heidelberg	Chicken (meat)	2013	USA	634	CDC 2020 [d]
Typhimurium	Chicks, ducklings (live)	2013	USA	356	CDC 2020 [d]
Enteritidis	Chicken (eggs)	2014	EU	>400	[14]
Multiple NTS [c]	Chicks, ducklings (live)	2014	USA	363	CDC 2020 [d]
Multiple NTS	Chicks, ducklings (live)	2015	USA	252	CDC 2020 [d]
Multiple NTS	Chicks, ducklings (live)	2016	USA	895	CDC 2020 [d]
Typhimurium	Chicken (egg)	2015–2016	Australia	272	[15]
Enteritidis	Chicken (eggs)	2016–present	EU	1656	ECDC 2020 [e]
Multiple NTS	Chicks, ducklings (live)	2017	USA	1120	CDC 2020 [d]
Typhimurium	Chicken (salad)	2018	USA	265	CDC 2020 [d]
Reading	Turkey	2018	USA	358	CDC 2020 [d]
Enteritidis	Chicken (processed meat)	2017–2019	Canada	584	Public Health Service 2020 [f]
Enteritidis	Chicks, ducklings (live)	2019	USA	1134	CDC 2020 [d]

[a] Number of reported incidences. [b] Estimated due to inadequate reporting. [c] More than 3 NTS serovars were involved. [d] According to the online data published by the Centers for Disease Control and Prevention in 2020 June (https://www.cdc.gov/Salmonella/outbreaks.html). [e] According to the online data published by the European Centre for Disease Control and Prevention in 2020, June (https://www.ecdc.europa.eu/en/infectious-diseases-and-public-health/salmonellosis/threats-and-outbreaks). [f] Public Health Services, Canada website (https://www.canada.ca/en/public-health/services/diseases/salmonellosis-salmonella.html). NTS: non-typhoidal *Salmonella*.

1.1. *Iron Homeostasis by Salmonella in a Nutshell: Regulation and Iron-Uptake Systems*

Iron is an indispensable element for *S. enterica*. Key enzymes involved in bacterial metabolism depend on iron as a cofactor including DNA synthesis and repair enzymes [16]. Due to its transitional nature, iron can be either Fe^{2+}/Fe^{3+} at physiological pH (7.2). In anaerobic environments, Fe^{2+} can be dominant over ferric iron, while Fe^{3+} can be abundant in aerobic conditions. *Salmonella* has established various mechanisms to internalize iron depending on its availability. In this review, we will discuss several important iron-uptake systems available in chicken-associated NTS strains (Figure 1). For more detail about iron homeostasis in bacteria in general, readers are directed to several references [16–21].

1.2. *Ferric Uptake Regulator (Fur)-Mediated Regulation of Iron Uptake, Storage and Utilization*

In addition to its innumerable beneficial effects, iron also catalyzes toxic metabolites such as superoxides, hydroxyl free radicals through Haber-Weiss and Fenton reactions in vivo which can damage bacterial DNA, iron-sulfur clusters, hence being harmful unless regulated [22,23]. The regulation is mainly under an auto-regulated protein called ferric uptake regulator (Fur) [24]. Fur acts as a repressor for most promoters related to iron uptake [25–27]. Under iron rich conditions, Fur binds to Fe^{2+}, which causes Fur dimerization and subsequent binding to a consensus DNA sequence called the "fur box" (GATAATGATAATCATTATC), often present in promoter-containing regions. Binding overlaps the RNA polymerase (RNAP) binding sequence in the promoter region of iron-regulated genes [28]. This, in turn, hinders transcription of genes by the RNAP. Under iron-depleted conditions, Fe^{2+} dissociates from the dimer, the blockade for RNAP is removed, and iron-regulated genes are expressed. Apart from serving as a direct transcriptional repressor, Fur positively regulates iron storage and iron utilization genes via small RNAs called RyhB (*E. coli*) or its homologues (RfrA/B in *Salmonella*) [29,30]. For an example, under iron-rich conditions Fur upregulates iron storage proteins called bacterioferritins in *E. coli* via RyhB [31]. First, Fur-Fe^{2+} represses *ryhB* transcription and downregulates RyhB accumulation in the cell. Low intracellular RyhB concentration in turn alleviates RyhB-mediated destruction of mRNA transcripts and leads to the upregulation of iron storage proteins.

The network of interacting partners by RyhB and its homologs have added more complexity to the Fur mediated iron regulation and interactosome of these RNAs are under active research [32].

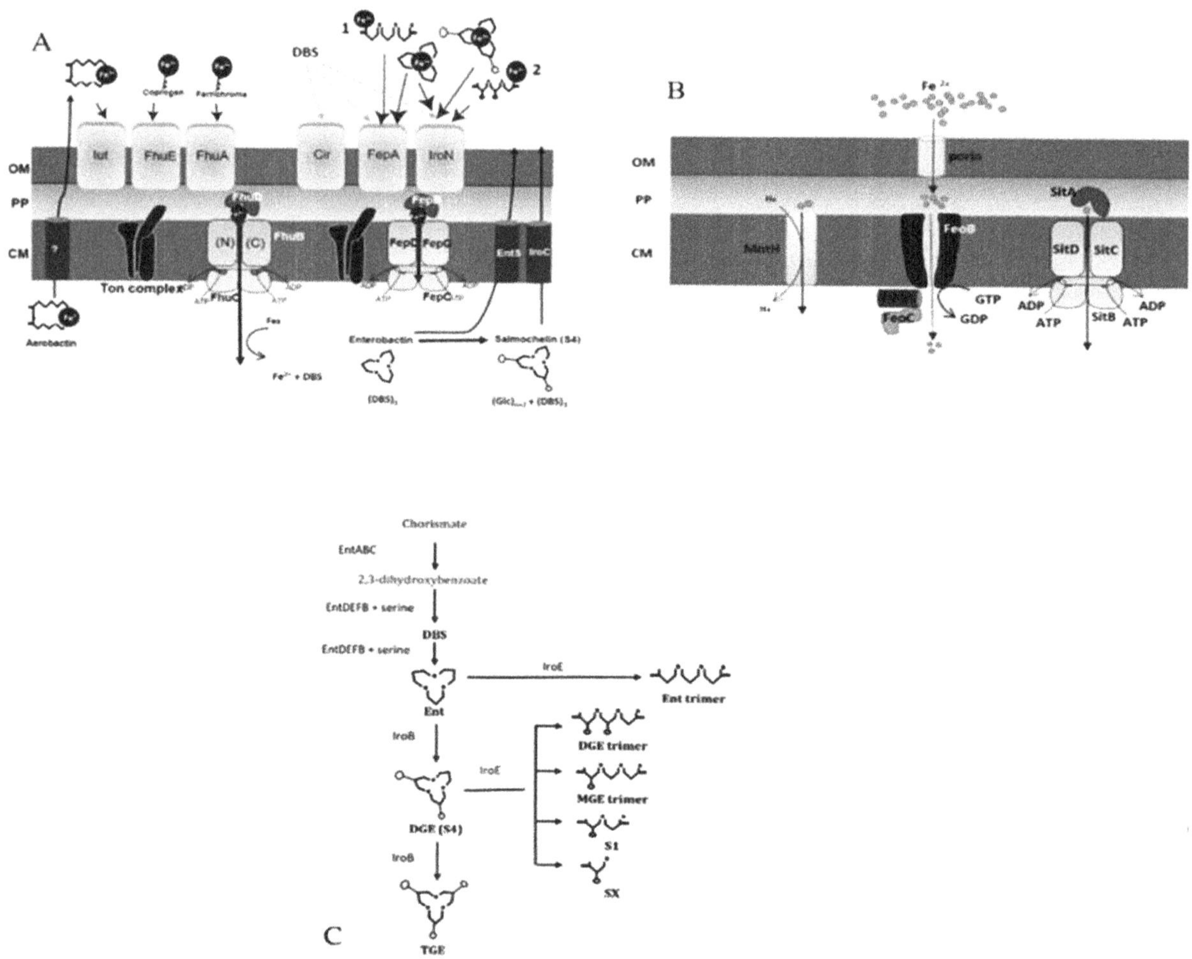

Figure 1. Schematic representation of iron-uptake systems in non-typhoidal Salmonella strains. (**A**) Fe^{3+} uptake systems. Enterobactin, salmochelin and aerobactin are secreted (e.g., through EntS and IroC) to sequester Fe^{3+} and then bind to their cognate receptors in the outer membrane (OM). Coprogen and ferrichrome are other ferric iron chelators present in the environment. Energy is generated through the proton motive force (PMF) in the cytoplasmic membrane (CM) and transduced to the receptor by the Ton complex (TonB-ExbB-ExbD). The energized receptor undergoes a conformational change which opens the pathway to mediate uptake of the iron-loaded siderophores into the periplasm (PP). The iron-liganded siderophores bind to periplasmic binding proteins (FhuD, FepB) which then shuttle them through ABC family permeases into the cytosol. 1,2 represent linearized forms of enterobactin and salmochelin respectively. (**B**) Fe^{2+} uptake systems. Ferrous iron in aqueous medium travels though porin channels in the OM according to the concentration gradient. FeoABC is specific for Fe^{2+} uptake. Both MntH and SitABCD are divalent metal transporters. (**C**) Forms of siderophores. Cyclic forms of enterobactin and salmochelin are hydrolyzed by the *iro* gene cluster to produce linearized forms of iron chelators.

1.3. Uptake of Ferric (Fe^{3+}) Iron via Siderophores

Fe^{3+} is insoluble and often sequestered by host proteins (i.e., hemoglobin, transferrin, lactoferrin) or bound in complexes ($Fe(OH)_3$) outside the host. *Salmonella* secrets high-affinity iron-binding molecules called siderophores (500–1000 da) to hijack Fe^{3+}. Two siderophores belonging to the catecholate type are well-characterized: enterobactin and salmochelin. Enterobactin is nature's superglue for Fe^{3+} which forms an incredibly stable complex with ferric ion at $K_f = 10^{49}$ (K_f = formation constant) [33]. Chemically it is designated as the cyclic trilactone of *N*-2,3-dihyroxybenzoyl-L-serine.

N-2,3-dihyroxybenzoyl L-serine (DBS) is the building block of enterobactin which undergoes cyclization to accommodate iron by six coordinated oxygen atoms in three DBS units. DBS itself can scavenge Fe^{3+} with low affinity [34]. Salmonella uses nonribosomal peptide synthesis pathways (NRPS) encoded by *entBCDE* (Figure 1C) to generate enterobactin in the cytoplasm which is then exported by EntS located in the inner membrane [35]. Except for some chicken-specific *Salmonella* serovars, all other chicken-associated-*Salmonella* produce enterobactin [36]. Enterobactin can be further linearized due to the action of hydrolase enzymes (IroE) located in the bacterial periplasm before secretion (Figure 1C). The linearized forms of the enterobactin (Ent-trimer, Ent-dimer) retain the ability to scavenge ferric iron, but with reduced affinity compared to its cyclic form ($K_f = 10^{43}$) [33]. Once the secreted enterobactin and linearized forms are iron-loaded, they are taken up by their cognate receptors in the Salmonella outer membrane. Cyclic and linearized forms of enterobactin (ex; Ent-trimer) specifically bind to FepA. Evidence has suggested that enterobactin break down products like DBS, can be transported via Cir, FepA and IroN once loaded with Fe^{3+} [37]. These receptors share sequence similarity and follow the same general structure [18]. They are composed of a 22 antiparallel stranded β-barrel (which forms the channel) and an *N*-terminal globular domain referred to as the "plug" or "cork". The energy generated by the proton motive force in the inner membrane is coupled to the outer membrane receptors via the TonB-ExbB-ExbD complex to achieve siderophore internalization (passage through the upper binding pocket), then migration through the channel (plug undergoes conformational changes) into the periplasm. Internalized iron is then released by degradation of enterobactin using Fes enzymes located in the cytoplasm.

Enterobactin can be glycosylated by a glycosyl transferase enzyme, IroB, to form salmochelin [38]. Glycosylation affixes glucose molecules to enterobactin thus forming the more hydrophilic salmochelin. It has been hypothesized that salmochelin is produced to counteract iron starvation mounted by the host. This has been supported by the observation that salmochelin is a better iron scavenger than enterobactin in presence of serum albumin and also it is not bound by the mammalian innate molecule lipocalin 2 (Lcn-2) which captures apo-enterobactin or Fe^{3+}-enterobactin to impede iron scavenging by bacteria [39,40]. Lcn-2 is secreted by phagocytic cells (macrophages, neutrophils) and epithelial cells during host's inflammatory response. Glycosylation of the enterobactin moiety sterically hinders the binding capacity of Lcn-2 and therefore salmochelin is considered a "stealth" siderophore. IroB can sequentially synthesize several versions of salmochelin termed mono glycosylated enterobactin (MGE), di-glycosylated enterobactin (DGE/S4) and tri-glycosylated enterobactin (TGE) [38,39]. Work done by Lin et al., 2005 has further demonstrated that the periplasmic enzyme IroE can linearize salmochelin to linear trimer (linearized TGE/S3-not shown in the Figure 1C), linear dimer (DGE/S2), MGE trimer, linear *C*-glycosylated $(DBS)_2$ (S1) and linear monomer (SX) in vitro [39]. Also, the authors showed that IroD, a cytoplasmic esterase, can degrade the salmochelin forms into its building blocks (DBS) thus releasing the iron into the bacterial cytoplasm [40]. Salmochelins have high specificity for outer membrane receptor IroN and are subjected to TonB-dependant uptake like other siderophores.

Some NTS serovars produce aerobactin, a mixed type of siderophore known as citrate-hydroxamate type. Aerobactin is synthesized by a NRPS pathway utilizing enzymes encoded in the *iucABCD* operon. During synthesis, L-lysine is first converted to N^6-acetyl-N^6-hydroxy-l-lysine and then complexed into a citric acid backbone [41]. The iron complex formation constant of aerobactin ($K_f = 10^{23}$) is weaker than that of enterobactin [42]. Aerobactin follows the same rule as catecholate-type siderophores regarding its uptake (Iut receptor) and TonB-dependant transport into the bacterial periplasm. Once in the periplasm, aerobactin is transported through the binding-protein-dependent ABC transport system FhuBCD [43]. FhuBCD also mediates the energy-dependant uptake of ferrichromes and coprogen from the environment (Figure 1A) [43].

A less common class of siderophores which can be found in *Salmonella* serovars are phenolate type siderophores such as yersiniabactin (Ybt). Ybt is abundantly produced in *Yersinia* species encoded by a genomic island called high pathogenicity island 1(HPI) [44]. HPI 1 is absent from most *Salmonella enterica* serovar subspecies 1 [44] and hence its distribution in *Salmonella* serovars is low. Seven proteins

(HMWP1, HMWP2, YbtD, YbtE, YbtS, YbtT and YbtU) have been described in Ybt synthesis from the precursor isochorismic acid in *Yersinia* species. The final product is a four-ring structure composed of salicylate, one thiazolidine and two thiazoline rings. Ybt shows a higher affinity for Fe^{3+} ($K_f = 10^{36}$) than aerobactin, hence it is a potent iron chelator. Once loaded with iron, yersiniabactin is taken up by the Psn/FyuA receptor in the outer membrane and then shuttled through the YbtPQ ABC transporter across the inner membrane (not shown in the figure).

1.4. Uptake of Ferrous Iron (Fe^{2+}) via FeoABC, SitABCD and MntH

Ferrous iron is water-soluble and can readily pass through the outer membrane porin proteins into the periplasm following the concentration gradient. Once in the periplasmic space, Salmonella can take up Fe^{2+} via 3 systems: FeoABC, SitABCD and MntH. FeoABC belongs to a family of transporters that have high specificity for Fe^{2+}. For the FeoABC system, the FeoB permease forms a channel in the inner membrane and FeoA and FeoC interact with FeoB in the cytoplasm. The *N*-terminal, cytoplasmic portion of FeoB contains a G-protein domain which can perform GTP binding and hydrolysis. Therefore, Feo-mediated Fe^{2+} uptake is coupled to GTP hydrolysis and signal transduction. For the latest structure and biology of the FeoABC system, readers are directed to two recent articles [45,46].

SitABCD is an ABC transporter family protein complex allowing the passage of primarily Mn^{2+} in alkaline pH but capable of transporting Fe^{2+} with low affinity [47]. Kehres et al., 2002 showed that SitABCD of Salmonella Typhimurium only transported Fe^{2+} when the concentration of Fe^{2+} reached 1 μM or higher in vitro [47]. MntH was also dominant in transporting Mn^{2+} rather than Fe^{2+}. It was evident that uptake of Mn^{2+} was independent of pH, while Fe^{2+} transport increased by the acidic pH [47]. Further, it was revealed that affinity for Fe^{2+} to MntH was much lower than to SitABCD and only transported ferrous iron when it reached a concentration of higher than 1 μM in vitro [47]. Since the free, labile iron level is believed to be extremely low in biological fluids ($<10^{-18}$M) and tissues, the role of SitABCD and MntH in ferrous iron transport is hypothesized to be of relatively minor significance compared to Feo-mediated iron uptake. The FeoABC system is recognized as the main ferrous iron transporter for many Enterobacteriaceae [48].

2. Emergence of Chicken-Associated Invasive NTS: The Iron Link

NTS strains are mainly asymptomatic colonizers in adult chickens, but strains of certain serovars can be fatal when infecting day-old chicks [49,50]. The major chicken-associated NTS serovars with potential to cause human epidemics are listed in Table 2. In countries belonging to the European Union (EU), the majority of breeders and layers were infected with *Salmonella* Enteritidis (SEn) while broilers were dominantly colonized by *Salmonella* Virchow (SVr) [51]. In contrast to the EU countries, *Salmonella* Kentucky (SKn) has been the predominant serovar isolated from poultry products in North America [10,52]. Generally, there is a high genetic synteny among NTS serovars (listed in Table 2) of chicken origin at core genomic levels [53]. Table 2 has only listed some the genetic differences which may be linked to virulence in chickens or humans.

Table 2. Most prevalent chicken-associated NTS serovars with public-health risk.

Salmonella Serovar	Genetic/Phenotypic Signatures	Role Related to Virulence in Chicken or Human	References
Kentucky (SKn)	(1) Colicin production (pColV) (2) Salmonella genomic island 1 (SGI1) (3) RpoS regulated gene cluster: csg (curli), prpBCDE (propionate catabolism) (4) Lack of Saf and Sef fimbria (5) Additional iron uptake carried in pColV; siderophores- aerobactin & salmochelin, *sit* operon (Mn^{2+}, Fe^{2+} uptake)	(1) Increased colonization in chicken gut (2) Multidrug resistant (MDR) including 3rd generation cephalosporin, ciprofloxacin resistant *, (3) Upregulated in chicken cecal explants (4) Decreased invasiveness in humans compared to other NTS (5) NDA (no data available)	[54–56]

Table 2. *Cont.*

Salmonella Serovar	Genetic/Phenotypic Signatures	Role Related to Virulence in Chicken or Human	References
Heidelberg (SHb)	(6) Type IV secretion (T4SS) (7) SopE (T3SS1 effector) duplication in the chromosome (8) Salmonella atypical fimbria (*safABCD*) (9) Additional iron uptake carried in pColV; siderophore-aerobactin	(6) Dissemination of antibiotics resistance and efficient survival in macrophages (7) Invasion into epithelial cells and induce inflammation (8) Only presented in the outbreak strain linked to human salmonellosis. (9) NDA	[55,57,58]
Typhimurium (STm)	(10) *Salmonella* genomic island 1 (SGI1) (11) *Salmonella* genomic island 4 (SGI4) (12) Plasmid encoded factors; *mig-5*, *rck*, *spv* (*Salmonella* plasmid virulence), *pef* , (13) Additional iron uptake in pColV; aerobactin, salmochelin *sit* operon (Mn^{2+}, Fe^{2+})	(10) Sequence type DT104 showed Increased egg contamination compared to SEn phage type 4, contains ACSSuT # drug-resistant phenotype (11) Heavy metal resistant in DT104 (12) colonization in chicken gut, systemic spread (13) NDA	[59–62]
Typhimurium mono phasic variant (STmv) (DT193/DT120)	(14) Phase 2 flagellin not expressed (*fljBA* operon) (15) SGI-4 (16) Lack of *Salmonella* plasmid virulence locus, (17) Lack of Gifsy prophages	(14) Predicted to be an adaptation related to the expansion of reservoir host (15) resistant to heavy metals copper and zinc (16) less invasive in humans (17) NDA	[59,63,64]
Enteritidis (SEn)	(18) pSLA5 plasmid (19) Plasmid encoded factors; *mig-5*, *rck*, *spv* (*Salmonella* plasmid virulence), *pef* (20) Peg fimbria	(18) Associated with recent outbreaks in the EU. (19) Colonization in chicken gut, systemic spread (20) Generally unique to Enteritidis. Facilitates cecal colonization in chickens	[65–68]
Virchow (SVr)	(21) *Salmonella* Typhi colonization factor: TcfA (22) Novel SopE effector	(21) TcfA fimbriae provides tissue tropism in invasion into human cells. Role in chickens unknown (22) Associated with invasive nature of SVQ1 strain linked to outbreaks in Australia	[53,69]
Montevideo (SMv)	(23) Typhoid-associated virulence factors; TcfA fimbria, cytolethal toxin B etc.	(23) Predicted to increase tissue tropism and invasions in humans. Role in chickens unknown	[53,70]
Infantis (SIn)	(24) Plasmid-encoded factors;(pESI like); • MDR; Extended spectrum beta lactamases (*bla*$_{CTX-M-65}$) • Additional ferric uptake system; yersiniabactin (*irp*), • Fimbria: *E coli* K88, Infantis plasmid fimbriae (*ipf*)	(24) Associated in human outbreaks. Also, plasmid-encoded fimbria were contributed a colonization in the gastrointestinal tract of chicks	[71–74]

* Global pandemic strain of SKn with ciprofloxacin resistant, ST198-X1-SGI1 originated from chickens. # ACSSuT = ampicillin, chloramphenicol, streptomycin, sulfamethoxazole and tetracycline.

The chicken host has been a hotspot for shaping new NTS pathotype strains that can cause extraintestinal diseases in humans due to bacteremia, often with antimicrobial resistant (AMR) phenotypes. NTS bacteremia can lead to severe inflammation within different organs, leading to organ dysfunction and sometimes death (Figure 2). In these more systemic infections, antibiotics are required for successful treatment. *Salmonella* Heidelberg (SHb) and SVr are among the top-four NTS serovars with highest invasiveness indices (proportion of bacteremia from total isolates) globally for which chickens act as a reservoir [75–78]. Apart from that, *Salmonella* Typhimurium (STm) and SEn are cumulatively responsible for the highest human epidemics globally with potential to cause blood-borne infections [79]. Comparative genomic analysis has predicted that *Salmonella* pathogenicity islands (SPI), adhesin molecules (fimbriae, invasins), secretion systems, virulence plasmid (spv), toxins, multidrug resistant genomic islands and colonization factors have a role in causing blood-borne infection in humans [52,53,57,58,80,81]. Another important virulence trait that has been overlooked in NTS serovars is iron uptake. As summarized in Table 2, there is a general trend in strains of important NTS serovars to acquire additional iron-uptake systems. Kajanchi et al. (2017) reported that a significant number of STm strains, isolated from chickens, turkeys and humans, carried ColV plasmids which encoded genes for divalent metal uptake (*sitABCD*) and Fe^{3+} uptake via synthesis, secretion and translocation of aerobactin (*iucABCD, iut*) [62]. The plasmid encoded *sitABCD* was phylogenetically distinct from the chromosomally encoded loci. The effect of having two *sitABCD* operons for clonal expansion and/or virulence is still unknown. ColV plasmids have been associated with SKn strains and to a lesser extent with SHb strains in the USA that were isolated from poultry [55]. For SKn, there was a significant fitness defect in colonizing the chicken cecum in strains lacking pColV [55]. In addition, systemic dissemination and the ability to cause splenic lesions was reduced in pColV null background compared to the pColV positive strain, indicating that genetic factors carried in pColV plasmids are important virulence determinants during extraintestinal disease [55]. SKn is an emerging pathogen which can cause blood-born infections in humans [82–84], thus ColV plasmid-encoded factors including iron uptake functions most likely contribute to overall virulence.

The aerobactin operon (*iucABCD*), also carried on pColV plasmids, is of particular interest, because normally its prevalence is low in most Salmonella [42]. Aerobactin-producing NTS serovars (SEn, STm, SVr,SIn etc) were highly associated with human salmonellosis caused by ingestion of contaminated poultry products in Spain [85]. In some reports, it has been documented that aerobactin production is exclusively linked to blood-born infection rather gastroenteritis, as aerobactin-producing NTS serovars were exclusively isolated from human blood [86,87]. In fact, some of the properties of aerobactin can provide NTS serovars a better survivability during systemic dissemination, even though affinity to Fe^{3+} of aerobactin is lower than most other siderophores. Some of these features include: higher transfer rate of Fe^{3+} from transferrin receptors to aerobactin in the serum, higher solubility, low wastage of resources during aerobactin production (recycled) and rapid secretion out of the cells to be available for ferric uptake compared to enterobactin, which tends to accumulate in the inner-membrane [42]. The iron in the mucosal surface of the gastrointestinal tract is mainly bound by lactoferrins which has a high affinity for iron ($K_f = 10^{20}$) like transferrin [88,89]. Therefore, secretion of additional siderophores such as aerobactin may provide NTS strains a competitive advantage for multiplication and invasion into the gastrointestinal tract. In addition, aerobactin is not bound by Lcn-2 which will provide a defense against Lcn-2-mediated iron starvation during inflammation. So, in the bottom line, aerobactin can be involved not only in the systemic phase of infection but also in enteric infection. The pColV plasmids are well-distributed among *E. coli* strains and it is believed that chicken-associated NTS strains may have acquired the pColV from an avian pathogenic *E. coli* (APEC) strain. APEC strains cause high morbidity and mortality in chickens (colibacillosis) due to their ability to cause septicemia [90]. Dozois et al., 2003 showed that among pathogen-specific gene clusters expressed in APEC strains, both aerobactin and salmochelin were important for virulence in chickens [91]. Further, significant reduction of colibacillosis-associated pathology was observed in an aerobactin-knockout APEC strain carrying ColV plasmids [92]. In a similar manner the hypervirulent *Klebsiella pneumoniae* strain solely uses aerobactin to confer its hypervirulent phenotype which leads to septicemia in humans [93]. By all these means, acquiring aerobactin production may indeed cause the chicken-associated NTS serovars to become more virulent once infected in humans. There are number of other genetic factors encoded on pColV plasmids which can contribute to virulence, including the *iss* gene associated with increased serum survival in APEC strains [94]. Therefore, experimental approaches will be necessary to study the role of aerobactin encoded on pColV regarding virulence of NTS serovars in chickens and humans.

A recently emerging poultry-associated multidrug resistant *Salmonella* Infantis (SIn) lineage, harbored yersiniabactin secretion systems *(irp)* on pESI like plasmids [71,95]. As mentioned earlier, yersiniabactin is rarely present in Salmonella strains and its role is unknown regarding the existence in chicken-associated NTS strains. Yersiniabactin can sequester copper iron apart from ferric, to form a stable complex (yersiniabactin-cupric) which resists proteasomal degradation. In a series of experiments conducted by Chaturvedi and colleagues, they were able to show that the yersiniabactin-cupric complex neutralized superoxide (super oxide dismutase-like activity) generated in phagosomes which gave uropathogenic *E coli* bacteria, a survival advantage in vitro and in vivo [96,97]. This new paradigm for the role of yersiniabactin in virulence is highly applicable to NTS serovars, because *Salmonella enterica* species do need to resist copper (Cu^{2+}) accumulation inside macrophages for the survival [98]. Once accumulated in the cytoplasm of macrophages, Cu^{2+} oxidized into a Cu^{1+} which is toxic to bacteria. So, co-expression of yersiniabactin and catecholate siderophores (enterobactin, salmochelin) in the SIn strain may provide a survival advantage by facilitating iron acquisition as well resistance to copper-mediated toxicity.

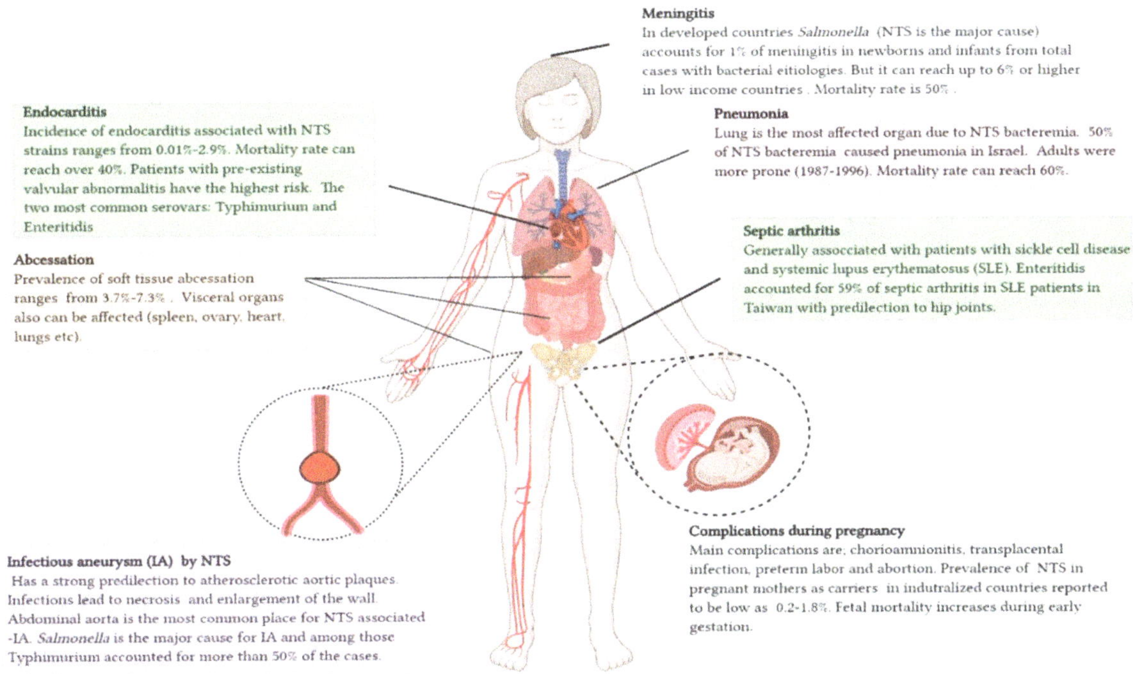

Figure 2. Bacteremia-induced complications by non-typhoidal *Salmonella*. Generally, 5% of gastroenteritis cases develop into bacteremia-associated complications in immunocompetent people. However the burden of NTS bacteremia is higher in immunocompromised patients and children under 5 years old (can reach up to 34%). Data related to epidemiology has been obtained from a variety of published case reports and outbreak analysis. [99–110].

The acquisition of siderophore secretion and metal iron-uptake systems in chicken-associated NTS serovars might be linked to their invasive phenotypes in humans but more studies are needed to confirm their role. Whether they are important for the pathogenesis in chickens remains a question to be answered.

3. Iron Uptake in NTS Virulence: Chicken vs. Mammalian Models

Most of our understanding related to the role of iron-regulated gene clusters in *Salmonella* pathogenesis has derived from experimental infection with *Salmonella* Typhimurium (STm) using mouse models and mammalian cell culture assays. Due to differences in how pathogens interact with avian environments, we cannot directly extrapolate this information to chickens [111,112]. The relationship of virulence with various iron-uptake systems in pathogenic bacteria including *Salmonella enterica* species has been extensively reviewed [16–21,113]. Unfortunately, limited data in chicken models and avian cell lines remains a barrier to understanding the host–pathogen interactions of the iron-uptake system in Salmonella serovars. Here we discuss the potential role of iron-uptake systems in NTS serovars towards infection and colonization in chickens compared to mammals. Some of the gaps in knowledge which need to be addressed in poultry are summarized in Figure 3.

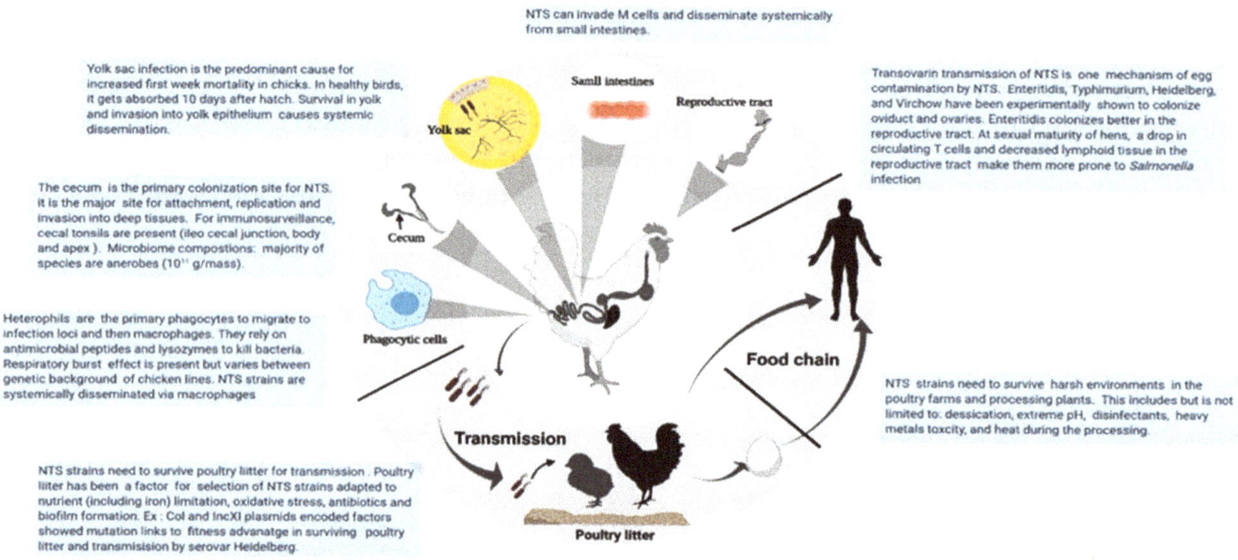

Figure 3. Interaction of non-typhoidal *Salmonella* strains with chicken and the environment. The role of iron-uptake systems during key steps of *Salmonella* life cycle illustrated here needs to be investigated in chicken models in future [50,114–122].

3.1. Feo-Mediated Fe^{2+} Uptake Involved in Rapid Colonization of the Gut and Systemic Spread

To identify differentially expressed gene profiles of STm isolated during colonization of the lumen of the chicken cecum (compared to in vitro cultures), Harvey et al., 2011, detected the upregulation of the *sitABCD* operon [123]. In contrast, the major Fe^{2+} uptake facilitator, the FeoABC system, was not differentially expressed during the same experiment. However, these researchers only assessed gene expression at 16 hours post-infection in newly hatched chicks so they may not have been able to capture the full spectrum of iron-regulated gene expression over time [123]. The *sitABCD* gene cluster was a major virulence factor in an avian pathogenic *E. coli* (APEC) strain causing colibacillosis in a chicken air sac model [124]. Evidence suggested that manganese uptake was more important than the Fe^{2+} uptake during extraintestinal phase in APEC strains [124]. In contrast, both Mn^{2+} and Fe^{2+} uptake contributed to the full virulence of STm to cause typhoid disease in mice [125]. Portillo et al., 1992 estimated that 1 μM of free Fe^{2+} prevailed inside the STm containing vacuole within Madin-Darby canine kidney cells and it was sufficient for replication, for at least 8 h of infection [126]. This suggested that Fe^{2+} iron uptake might be more important than Fe^{3+} in the initial stages of STm establishment in the gastrointestinal tract. Supporting this hypothesis, Tsolis et al., 1996, showed that the lack of the Feo system significantly reduced the fecal shedding of STm in mice (C57BL/6) at day 4 post-challenge while a Fe^{3+} uptake null strain was recovered at a level similar to the wildtype [127]. In line with these findings, Costa et al., 2017 showed that Feo-mediated iron uptake provided a fitness advantage for STm, during gastrointestinal colonization (fecal shedding) via intragastrical route in a streptomycin-pretreated mouse (C57BL/6) colitis model at 2 days post-infection [128].

Similar to mammals, chickens mediate Fe^{2+} egress from macrophages by expressing NRAMP-1 (Natural Resistance-Associated Protein 1) in the phagosomal membrane [129]. The action of NRAMP-1 is thought to limit the free, labile iron pool available to intracellular pathogens [130]. Thus, it is very likely that Feo-mediated ferrous iron uptake plays a crucial role for Salmonella to establish systemic infections in chicken. NRAMP-1 expression has been linked to Salmonella-resistance in certain chicken genetic lines (White Leghorn W1) [131]. The susceptible chicken line (CC) had a conservative mutation in the amino acid residue located at 223 ($Arg^{223} \rightarrow Gln^{223}$) of NRAMP-1, which was highly predictive of a functional anomaly in the NRAMP- 1 protein [131]. Consistent with this finding, authors observed that only 15% birds survived to a parenteral challenge of STm in the susceptible chicken line (CC) 7 days post-infection while almost all birds survived in the resistant chicken line [131]. However, the mortality rate of the susceptible chicken line was comparable to the resistant chicken line beyond day 7 post-infection irrespective of the NRAMP-1 status [131]. This reflected that Fe^{2+} starvation in presence of a functional NRAMP-1 certainly did limit rapid systemic spread of the STm in chicken but bacteria somehow adopted the new iron status in chicken and survived, pertaining their virulence during persistent infection. Future studies are needed to examine the iron distribution during *Salmonella* pathogenesis in chicken (cecal colonization and extraintestinal dissemination) and how this will shape overall regulation of iron-uptake systems in NTS serovars.

While further experiments are warranted to investigate the role of Fe^{2+}uptake in relationship to the NRAMP-1 status in chicken lines, mouse models of infections have provided some insight into the interplay between NRAMP-1 and Feo-mediated iron uptake. Feo-mediated iron uptake provided a competitive advantage during persistent infection of STm (SL1344-calf virulent isolate) in both NRAMP-positive and -negative backgrounds of mice [132]. Authors observed that a Δ*feo* STm strain was significantly reduced in its ability to colonize deeper tissue in the gut such as Peyer's patches (PP), mesenteric lymph nodes (MLN), as well as liver and spleen during a mixed infection [132]. Mice were orally challenged resembling natural infection with *Salmonella*. In the same study, it was documented that the lack of Feo-mediated Fe^{2+} uptake affected the overall iron homeostasis in a STm strain during a single infection challenge model [132]. The study revealed that the Δ*feo* STm strain compensated the requirement of iron by upregulating siderophore-mediated Fe^{3+} uptake (enterobactin, salmochelin) systems during systemic infection (liver and spleen) [132]. Interestingly, this upregulation of siderophore-mediated ferric uptake resulted in increased bacterial burden in the liver and spleen during persistent infection in $NRAMP^{+/+}$ mice [132]. There are growing numbers of evidence indicating that Salmonella preferentially resided in hemo-phagocytosed macrophages in the liver and spleen during infection [133–135]. One plausible explanation for this might be the abundant source of iron that Salmonella can exploit during degradation of erythrocytes (Fe^{3+}/Fe^{2+}) in those macrophages. Hence hypersecretion of siderophores may benefit growing *Salmonella* under such conditions. Expression of iron-uptake systems certainly may differ among different types of tissues the bacterium has to encounter or might vary due to host responses. For example, transferrin-bound iron (Fe^{3+}) in the intestines provides a good source of iron for Salmonella and the uptake can be facilitated by the stress-induced norepinephrine hormone which is produced abundantly in the mesenteric organs both in chickens and mice [136].

Highlights-1:

(i) Feo-mediated ferrous iron uptake is important for rapid colonization by and systemic spread of *Salmonella* Typhimurium in $NRAMP^{+/+}$ mice. We predict the same in chicken–NTS interaction.

(ii) Feo may not be essential for persistent infection in mouse models due to redundancy of various iron-uptake systems. This includes Mn^{2+} uptake via SitABCD and MntH, and uptake of siderophores.

(iii) NTS predilects to iron-rich hemophagocytes during systemic infection.

3.2. Siderophore Synthesis Is Important During Persistent Infection and Bacteremia

Iron restriction is well-studied related to antimicrobial properties of egg white in vitro [137–142]. Kang et al., 2006, showed that a Δ*entF* strain of SEn which was unable to produce a catecholate siderophore, was significantly attenuated in its ability to survive in egg albumen in vitro which suggested that siderophore production is an important virulence determinant during internal contamination of the eggs [143]. The egg is enriched with a variety of iron chelators such as ovotransferrin (in egg white) and phosphovitin (in yolk) hence it is very likely that potent ferric hijacking systems will benefit *Salmonella* in colonizing the eggs during transovarian transmission. Van Immerseel et al., 2010, proposed the hypothesis that stress-induced survival mechanisms governed by SEn led to egg-associated human outbreaks due to the fact that eggs possessed an arsenal of antimicrobial properties [144]. However, in-vivo gene expression studies did not identify iron-uptake systems as differentially expressed gene clusters during oviduct colonization or egg contamination [145,146]. Gene expression studies have been conducted using an intravenous challenge model which is an unnatural route of infection in hens. So, it might be possible that gene expression of *Salmonella* during intravenous challenge might be different compared to oral infection in hens. Siderophore-mediated ferric iron uptake has not been identified as a major virulence determinant during colonization in the gut and systemic infection in chicken, so far. There are not enough studies performed using iron-homeostasis-related mutants of Salmonella to investigate their role in infection, colonization and transmission in a chicken model. In a series of experiments executed by Rabsch et al., 2003, it was proposed that siderophore degradation product such as *N*-2,3-dihyroxybenzoyl-L-serine (DBS) will be more important in colonization and systemic spread in the absence of an active siderophore uptake system in chicken [37]. The authors confirmed this hypothesis in a mouse model of infection (intragastric route) using a Δ*fepA* Δ*iroN* Δ*cir* strain of STm (SL1344) which was significantly attenuated in colonization of the cecum and systemic spread, which in contrast was not observed in a Δ*fepA* Δ*iroN* mutant (enterobactin and salmochelin uptake deficient). In a chicken model, SEn strains carrying *fepA iroN* mutation profiles behaved similarly as in mice indicating that siderophore uptake was not essential during early colonization events [37]. Interestingly, the authors concluded that in BALB/c mice who are intrinsically susceptible to *Salmonella* infection, salmochelin was not important to cause infection. All these data have to be used cautiously due to following reasons; (i) *N*-2,3-dihyroxybenzoyl-L-serine (DBS) is not occurring naturally in the environment. It needs to be synthesized (*entABCDE*) or liberated as a byproduct due to action of Fes and IroE (Figure 1) on enterobactin/salmochelin. So, if DBSs are important so is the siderophore synthesis. When uptake routes are blocked spontaneous breakdown of siderophores can be a rapid process. (ii) At a given time, siderophores and its degraded products (enterobactin, salmochelins, Ent-trimer, Ent-dimer, DGE-trimer, DBS etc.) can be present and this cocktail may have a biological role in vivo. For example, degradation to more soluble form such as DBS, enables *Salmonella* to internalize iron rapidly. The mixture of derivatives might also exhaust the immune system in mounting an effective antibody response (antibodies against one particular siderophore derivative will spare others in the mixture) [147,148]. (iii) The genetic background of the host organism will have a major effect on the outcome of animal experiments. For example, the importance of iron-uptake systems described in mice that are genetically susceptible or resistant to Salmonella has been contrasting [149,150]. This will most likely be applicable to chickens as well (Salmonella-resistant and -susceptible chicken lines). Another crucial factor is the age of the birds: e.g., chicks (weak immune system) vs. adult chickens.

Fe^{3+} uptake via FepB (periplasmic binding protein for some catecholate type siderophores) has been identified as an absolute requirement for the persistent infection in mice (Sv129S6-Nramp1$^{+/+}$) with STm (SL1344) [151]. FepB is needed to shuttle Fe^{3+} bound to enterobactin, salmochelin or DBS (2,3-dihydrobenzoic acids), from the periplasm to the inner membrane transport components (Figure 1A). The Δ*fepB* of STm dramatically lowered the bacterial recovery below the detection limit in most of the tissues examined in mice (cecum, MLN, PP, liver and spleen) [151]. Most importantly, the authors in these studies showed that siderophore synthesis (enterobactin, salmochelin) played a significant role in gastrointestinal colonization and systemic spread during persistent infection [151].

Salmochelin synthesis and export have been identified as major virulence factors during bacteremia in mice (C3H, Nramp^{+}) measured by mortality after intraperitoneal injection of STm [152]. Parenteral injection of STm carrying a mutation in *tonB* which completely blocked all siderophore uptake has previously been shown to significantly increase the LD50 in mice compared to the challenge with wildtype STm [127]. Further, in a study which analyzed differentially expressed genes in STm-SL1344 by transcriptomic and proteomics techniques, enterobactin synthesis and uptake genes were highly upregulated during systemic infection in a mouse (C57BL/6) model [153]. Most interesting finding of that study was, in addition to enterobactin, salmochelin-related genes were upregulated in immune-deficient mice background (deficient in ROS generation) but not in wildtype mice background [153]. In the same study high bacterial growth has been observed in spleen of immune-deficient mice which may have been linked to a high demand of iron for growth of STm [153]. It is well-documented that salmochelin provides a defense against Lcn-2-mediated enterobactin chelation by the host during inflammation (mouse colitis model) [154]. Hence it is possible that mice with deficiency in respiratory burst effect, may rely on antimicrobial mechanisms such as more Lcn-2 secretion to limit *Salmonella* replication in phagocytic cells. Also, serum is considered as an extremely low iron compartment for pathogens in vertebrates [155]. Serum iron is mostly bound to transferrin, albumin and ferritins. In the presence of serum albumin, enterobactin is not considered as an efficient iron chelator as it is rapidly cleared [156,157]. Hence secretion of stealth siderophores (aerobactin, salmochelin and yersiniabactin) will be beneficial for NTS serovars during bacteremia.

The extracellular fatty acid-binding protein (ExFABP) of chickens has been identified as the chicken equivalent of Lcn-2 [158]. Its overall structure is similar to Lcn-2 yet it has a more extended positively charged calyx (which is the binding pocket for ligands) with two binding specificities: one for siderophores and the other for lysophosphatidic acid [158]. Interestingly, the calyx of Ex-FABP accommodates one form of salmochelin, mono- glycosylated enterobactin (MGE/S1) which is not normally bound by Lcn-2 [158]. Lcn-2 cannot bind to any salmochelin derivatives. So, the "chicken lipochalin-2" seems to be more potent in withholding iron compared to Lcn-2 during *Salmonella* infection. There is ample evidence for expression of Ex-FABP in the cecum associated with inflammation of day-old chicks when infected by NTS [159,160]. Chicken egg white which has antibacterial properties against *Salmonella* in vitro also contains Ex-FABP [145]. Adult chickens generate a more tolerogenic response towards non-typhoidal *Salmonella* (NTS) infection [161,162]. The inflammation induced in adult chicken is transient yet sufficient enough to contain the bacteria in the gut while some may spread systemically to colonize spleen and liver. Significant inflammation in the liver and spleen has not been observed in more mature birds except for follicular lesion [161]. The lack of marked inflammatory response in adult chicken towards NTS infection is an indication that some of the stealth siderophore secretion might not be essential during the colonization process compared to mammals.

Highlights-2:

(i) Ferric iron uptake mechanisms are important for persistent infection.We predict similar results for chicken as those found in mouse models because bioavailability of iron is expected to be low in most compartments of the host.
(ii) Aerobactin, salmochelin and yersiniabactin provide a serum resistance during bacteremia and systemic infection. This may explain the siderophore link towards chicken-associated virulent NTS serovars.
(iii) The role of stealth siderophores of NTS in adult chickens during colonization may be nonessential due to tolerogenic response.

4. Opening the Pandora's Box of Gallus-Iron-*Salmonella* Interaction

Iron uptake is a primary virulence factor for *Salmonella*. But how each iron-uptake system partakes in pathogenesis in a chicken model still needs a thorough investigation. This is intriguing because chickens are the major reservoir for Salmonella; yet we know least about its interactions with the host. We want to highlight some of the important aspects which need to be addressed in future experiments using chickens as model related to the Gallus-Iron-Salmonella interaction. This will certainly lay a platform to discuss the potential for developing therapeutics targeted at iron homeostasis in *Salmonella*.

4.1. Nutritional Immunity Status in Chicken during Salmonella Infection

Nutritional immunity is defined as part of the host's innate immune response to withhold essential nutrients, including iron, from invading pathogens [163]. The interplay between iron-withholding mechanisms in chicken and iron homeostasis in Salmonella during pathogenesis is largely unknown. The interaction between siderophores and extracellular fatty acid binding protein (ExFABP), which is part of chicken-iron-withholding strategy, has recently been well-documented in eggs [164]. A study revealed that SEn has to synthesize stealth siderophores such as salmochelin to overcome iron starvation induced by ExFABP (chelation of Fe^{3+}-enterobactin) in egg white in vitro [164]. Ovotransferrin, synthesized by oviduct cells, is a transferrin family protein which transports iron into the growing embryo. It is the major constituter of egg albumin. The iron complex formation constant of ovotransferrin (iron affinity of the C lobe is 10^{18} and N lobe is 10^{14}) is low compared to most siderophores secreted by Salmonella hence iron restriction is not the major mechanism behind its antibacterial effect [165]. Egg yolk is the major iron store for growing embryos and almost all iron is bound to phosvitin. The affinity of phosvitin to iron is comparable to ovotransferrin ($K_f = 10^{18}$) [166]. So, Salmonella can rely on enterobactin ($K_f = 10^{49}$) rather on the expression of stealth siderophore to hijack iron from phosvitins, unless ExFABP is expressed in sufficient amounts. However, currently there is no evidence that stealth siderophores are indeed expressed to counteract ExFABP-mediated nutritional immunity in chickens during colonization in various tissue in vivo.

Adaptation to an iron-deficiency status in humans plays an important role in resistance to bacterial and viral infections [167]. The response is also termed as hypoferremia of inflammation or anemia of inflammation (AI). The key player for hypoferremic response is recognized as hepcidin, the master regulator for iron metabolism in humans and it is believed to be hepcidin independent in chickens (chicken genome seems to lack hepcidin up to date) [168–170]. Inflammation caused by pathogenic invasion induces hepcidin secretion from liver [171]. Hepcidin mediates ferroportin (Fpn) degradation which inhibits iron efflux from macrophages and iron absorption from intestines [172]. Fpn degradation also affects hepatocytes which increases their ferritin levels and the ability to store accumulated iron. All these mechanisms lead to a significant drop in the serum iron level (hypoferremia). The low level of iron in the serum may limit bacteremia, yet current evidence suggested that the burden of NTS increased in systemic infection-related sites such as the spleen during hypoferremic response in mice [173–175]. Similarly, infection with chicken-specific serovars such as *Salmonella* Gallinarum and *Salmonella* Pullorum led to anemia of inflammation (AI) in chicken with increased bacterial burden in spleen and liver [176]. The increased *Salmonella* colonization in the "systemic sites" correlated with a spike in the iron content both in mice and chickens. The reason for such a spike of iron in spleen can be partly due to the accelerated red blood cell turnover rate triggered by inflammation induced hypoferremia response. It has been documented that in mammals the half-life of red blood cells decreased dramatically during AI response and led to increased destruction of red blood cells by macrophages in spleen and liver [177]. Since Salmonella can profit from the iron abundancy (Fe^{2+}/Fe^{3+}) in hemophagocytic cells [132], they may preferentially rely on a specific iron uptake system during AI. Supporting this hypothesis, the African lineage of iNTS (invasive NTS) strain *Salmonella* Typhimurium 313 (ST313) appears not to rely on salmochelin-mediated Fe^{3+} uptake during systemic infection in mice [178]. There is a strong association of African linage of iNTS strains with malaria parasites which increase intracellular iron levels in macrophages [179]. An abundance of the Fe^{2+} pool may have inherently adapted the ST313 to reduce the expression of stealth siderophore uptake systems which are a metabolically demanding process to produce. There is currently no experimental data indicating the occurrence of AI in chicken during NTS infection. Broader host range serovars such as NTS strains colonize mainly the gastrointestinal tract without overt inflammation in adult birds. In such a situation, AI will not be profound. Virulence of NTSs varies according to serovars and chicken susceptibility depends on their genetic background and the age of the birds. For example, NTS such as STm and SEn do cause systemic inflammation during enteric infection in young chickens. They are also capable of infecting the yolk sac in young birds leading to the development of omphalitis. Yolk sac infections result in high mortality due to septicemia [180]. The role of iron-uptake systems of NTS, when the host undergoes hypoferremia needs to be investigated in a chicken model of infection. It will be especially important to examine iron distribution in compartments such as blood, liver, spleen and gastrointestinal tract of chickens following infection. Research on iron-regulated gene expression combined with proteomic studies is needed to assess how each iron-uptake system is regulated in parallel to anemia of inflammation.

4.2. Non-Canonical Function of Siderophores: Defense against Respiratory Burst and Immunomodulatory Function

There are growing number of evidences suggesting that siderophores have other biological functions apart from Fe^{3+} uptake [181]. One such alternative function is defense against oxidative stress provided by catecholate siderophores [182–184]. The mechanism behind the enterobactin-mediated defense against reactive oxygen species is currently been investigated. One of the mechanisms suggested that Ent-trimer (Figure 1C) which is the linearized molecule of enterobactin, participates in ROS scavenging by providing hydroxyl groups from the freed end of the backbone [185]. Generation of a robust respiratory burst is a key mechanism to kill Salmonella inside phagocytic cells [186]. In this regard, catecholate siderophore production will provide a survival advantage inside macrophages which is a major replication niche during systemic dissemination and colonization. Also, it may be plausible that synthesis of catecholate siderophores will be important irrespective of iron limitation inside phagocytic cells because of their diverse functions apart from iron scavenging. Some of the phagocytic cells in the chicken immune system do not induce a strong respiratory burst effect to *Salmonella*. The chicken lacks neutrophils yet has heterophils that are functionally equivalent to neutrophils. Heterophils are unable to synthesize myeloperoxidases and rely on a repertoire of antimicrobial peptides to kill bacteria instead of respiratory burst [114,187,188]. It has been documented that enterobactin inhibited the myeloperoxidases activity in *E coli* and provided a survival advantage in inflamed gut [184]. Hence it is important to investigate the interplay between enterobactin and heterophils during gastrointestinal colonization. Macrophages from Salmonella-resistant chicken lines *(SALI)* showed more pronounced respiratory burst effect while susceptible and inbred lines had low, variable level respectively [189]. So future experiments are warranted in chickens to investigate the role of siderophore-mediated defense against reactive oxygen and nitrogen species.

Holden et al., 2016, showed that siderophores produced by *Klebsiella pneumoniae* (enterobactin, salmochelin and yersiniabactin) can induce inflammation in lung epithelial tissue by stabilizing the hypoxia inducible factor-1α (HIF-1α) in C57BL/6 mice [190]. In a previous study, Holden et al., 2014, showed that enterobactin together with Lcn-2 can potentiate the induction of pro-inflammatory cytokines in cultured murine lung epithelial cells through chelation of iron [191]. These data are highly suggestive that siderophores can mount an inflammation in vivo. Inflammatory cytokines liberated will help to attract macrophages and dendritic cells to the infective loci and subsequent systemic spread. It will be interesting to investigate whether siderophores facilitate systemic infection by induction of inflammation at different colonization sites in chicken by NTS serovars. Enterobactin-mediated iron chelation has been documented to polarize the macrophage from M1 phenotype to M2 phenotype in bone-marrow-derived cells [192]. M2 phenotype of macrophages will safeguard intracellular pathogen such as Salmonella by avoiding generating an oxidative killing mechanism [193]. Chicken has low number of resident macrophages in organs and relies on bone-marrow-derived monocytes to migrate to the inflammatory loci for pathogen control [187]. Presence of distinct M1 (killing/towards inflammatory) and M2 (healing/towards adaptive response) phenotypes [194] of chicken macrophages is yet to be fully elucidated. Further studies are needed to unravel how *Salmonella* mediates iron homeostasis in infected chicken macrophages as this microenvironment may impose a different iron status during polarization [195].

5. Concluding Remarks

Our understanding of iron in infection and immunity remains close to its infancy due to the complex nature of the interaction and ever-growing *Salmonella* serovars found in nature. Concerning chickens as a reservoir, it will be pivotal to understand how iron-regulated genes of *Salmonella* are expressed during pathogenesis in a chicken model of infection (Figure 3). Enhanced detection of in vivo siderophore production during colonization in different chicken host niches in situ will be key in understanding their role in the future. Experiments are needed to address how iron metabolism and homeostasis in the chicken are regulated in response to NTS infection. There are other metal uptake systems ($Mn2^+$, Cu, $Zn2^+$) apart from iron uptake which are not well-characterized in a chicken model regarding their role in NTS colonization. We believe that these efforts to understand the involvement of iron homeostasis in pathogenesis of NTS will pave the way for the development of a successful therapeutic strategy in the poultry industry to limit chicken-associated *Salmonella* "spillovers" to humans and the environment.

Author Contributions: D.H.W. and W.K. designed the study, collected data and created the figures; D.H.W., W.K., B.A. and A.P.W. wrote the manuscript. Figures are created with BioRenders.com (https://biorender.com/) subscribed to D.H.W. All authors have read and agreed to the published version of the manuscript.

Acknowledgments: We thank Po-King S. Lam, Colette Wheler and Arshud Dar for fruitful discussions. Work in the laboratory of W.K. was supported through funds from the Chicken Farmers of Canada (CFC), the Canadian Poultry Research Council (CPRC), the Saskatchewan Chicken Industry Development Fund (SCIDF), the Canadian Poultry Research Council/Agri-Food (Canada), Egg Farmers of Alberta (EFA), the Department of Alberta Agriculture and Forestry (AAF), the Saskatchewan Ministry of Agriculture—Agriculture Development Fund (ADF) and Egg Farmers of Canada (EFC). This report was published with the permission of the Director of VIDO-InterVac as journal series number 898.

References

1. Ryan, M.P.; O'Dwyer, J.; Adley, C.C. Evaluation of the complex nomenclature of the clinically and veterinary significant pathogen Salmonella. *Biomed Res. Int.* **2017**, *2017*. [CrossRef] [PubMed]
2. Tindall, B.; Grimont, P.; Garrity, G.; Euzeby, J. Nomenclature and taxonomy of the genus Salmonella. *Int. J. Syst. Evol. Microbiol.* **2005**, *55*, 521–524. [CrossRef] [PubMed]
3. Grimont, P.A.; Weill, F.-X. Antigenic formulae of the Salmonella serovars. *Who Collab. Cent. Ref. Res. Salmonella* **2007**, *9*, 1–166.
4. Giammanco, G.M.; Pignato, S.; Mammina, C.; Grimont, F.; Grimont, P.A.; Nastasi, A.; Giammanco, G. Persistent endemicity of Salmonella bongori 48: z35: In southern Italy: Molecular characterization of human, animal, and environmental isolates. *J. Clin. Microbiol.* **2002**, *40*, 3502–3505. [CrossRef] [PubMed]
5. Aleksic, S.; Heinzerling, F.; Bockemühl, J. Human infection caused by salmonellae of subspecies II to VI in Germany, 1977–1992. *Z. Bakteriol.* **1996**, *283*, 391–398. [CrossRef]
6. Desai, P.T.; Porwollik, S.; Long, F.; Cheng, P.; Wollam, A.; Clifton, S.W.; Weinstock, G.M.; McClelland, M. Evolutionary genomics of Salmonella enterica subspecies. *MBio* **2013**, *4*, e00579-12. [CrossRef]
7. Porwollik, S.; Wong, R.M.-Y.; McClelland, M. Evolutionary genomics of Salmonella: Gene acquisitions revealed by microarray analysis. *Proc. Natl. Acad. Sci. USA* **2002**, *99*, 8956–8961. [CrossRef]
8. Fricke, W.F.; Mammel, M.K.; McDermott, P.F.; Tartera, C.; White, D.G.; LeClerc, J.E.; Ravel, J.; Cebula, T.A. Comparative genomics of 28 Salmonella enterica isolates: Evidence for CRISPR-mediated adaptive sublineage evolution. *J. Bacteriol.* **2011**, *193*, 3556–3568. [CrossRef]
9. Li, M.; Havelaar, A.H.; Hoffmann, S.; Hald, T.; Kirk, M.D.; Torgerson, P.R.; Devleesschauwer, B. Global disease burden of pathogens in animal source foods, 2010. *PLoS ONE* **2019**, *14*, e0216545. [CrossRef]
10. Ferrari, R.G.; Rosario, D.K.; Cunha-Neto, A.; Mano, S.B.; Figueiredo, E.E.; Conte-Junior, C.A. Worldwide epidemiology of Salmonella serovars in animal-based foods: A meta-analysis. *Appl. Environ. Microbiol.* **2019**, *85*, e00591-19. [CrossRef]
11. Borges, K.A.; Furian, T.Q.; De Souza, S.N.; Tondo, E.C.; Streck, A.F.; Salle, C.T.P.; de Souza Moraes, H.L.; Do Nascimento, V.P. Spread of a major clone of Salmonella enterica serotype Enteritidis in poultry and in salmonellosis outbreaks in Southern Brazil. *J. Food Prot.* **2017**, *80*, 158–163. [CrossRef] [PubMed]
12. Wei, S.-H.; Huang, A.S.; Liao, Y.-S.; Liu, Y.-L.; Chiou, C.-S. A large outbreak of salmonellosis associated with sandwiches contaminated with multiple bacterial pathogens purchased via an online shopping service. *Foodborne Pathog. Dis.* **2014**, *11*, 230–233. [CrossRef] [PubMed]

13. Kinross, P.; Van Alphen, L.; Urtaza, J.M.; Struelens, M.; Takkinen, J.; Coulombier, D.; Mäkelä, P.; Bertrand, S.; Mattheus, W.; Schmid, D. Multidisciplinary investigation of a multicountry outbreak of Salmonella Stanley infections associated with turkey meat in the European Union, August 2011 to January 2013. *Eurosurveillance* **2014**, *19*, 20801. [CrossRef] [PubMed]
14. Hörmansdorfer, S.; Messelhäußer, U.; Rampp, A.; Schönberger, K.; Dallman, T.; Allerberger, F.; Kornschober, C.; Sing, A.; Wallner, P.; Zapf, A. Re-evaluation of a 2014 multi-country European outbreak of Salmonella Enteritidis phage type 14b using recent epidemiological and molecular data. *Euro Surveill.* **2017**, *22*, 17-00196. [CrossRef] [PubMed]
15. Ford, L.; Wang, Q.; Stafford, R.; Ressler, K.-A.; Norton, S.; Shadbolt, C.; Hope, K.; Franklin, N.; Krsteski, R.; Carswell, A. Seven Salmonella Typhimurium outbreaks in Australia linked by trace-back and whole genome sequencing. *Foodborne Pathog. Dis.* **2018**, *15*, 285–292. [CrossRef]
16. Andrews, S.C.; Robinson, A.K.; Rodríguez-Quiñones, F. Bacterial iron homeostasis. *FEMS Microbiol. Rev.* **2003**, *27*, 215–237. [CrossRef]
17. Wooldridge, K.G.; Williams, P.H. Iron uptake mechanisms of pathogenic bacteria. *FEMS Microbiol. Rev.* **1993**, *12*, 325–348. [CrossRef]
18. Krewulak, K.D.; Vogel, H.J. Structural biology of bacterial iron uptake. *Biochim. Biophys. Acta Biomembr.* **2008**, *1778*, 1781–1804. [CrossRef]
19. Ratledge, C.; Dover, L.G. Iron metabolism in pathogenic bacteria. *Ann. Rev. Microbiol.* **2000**, *54*, 881–941. [CrossRef]
20. Miethke, M.; Marahiel, M.A. Siderophore-based iron acquisition and pathogen control. *Microbiol. Mol. Biol. Rev.* **2007**, *71*, 413–451. [CrossRef]
21. Sheldon, J.R.; Heinrichs, D.E. Recent developments in understanding the iron acquisition strategies of gram positive pathogens. *FEMS Microbiol. Rev.* **2015**, *39*, 592–630. [CrossRef] [PubMed]
22. Imlay, J.A. Oxidative Stress. *Ecosal Plus* **2009**, *3*. [CrossRef] [PubMed]
23. Liochev, S.I.; Fridovich, I. The Haber-Weiss cycle—70 years later: An alternative view. *Redox Rep.* **2002**, *7*, 55–57. [CrossRef] [PubMed]
24. Stojiljkovic, I.; Hantke, K. Functional domains of theescherichia coli ferric uptake regulator protein (fur). *Mol. Gen. Genet.* **1995**, *247*, 199–205. [CrossRef]
25. Bagg, A.; Neilands, J. Ferric uptake regulation protein acts as a repressor, employing iron (II) as a cofactor to bind the operator of an iron transport operon in Escherichia coli. *Biochemistry* **1987**, *26*, 5471–5477. [CrossRef]
26. Tsolis, R.M.; Bäumler, A.J.; Stojiljkovic, I.; Heffron, F. Fur regulon of Salmonella typhimurium: Identification of new iron-regulated genes. *J. Bacteriol.* **1995**, *177*, 4628–4637. [CrossRef]
27. Foster, J.W.; Hall, H.K. Effect of Salmonella typhimurium ferric uptake regulator (fur) mutations on iron-and pH-regulated protein synthesis. *J. Bacteriol.* **1992**, *174*, 4317–4323. [CrossRef]
28. Carpenter, B.M.; Whitmire, J.M.; Merrell, D.S. This is not your mother's repressor: The complex role of fur in pathogenesis. *Infect. Immun.* **2009**, *77*, 2590–2601. [CrossRef]
29. Oglesby-Sherrouse, A.G.; Murphy, E.R. Iron-responsive bacterial small RNAs: Variations on a theme. *Metallomics* **2013**, *5*, 276–286. [CrossRef]
30. Kim, J.N.; Kwon, Y.M. Genetic and phenotypic characterization of the RyhB regulon in Salmonella Typhimurium. *Microbiol. Res.* **2013**, *168*, 41–49. [CrossRef]
31. Massé, E.; Gottesman, S. A small RNA regulates the expression of genes involved in iron metabolism in Escherichia coli. *Proc. Natl. Acad. Sci. USA* **2002**, *99*, 4620–4625. [CrossRef] [PubMed]
32. Figueroa-Bossi, N.; Bossi, L. Sponges and predators in the small RNA world. Regulating with RNA in Bacteria and Archaea. *microbiolspec* **2018**, *6*. [CrossRef]
33. Scarrow, R.C.; Ecker, D.J.; Ng, C.; Liu, S.; Raymond, K.N. Iron (III) coordination chemistry of linear dihydroxyserine compounds derived from enterobactin. *Inorg. Chem.* **1991**, *30*, 900–906. [CrossRef]
34. Hantke, K. Dihydroxybenzolyserine—a siderophore for E. coli. *FEMS Microbiol. Lett.* **1990**, *67*, 5–8.
35. Raymond, K.N.; Dertz, E.A.; Kim, S.S. Enterobactin: An archetype for microbial iron transport. *Proc. Natl. Acad. Sci. USA* **2003**, *100*, 3584–3588. [CrossRef] [PubMed]
36. Langridge, G.C.; Fookes, M.; Connor, T.R.; Feltwell, T.; Feasey, N.; Parsons, B.N.; Seth-Smith, H.M.; Barquist, L.; Stedman, A.; Humphrey, T. Patterns of genome evolution that have accompanied host adaptation in Salmonella. *Proc. Natl. Acad. Sci. USA* **2015**, *112*, 863–868. [CrossRef]

37. Rabsch, W.; Methner, U.; Voigt, W.; Tschäpe, H.; Reissbrodt, R.; Williams, P.H. Role of receptor proteins for enterobactin and 2, 3-dihydroxybenzoylserine in virulence of Salmonella enterica. *Infect. Immun.* **2003**, *71*, 6953–6961. [CrossRef]
38. Hantke, K.; Nicholson, G.; Rabsch, W.; Winkelmann, G. Salmochelins, siderophores of Salmonella enterica and uropathogenic Escherichia coli strains, are recognized by the outer membrane receptor IroN. *Proc. Natl. Acad. Sci. USA* **2003**, *100*, 3677–3682. [CrossRef]
39. Lin, H.; Fischbach, M.A.; Liu, D.R.; Walsh, C.T. In vitro characterization of salmochelin and enterobactin trilactone hydrolases IroD, IroE, and Fes. *J. Am. Chem. Soc.* **2005**, *127*, 11075–11084. [CrossRef]
40. Bister, B.; Bischoff, D.; Nicholson, G.J.; Valdebenito, M.; Schneider, K.; Winkelmann, G.; Hantke, K.; Süssmuth, R.D. The structure of salmochelins: C-glucosylated enterobactins of Salmonella enterica §. *Biometals* **2004**, *17*, 471–481. [CrossRef]
41. Oves-Costales, D.; Kadi, N.; Challis, G.L. The long-overlooked enzymology of a nonribosomal peptide synthetase-independent pathway for virulence-conferring siderophore biosynthesis. *Chem. Commun.* **2009**, *43*, 6530–6541. [CrossRef] [PubMed]
42. De Lorenzo, V.; Martinez, J. Aerobactin production as a virulence factor: A reevaluation. *Eur. J. Clin. Microbiol. Infect. Dis.* **1988**, *7*, 621–629. [CrossRef] [PubMed]
43. Köster, W. ABC transporter-mediated uptake of iron, siderophores, heme and vitamin B12. *Res. Microbiol.* **2001**, *152*, 291–301. [CrossRef]
44. Oelschlaeger, T.; Zhang, D.; Schubert, S.; Carniel, E.; Rabsch, W.; Karch, H.; Hacker, J. The high-pathogenicity island is absent in human pathogens of Salmonella enterica subspecies I but present in isolates of subspecies III and VI. *J. Bacteriol.* **2003**, *185*, 1107–1111. [CrossRef] [PubMed]
45. Lau, C.K.; Krewulak, K.D.; Vogel, H.J. Bacterial ferrous iron transport: The Feo system. *FEMS Microbiol. Rev.* **2016**, *40*, 273–298. [CrossRef]
46. Sestok, A.E.; Linkous, R.O.; Smith, A.T. Toward a mechanistic understanding of Feo-mediated ferrous iron uptake. *Metallomics* **2018**, *10*, 887–898. [CrossRef]
47. Kehres, D.G.; Janakiraman, A.; Slauch, J.M.; Maguire, M.E. SitABCD is the alkaline Mn2+ transporter of Salmonella enterica serovar Typhimurium. *J. Bacteriol.* **2002**, *184*, 3159–3166. [CrossRef]
48. Cartron, M.L.; Maddocks, S.; Gillingham, P.; Craven, C.J.; Andrews, S.C. Feo–transport of ferrous iron into bacteria. *Biometals* **2006**, *19*, 143–157. [CrossRef]
49. Dhillon, A.; Alisantosa, B.; Shivaprasad, H.; Jack, O.; Schaberg, D.; Bandli, D. Pathogenicity of Salmonella enteritidis phage types 4, 8, and 23 in broiler chicks. *Avian Dis.* **1999**, *43*, 506–515. [CrossRef]
50. Roy, P.; Dhillon, A.; Shivaprasad, H.; Schaberg, D.; Bandli, D.; Johnson, S. Pathogenicity of different serogroups of avian salmonellae in specific-pathogen-free chickens. *Avian Dis.* **2001**, *45*, 922–937. [CrossRef]
51. Hazards, E.P.o.B.; Koutsoumanis, K.; Allende, A.; Alvarez-Ordóñez, A.; Bolton, D.; Bover-Cid, S.; Chemaly, M.; De Cesare, A.; Herman, L.; Hilbert, F. Salmonella control in poultry flocks and its public health impact. *EFSA J.* **2019**, *17*, e05596.
52. Shah, D.H.; Paul, N.C.; Sischo, W.C.; Crespo, R.; Guard, J. Population dynamics and antimicrobial resistance of the most prevalent poultry-associated Salmonella serotypes. *Poult. Sci.* **2017**, *96*, 687–702. [CrossRef] [PubMed]
53. Suez, J.; Porwollik, S.; Dagan, A.; Marzel, A.; Schorr, Y.I.; Desai, P.T.; Agmon, V.; McClelland, M.; Rahav, G.; Gal-Mor, O. Virulence gene profiling and pathogenicity characterization of non-typhoidal Salmonella accounted for invasive disease in humans. *PLoS ONE* **2013**, *8*, e58449. [CrossRef] [PubMed]
54. Waters, V.L.; Crosa, J.H. Colicin V virulence plasmids. *Microbiol. Mol. Biol. Rev.* **1991**, *55*, 437–450. [CrossRef]
55. Johnson, T.J.; Thorsness, J.L.; Anderson, C.P.; Lynne, A.M.; Foley, S.L.; Han, J.; Fricke, W.F.; McDermott, P.F.; White, D.G.; Khatri, M. Horizontal gene transfer of a ColV plasmid has resulted in a dominant avian clonal type of Salmonella enterica serovar Kentucky. *PLoS ONE* **2010**, *5*, e15524. [CrossRef] [PubMed]
56. Cheng, Y.; Pedroso, A.A.; Porwollik, S.; McClelland, M.; Lee, M.D.; Kwan, T.; Zamperini, K.; Soni, V.; Sellers, H.S.; Russell, S.M. rpoS-Regulated core genes involved in the competitive fitness of Salmonella enterica serovar Kentucky in the intestines of chickens. *Appl. Environ. Microbiol.* **2015**, *81*, 502–514. [CrossRef]
57. Hoffmann, M.; Zhao, S.; Pettengill, J.; Luo, Y.; Monday, S.R.; Abbott, J.; Ayers, S.L.; Cinar, H.N.; Muruvanda, T.; Li, C. Comparative genomic analysis and virulence differences in closely related Salmonella enterica serotype Heidelberg isolates from humans, retail meats, and animals. *Genome Biol. Evol.* **2014**, *6*, 1046–1068. [CrossRef]

58. Dhanani, A.S.; Block, G.; Dewar, K.; Forgetta, V.; Topp, E.; Beiko, R.G.; Diarra, M.S. Genomic comparison of non-typhoidal Salmonella enterica serovars Typhimurium, Enteritidis, Heidelberg, Hadar and Kentucky isolates from broiler chickens. *PLoS ONE* **2015**, *10*, e0128773. [CrossRef]

59. Branchu, P.; Bawn, M.; Kingsley, R.A. Genome variation and molecular epidemiology of Salmonella enterica serovar typhimurium pathovariants. *Infect. Immun.* **2018**, *86*, e00079-18. [CrossRef]

60. Mulvey, M.R.; Boyd, D.A.; Olson, A.B.; Doublet, B.; Cloeckaert, A. The genetics of Salmonella genomic island 1. *Microbes Infect.* **2006**, *8*, 1915–1922. [CrossRef]

61. Guiney, D.G.; Fierer, J. The role of the spv genes in Salmonella pathogenesis. *Front. Microbiol.* **2011**, *2*, 129. [CrossRef] [PubMed]

62. Khajanchi, B.K.; Hasan, N.A.; Choi, S.Y.; Han, J.; Zhao, S.; Colwell, R.R.; Cerniglia, C.E.; Foley, S.L. Comparative genomic analysis and characterization of incompatibility group FIB plasmid encoded virulence factors of Salmonella enterica isolated from food sources. *BMC Genom.* **2017**, *18*, 570. [CrossRef] [PubMed]

63. Petrovska, L.; Mather, A.E.; AbuOun, M.; Branchu, P.; Harris, S.R.; Connor, T.; Hopkins, K.L.; Underwood, A.; Lettini, A.A.; Page, A. Microevolution of monophasic Salmonella typhimurium during epidemic, United Kingdom, 2005–2010. *Emerg. Infect. Dis.* **2016**, *22*, 617. [CrossRef] [PubMed]

64. Huehn, S.; Bunge, C.; Junker, E.; Helmuth, R.; Malorny, B. Poultry-associated Salmonella enterica subsp. enterica serovar 4, 12: d:– reveals high clonality and a distinct pathogenicity gene repertoire. *Appl. Environ. Microbiol.* **2009**, *75*, 1011–1020. [CrossRef]

65. Thomson, N.R.; Clayton, D.J.; Windhorst, D.; Vernikos, G.; Davidson, S.; Churcher, C.; Quail, M.A.; Stevens, M.; Jones, M.A.; Watson, M. Comparative genome analysis of Salmonella Enteritidis PT4 and Salmonella Gallinarum 287/91 provides insights into evolutionary and host adaptation pathways. *Genome Res.* **2008**, *18*, 1624–1637. [CrossRef]

66. Wuyts, V.; Denayer, S.; Roosens, N.H.; Mattheus, W.; Bertrand, S.; Marchal, K.; Dierick, K.; De Keersmaecker, S.C. Whole genome sequence analysis of Salmonella Enteritidis PT4 outbreaks from a national reference laboratory's viewpoint. *PLoS Curr.* **2015**. [CrossRef]

67. Silva, C.A.; Blondel, C.J.; Quezada, C.P.; Porwollik, S.; Andrews-Polymenis, H.L.; Toro, C.S.; Zaldívar, M.; Contreras, I.; McClelland, M.; Santiviago, C.A. Infection of mice by Salmonella enterica serovar Enteritidis involves additional genes that are absent in the genome of serovar Typhimurium. *Infect. Immun.* **2012**, *80*, 839–849. [CrossRef]

68. Clayton, D.J.; Bowen, A.J.; Hulme, S.D.; Buckley, A.M.; Deacon, V.L.; Thomson, N.R.; Barrow, P.A.; Morgan, E.; Jones, M.A.; Watson, M. Analysis of the role of 13 major fimbrial subunits in colonisation of the chicken intestines by Salmonella enterica serovar Enteritidis reveals a role for a novel locus. *BMC Microbiol.* **2008**, *8*, 228. [CrossRef]

69. Bachmann, N.L.; Petty, N.K.; Zakour, N.L.B.; Szubert, J.M.; Savill, J.; Beatson, S.A. Genome analysis and CRISPR typing of Salmonella enterica serovar Virchow. *BMC Genom.* **2014**, *15*, 389. [CrossRef]

70. Nguyen, S.V.; Harhay, D.M.; Bono, J.L.; Smith, T.P.; Fields, P.I.; Dinsmore, B.A.; Santovenia, M.; Wang, R.; Bosilevac, J.M.; Harhay, G.P. Comparative genomics of Salmonella enterica serovar Montevideo reveals lineage-specific gene differences that may influence ecological niche association. *Microb. Genom.* **2018**, *4*, e000202. [CrossRef]

71. Franco, A.; Leekitcharoenphon, P.; Feltrin, F.; Alba, P.; Cordaro, G.; Iurescia, M.; Tolli, R.; D'Incau, M.; Staffolani, M.; Di Giannatale, E. Emergence of a clonal lineage of multidrug-resistant ESBL-producing Salmonella Infantis transmitted from broilers and broiler meat to humans in Italy between 2011 and 2014. *PLoS ONE* **2015**, *10*, e0144802. [CrossRef] [PubMed]

72. Bogomazova, A.N.; Gordeeva, V.D.; Krylova, E.V.; Soltynskaya, I.V.; Davydova, E.E.; Ivanova, O.E.; Komarov, A.A. Mega-plasmid found worldwide confers multiple antimicrobial resistance in Salmonella Infantis of broiler origin in Russia. *Int. J. Food Microbiol.* **2019**, *319*, 108497. [CrossRef] [PubMed]

73. Aviv, G.; Elpers, L.; Mikhlin, S.; Cohen, H.; Vitman Zilber, S.; Grassl, G.A.; Rahav, G.; Hensel, M.; Gal-Mor, O. The plasmid-encoded Ipf and Klf fimbriae display different expression and varying roles in the virulence of Salmonella enterica serovar Infantis in mouse vs. avian hosts. *PLoS Pathog.* **2017**, *13*, e1006559. [CrossRef] [PubMed]

74. Alba, P.; Leekitcharoenphon, P.; Carfora, V.; Amoruso, R.; Cordaro, G.; Di Matteo, P.; Ianzano, A.; Iurescia, M.; Diaconu, E.L.; Study Group, E.-E.-A.N. Molecular epidemiology of Salmonella Infantis in Europe: Insights into the success of the bacterial host and its parasitic pESI-like megaplasmid. *Microb. Genom.* **2020**, *6*, e000365. [CrossRef] [PubMed]
75. Foley, S.; Lynne, A.; Nayak, R. Salmonella challenges: Prevalence in swine and poultry and potential pathogenicity of such isolates. *J. Anim. Sci.* **2008**, *86*, E149–E162. [CrossRef] [PubMed]
76. Salisbury, A.-M.; Leeming, G.; Nikolaou, G.; Kipar, A.; Wigley, P. Salmonella Virchow infection of the chicken elicits cellular and humoral systemic and mucosal responses, but limited protection to homologous or heterologous re-challenge. *Front. Vet. Sci.* **2014**, *1*, 6. [CrossRef]
77. Stanaway, J.D.; Parisi, A.; Sarkar, K.; Blacker, B.F.; Reiner, R.C.; Hay, S.I.; Nixon, M.R.; Dolecek, C.; James, S.L.; Mokdad, A.H. The global burden of non-typhoidal salmonella invasive disease: A systematic analysis for the Global Burden of Disease Study 2017. *Lancet Infect. Dis.* **2019**, *19*, 1312–1324. [CrossRef]
78. Jones, T.F.; Ingram, L.A.; Cieslak, P.R.; Vugia, D.J.; Tobin-D'Angelo, M.; Hurd, S.; Medus, C.; Cronquist, A.; Angulo, F.J. Salmonellosis outcomes differ substantially by serotype. *J. Infect. Dis.* **2008**, *198*, 109–114. [CrossRef]
79. Rabsch, W.; Tschäpe, H.; Bäumler, A.J. Non-typhoidal salmonellosis: Emerging problems. *Microbes Infect.* **2001**, *3*, 237–247. [CrossRef]
80. Foley, S.L.; Nayak, R.; Hanning, I.B.; Johnson, T.J.; Han, J.; Ricke, S.C. Population dynamics of Salmonella enterica serotypes in commercial egg and poultry production. *Appl. Environ. Microbiol.* **2011**, *77*, 4273–4279. [CrossRef]
81. den Bakker, H.C.; Switt, A.I.M.; Govoni, G.; Cummings, C.A.; Ranieri, M.L.; Degoricija, L.; Hoelzer, K.; Rodriguez-Rivera, L.D.; Brown, S.; Bolchacova, E. Genome sequencing reveals diversification of virulence factor content and possible host adaptation in distinct subpopulations of Salmonella enterica. *BMC Genom.* **2011**, *12*, 425. [CrossRef]
82. Lo-Ten-Foe, J.; Van Oers, J.; Kotsopoulos, A.; Buiting, A. Pulmonary colonization with Salmonella enterica serovar Kentucky in an intensive care unit. *J. Hosp. Infect.* **2007**, *67*, 105–107. [CrossRef] [PubMed]
83. Neelambike, S.; Shivappa, S.G. A Fatal Case of Acute Gastroenteritis with Sepsis due to Salmonella enterica Serovar Kentucky in an Immunocompetent Patient: A Case Report. *J. Clin. Diagn. Res.* **2019**, *13*, 1–2. [CrossRef]
84. Collard, J.-M.; Place, S.; Denis, O.; Rodriguez-Villalobos, H.; Vrints, M.; Weill, F.-X.; Baucheron, S.; Cloeckaert, A.; Struelens, M.; Bertrand, S. Travel-acquired salmonellosis due to Salmonella Kentucky resistant to ciprofloxacin, ceftriaxone and co-trimoxazole and associated with treatment failure. *J. Antimicrob. Chemother.* **2007**, *60*, 190–192. [CrossRef] [PubMed]
85. Carramiñana, J.J.; Yangüela, J.; Blanco, D.; Rota, C.; Agustín, A.I.; Herrera, A. Potential virulence determinants of Salmonella serovars from poultry and human sources in Spain. *Vet. Microbiol.* **1997**, *54*, 375–383. [CrossRef]
86. Visca, P.; Filetici, E.; Anastasio, M.; Vetriani, C.; Fantasia, M.; Orsi, N. Siderophore production by Salmonella species isolated from different sources. *FEMS Microbiol. Lett.* **1991**, *79*, 225–232. [CrossRef]
87. Rabsch, W.; Reissbrodt, R. Investigations of Salmonella strains from different clinical-epidemiological origin with phenolate and hydroxamate (aerobactin)–siderophore bioassays. *J. Hyg. Epidemiol. Microbiol. Immunol.* **1988**, *32*, 353–360. [PubMed]
88. Baker, E.N.; Anderson, B.F.; Baker, H.M.; Day, C.L.; Haridas, M.; Norris, G.E.; Rumball, S.V.; Smith, C.A.; Thomas, D.H. Three-dimensional structure of lactoferrin in various functional states. *Adv. Exp. Med. Biol.* **1994**, *357*, 1–12. [CrossRef]
89. Kell, D.B.; Heyden, E.L.; Pretorius, E. The Biology of Lactoferrin, an Iron-Binding Protein That Can Help Defend Against Viruses and Bacteria. *Front. Immunol.* **2020**, *11*, 1221. [CrossRef]
90. Dho-Moulin, M.; Fairbrother, J.M. Avian pathogenic Escherichia coli (APEC). *Vet. Res. BioMed Central* **1999**, *30*, 299–316.
91. Dozois, C.M.; Daigle, F.; Curtiss, R. Identification of pathogen-specific and conserved genes expressed in vivo by an avian pathogenic Escherichia coli strain. *Proc. Natl. Acad. Sci. USA* **2003**, *100*, 247–252. [CrossRef] [PubMed]
92. Ling, J.; Pan, H.; Gao, Q.; Xiong, L.; Zhou, Y.; Zhang, D.; Gao, S.; Liu, X. Aerobactin synthesis genes iucA and iucC contribute to the pathogenicity of avian pathogenic Escherichia coli O2 strain E058. *PLoS ONE* **2013**, *8*, e57794. [CrossRef] [PubMed]

93. Russo, T.A.; Olson, R.; MacDonald, U.; Beanan, J.; Davidson, B.A. Aerobactin, but not yersiniabactin, salmochelin, or enterobactin, enables the growth/survival of hypervirulent (hypermucoviscous) Klebsiella pneumoniae ex vivo and in vivo. *Infect. Immun.* **2015**, *83*, 3325–3333. [CrossRef]
94. Nolan, L.K.; Horne, S.; Giddings, C.; Foley, S.; Johnson, T.; Lynne, A.; Skyberg, J. Resistance to serum complement, iss, and virulence of avian Escherichia coli. *Vet. Res. Commun.* **2003**, *27*, 101–110. [CrossRef] [PubMed]
95. Aviv, G.; Tsyba, K.; Steck, N.; Salmon-Divon, M.; Cornelius, A.; Rahav, G.; Grassl, G.A.; Gal-Mor, O. A unique megaplasmid contributes to stress tolerance and pathogenicity of an emergent S almonella enterica serovar Infantis strain. *Environ. Microbiol.* **2014**, *16*, 977–994. [CrossRef] [PubMed]
96. Chaturvedi, K.S.; Hung, C.S.; Giblin, D.E.; Urushidani, S.; Austin, A.M.; Dinauer, M.C.; Henderson, J.P. Cupric yersiniabactin is a virulence-associated superoxide dismutase mimic. *ACS Chem. Biol.* **2014**, *9*, 551–561. [CrossRef]
97. Chaturvedi, K.S.; Hung, C.S.; Crowley, J.R.; Stapleton, A.E.; Henderson, J.P. The siderophore yersiniabactin binds copper to protect pathogens during infection. *Nat. Chem. Biol.* **2012**, *8*, 731–736. [CrossRef]
98. Osman, D.; Waldron, K.J.; Denton, H.; Taylor, C.M.; Grant, A.J.; Mastroeni, P.; Robinson, N.J.; Cavet, J.S. Copper homeostasis in Salmonella is atypical and copper-CueP is a major periplasmic metal complex. *J. Biol. Chem.* **2010**, *285*, 25259–25268. [CrossRef]
99. Guerrero, M.L.F.; Aguado, J.M.; Arribas, A.; Lumbreras, C.; de Gorgolas, M. The spectrum of cardiovascular infections due to Salmonella enterica: A review of clinical features and factors determining outcome. *Medicine* **2004**, *83*, 123–138. [CrossRef]
100. Shimoni, Z.; Pitlik, S.; Leibovici, L.; Samra, Z.; Konigsberger, H.; Drucker, M.; Agmon, V.; Ashkenazi, S.; Weinberger, M. Nontyphoid Salmonella bacteremia: Age-related differences in clinical presentation, bacteriology, and outcome. *Clin. Infect. Dis.* **1999**, *28*, 822–827. [CrossRef]
101. Acheson, D.; Hohmann, E.L. Nontyphoidal salmonellosis. *Clin. Infect. Dis.* **2001**, *32*, 263–269. [CrossRef] [PubMed]
102. Hall, R.L.; Partridge, R.; Venkatraman, N.; Wiselka, M. Invasive non-typhoidal Salmonella infection with multifocal seeding in an immunocompetent host: An emerging disease in the developed world. *Case Rep.* **2013**, *2013*, bcr2012008230. [CrossRef] [PubMed]
103. Brnčić, N.; Gorup, L.; Strčić, M.; Abram, M.; Mustač, E. Breast abscess in a man due to Salmonella enterica serotype Enteritidis. *J. Clin. Microbiol.* **2012**, *50*, 192–193. [CrossRef]
104. Hibbert, B.; Costiniuk, C.; Hibbert, R.; Joseph, P.; Alanazi, H.; Simard, T.; Dennie, C.; Angel, J.B.; O'Brien, E.R. Cardiovascular complications of Salmonella enteritidis infection. *Can. J. Cardiol.* **2010**, *26*, e323–e325. [CrossRef]
105. Schloesser, R.L.; Schaefer, V.; Groll, A.H. Fatal transplacental infection with non-typhoidal Salmonella. *Scand. J. Infect. Dis.* **2004**, *36*, 773–774. [CrossRef] [PubMed]
106. Ispahani, P.; Slack, R. Enteric fever and other extraintestinal salmonellosis in University Hospital, Nottingham, UK, between 1980 and 1997. *Eur. J. Clin. Microbiol. Infect. Dis.* **2000**, *19*, 679–687. [CrossRef] [PubMed]
107. Huang, J.-L.; Hung, J.-J.; Wu, K.-C.; Lee, W.-I.; Chan, C.-K.; Ou, L.-S. Septic arthritis in patients with systemic lupus erythematosus: Salmonella and nonsalmonella infections compared. *Semin Arthritis Rheum.* **2006**, *36*, 61–67. [CrossRef] [PubMed]
108. Hakim, S.; Davila, F.; Amin, M.; Hader, I.; Cappell, M.S. Infectious aortitis: A life-threatening endovascular complication of nontyphoidal salmonella bacteremia. *Case Rep. Med.* **2018**, *2018*, 6845617. [CrossRef]
109. Laohapensang, K.; Rutherford, R.B.; Arworn, S. Infected aneurysm. *Ann. Vasc. Dis.* **2010**, *3*, 16–23. [CrossRef]
110. Wu, H.-M.; Huang, W.-Y.; Lee, M.-L.; Yang, A.D.; Chaou, K.-P.; Hsieh, L.-Y. Clinical features, acute complications, and outcome of Salmonella meningitis in children under one year of age in Taiwan. *BMC Infect. Dis.* **2011**, *11*, 30. [CrossRef]
111. Kaiser, P. Advances in avian immunology—prospects for disease control: A review. *Avian Pathol.* **2010**, *39*, 309–324. [CrossRef]
112. Davison, F. The importance of the avian immune system and its unique features. *Avian Immunol.* **2014**, 1–9. [CrossRef]
113. Agoro, R.; Mura, C. Iron Supplementation Therapy, A Friend and Foe of Mycobacterial Infections? *Pharmaceuticals* **2019**, *12*, 75. [CrossRef] [PubMed]

114. Penniall, R.; Spitznagel, J.K. Chicken neutrophils: Oxidative metabolism in phagocytic cells devoid of myeloperoxidase. *Proc. Natl. Acad. Sci. USA* **1975**, *72*, 5012–5015. [CrossRef] [PubMed]
115. Clench, M.H.; Mathias, J.R. The avian cecum: A review. *Wilson Bull.* **1995**, *107*, 93–121.
116. Foley, S.L.; Johnson, T.J.; Ricke, S.C.; Nayak, R.; Danzeisen, J. Salmonella pathogenicity and host adaptation in chicken-associated serovars. *Microbiol. Mol. Biol. Rev.* **2013**, *77*, 582–607. [CrossRef]
117. Gantois, I.; Eeckhaut, V.; Pasmans, F.; Haesebrouck, F.; Ducatelle, R.; Van Immerseel, F. A comparative study on the pathogenesis of egg contamination by different serotypes of Salmonella. *Avian Pathol.* **2008**, *37*, 399–406. [CrossRef]
118. Desmidt, M.; Ducatelle, R.; Haesebrouck, F. Pathogenesis of Salmonella enteritidis phage type four after experimental infection of young chickens. *Vet. Microbiol.* **1997**, *56*, 99–109. [CrossRef]
119. Johnston, C.E.; Hartley, C.; Salisbury, A.-M.; Wigley, P. Immunological changes at point-of-lay increase susceptibility to Salmonella enterica Serovar enteritidis infection in vaccinated chickens. *PLoS ONE* **2012**, *7*, e48195. [CrossRef]
120. Oladeinde, A.; Cook, K.; Orlek, A.; Zock, G.; Herrington, K.; Cox, N.; Plumblee Lawrence, J.; Hall, C. Hotspot mutations and ColE1 plasmids contribute to the fitness of Salmonella Heidelberg in poultry litter. *PLoS ONE* **2018**, *13*, e0202286. [CrossRef]
121. Wigley, P.; Hulme, S.; Rothwell, L.; Bumstead, N.; Kaiser, P.; Barrow, P. Macrophages isolated from chickens genetically resistant or susceptible to systemic salmonellosis show magnitudinal and temporal differential expression of cytokines and chemokines following Salmonella enterica challenge. *Infect. Immun.* **2006**, *74*, 1425–1430. [CrossRef] [PubMed]
122. Andino, A.; Hanning, I. Salmonella enterica: Survival, colonization, and virulence differences among serovars. *Sci. World J.* **2015**, *2015*, 520179. [CrossRef]
123. Harvey, P.; Watson, M.; Hulme, S.; Jones, M.; Lovell, M.; Berchieri, A.; Young, J.; Bumstead, N.; Barrow, P. Salmonella enterica serovar typhimurium colonizing the lumen of the chicken intestine grows slowly and upregulates a unique set of virulence and metabolism genes. *Infect. Immun.* **2011**, *79*, 4105–4121. [CrossRef] [PubMed]
124. Sabri, M.; Caza, M.; Proulx, J.; Lymberopoulos, M.H.; Brée, A.; Moulin-Schouleur, M.; Curtiss, R.; Dozois, C.M. Contribution of the SitABCD, MntH, and FeoB metal transporters to the virulence of avian pathogenic Escherichia coli O78 strain χ7122. *Infect. Immun.* **2008**, *76*, 601–611. [CrossRef] [PubMed]
125. Boyer, E.; Bergevin, I.; Malo, D.; Gros, P.; Cellier, M. Acquisition of Mn (II) in addition to Fe (II) is required for full virulence of Salmonella enterica serovar Typhimurium. *Infect. Immun.* **2002**, *70*, 6032–6042. [CrossRef] [PubMed]
126. Portillo, F.G.d.; Foster, J.W.; Maguire, M.E.; Finlay, B.B. Characterization of the micro-environment of Salmonella typhimurium–containing vacuoles within MDCK epithelial cells. *Mol. Microbiol.* **1992**, *6*, 3289–3297. [CrossRef]
127. Tsolis, R.M.; Bäumler, A.J.; Heffron, F.; Stojiljkovic, I. Contribution of TonB-and Feo-mediated iron uptake to growth of Salmonella typhimurium in the mouse. *Infect. Immun.* **1996**, *64*, 4549–4556. [CrossRef] [PubMed]
128. Costa, L.F.; Mol, J.P.; Silva, A.P.C.; Macêdo, A.A.; Silva, T.M.; Alves, G.E.; Winter, S.; Winter, M.G.; Velazquez, E.M.; Byndloss, M.X. Iron acquisition pathways and colonization of the inflamed intestine by Salmonella enterica serovar Typhimurium. *Int. J. Med Microbiol.* **2016**, *306*, 604–610. [CrossRef]
129. Liu, W.; Kaiser, M.; Lamont, S. Natural resistance-associated macrophage protein 1 gene polymorphisms and response to vaccine against or challenge with Salmonella enteritidis in young chicks. *Poult. Sci.* **2003**, *82*, 259–266. [CrossRef]
130. Forbes, J.R.; Gros, P. Divalent-metal transport by NRAMP proteins at the interface of host–pathogen interactions. *Trends Microbiol.* **2001**, *9*, 397–403. [CrossRef]
131. Hu, J.; Bumstead, N.; Barrow, P.; Sebastiani, G.; Olien, L.; Morgan, K.; Malo, D. Resistance to salmonellosis in the chicken is linked to NRAMP1 and TNC. *Genome Res.* **1997**, *7*, 693–704. [CrossRef] [PubMed]
132. Nagy, T.A.; Moreland, S.M.; Detweiler, C.S. S almonella acquires ferrous iron from haemophagocytic macrophages. *Mol. Microbiol.* **2014**, *93*, 1314–1326.
133. Pilonieta, M.C.; Moreland, S.M.; English, C.N.; Detweiler, C.S. Salmonella enterica infection stimulates macrophages to hemophagocytose. *mBio* **2014**, *5*, e02211-14. [CrossRef] [PubMed]
134. Nix, R.N.; Altschuler, S.E.; Henson, P.M.; Detweiler, C.S. Hemophagocytic macrophages harbor Salmonella enterica during persistent infection. *PLoS Pathog* **2007**, *3*, e193. [CrossRef]

135. Sánchez-Moreno, P.; Olbrich, P.; Falcón-Neyra, L.; Lucena, J.M.; Aznar, J.; Neth, O. Typhoid fever causing haemophagocytic lymphohistiocytosis in a non-endemic country–first case report and review of the current literature. *Enferm. Infecc. Microbiol. Clin.* **2019**, *37*, 112–116. [CrossRef] [PubMed]
136. Williams, P.; Rabsch, W.; Methner, U.; Voigt, W.; Tschäpe, H.; Reissbrodt, R. Catecholate receptor proteins in Salmonella enterica: Role in virulence and implications for vaccine development. *Vaccine* **2006**, *24*, 3840–3844. [CrossRef]
137. Wellman-Labadie, O.; Picman, J.; Hincke, M. Comparative antibacterial activity of avian egg white protein extracts. *Br. Poult. Sci.* **2008**, *49*, 125–132. [CrossRef]
138. Baron, F.; Gautier, M.; Brule, G. Factors involved in the inhibition of growth of Salmonella enteritidis in liquid egg white. *J. Food Prot.* **1997**, *60*, 1318–1323. [CrossRef]
139. Kang, H.; Loui, C.; Clavijo, R.; Riley, L.; Lu, S. Survival characteristics of Salmonella enterica serovar Enteritidis in chicken egg albumen. *Epidemiol. Infect.* **2006**, *134*, 967–976. [CrossRef]
140. Réhault-Godbert, S.; Guyot, N.; Nys, Y. The golden egg: Nutritional value, bioactivities, and emerging benefits for human health. *Nutrients* **2019**, *11*, 684. [CrossRef]
141. Qin, X.; He, S.; Zhou, X.; Cheng, X.; Huang, X.; Wang, Y.; Wang, S.; Cui, Y.; Shi, C.; Shi, X. Quantitative proteomics reveals the crucial role of YbgC for Salmonella enterica serovar Enteritidis survival in egg white. *Int. J. Food Microbiol.* **2019**, *289*, 115–126. [CrossRef] [PubMed]
142. Julien, L.A.; Baron, F.; Bonnassie, S.; Nau, F.; Guérin, C.; Jan, S.; Andrews, S.C. The anti-bacterial iron-restriction defence mechanisms of egg white; the potential role of three lipocalin-like proteins in resistance against Salmonella. *BioMetals* **2019**, *32*, 453–467. [CrossRef] [PubMed]
143. Sattar Khan, M.; Nakamura, S.; Ogawa, M.; Akita, E.; Azakami, H.; Kato, A. Bactericidal action of egg yolk phosvitin against Escherichia coli under thermal stress. *J. Agric. Food Chem.* **2000**, *48*, 1503–1506. [CrossRef] [PubMed]
144. Van Immerseel, F. Stress-induced survival strategies enable Salmonella Enteritidis to persistently colonize the chicken oviduct tissue and cope with antimicrobial factors in egg white: A hypothesis to explain a pandemic. *Gut Pathog.* **2010**, *2*, 23. [CrossRef]
145. Raspoet, R.; Appia-Ayme, C.; Shearer, N.; Martel, A.; Pasmans, F.; Haesebrouck, F.; Ducatelle, R.; Thompson, A.; Van Immerseel, F. Microarray-based detection of Salmonella enterica serovar Enteritidis genes involved in chicken reproductive tract colonization. *Appl. Environ. Microbiol.* **2014**, *80*, 7710–7716. [CrossRef]
146. Gantois, I.; Ducatelle, R.; Pasmans, F.; Haesebrouck, F.; Van Immerseel, F. Salmonella enterica serovar Enteritidis genes induced during oviduct colonization and egg contamination in laying hens. *Appl. Environ. Microbiol.* **2008**, *74*, 6616–6622. [CrossRef]
147. Luo, M.; Lin, H.; Fischbach, M.A.; Liu, D.R.; Walsh, C.T.; Groves, J.T. Enzymatic tailoring of enterobactin alters membrane partitioning and iron acquisition. *ACS Chem. Biol.* **2006**, *1*, 29–32. [CrossRef]
148. Moore, D.G.; Yancey, R.; Lankford, C.; Earhart, C. Bacteriostatic enterochelin-specific immunoglobulin from normal human serum. *Infect. Immun.* **1980**, *27*, 418–423. [CrossRef]
149. Benjamin, W.; Turnbough, C.; Posey, B.; Briles, D. The ability of Salmonella typhimurium to produce the siderophore enterobactin is not a virulence factor in mouse typhoid. *Infect. Immun.* **1985**, *50*, 392–397. [CrossRef]
150. Yancey, R.J.; Breeding, S.; Lankford, C. Enterochelin (enterobactin): Virulence factor for Salmonella typhimurium. *Infect. Immun.* **1979**, *24*, 174–180. [CrossRef]
151. Nagy, T.A.; Moreland, S.M.; Andrews-Polymenis, H.; Detweiler, C.S. The ferric enterobactin transporter Fep is required for persistent Salmonella enterica serovar typhimurium infection. *Infect. Immun.* **2013**, *81*, 4063–4070. [CrossRef]
152. Crouch, M.L.V.; Castor, M.; Karlinsey, J.E.; Kalhorn, T.; Fang, F.C. Biosynthesis and IroC-dependent export of the siderophore salmochelin are essential for virulence of Salmonella enterica serovar Typhimurium. *Mol. Microbiol.* **2008**, *67*, 971–983. [CrossRef] [PubMed]
153. Oshota, O.; Conway, M.; Fookes, M.; Schreiber, F.; Chaudhuri, R.R.; Yu, L.; Morgan, F.J.; Clare, S.; Choudhary, J.; Thomson, N.R. Transcriptome and proteome analysis of Salmonella enterica serovar Typhimurium systemic infection of wild type and immune-deficient mice. *PLoS ONE* **2017**, *12*, e0181365. [CrossRef] [PubMed]
154. Raffatellu, M.; George, M.D.; Akiyama, Y.; Hornsby, M.J.; Nuccio, S.-P.; Paixao, T.A.; Butler, B.P.; Chu, H.; Santos, R.L.; Berger, T. Lipocalin-2 resistance confers an advantage to Salmonella enterica serotype Typhimurium for growth and survival in the inflamed intestine. *Cell Host Microbe* **2009**, *5*, 476–486. [CrossRef] [PubMed]

155. Anderson, G.J.; Frazer, D.M. Current understanding of iron homeostasis. *Am. J. Clin. Nutr.* **2017**, *106*, 1559S–1566S. [CrossRef] [PubMed]
156. Konopka, K.; Bindereif, A.; Neilands, J. Aerobactin-mediated utilization of transferrin iron. *Biochemistry* **1982**, *21*, 6503–6508. [CrossRef]
157. Montgomerie, J.; Bindereif, A.; Neilands, J.; Kalmanson, G.; Guze, L. Association of hydroxamate siderophore (aerobactin) with Escherichia coli isolated from patients with bacteremia. *Infect. Immun.* **1984**, *46*, 835–838. [CrossRef]
158. Correnti, C.; Clifton, M.C.; Abergel, R.J.; Allred, B.; Hoette, T.M.; Ruiz, M.; Cancedda, R.; Raymond, K.N.; Descalzi, F.; Strong, R.K. Galline Ex-FABP is an antibacterial siderocalin and a lysophosphatidic acid sensor functioning through dual ligand specificities. *Structure* **2011**, *19*, 1796–1806. [CrossRef]
159. Matulova, M.; Varmuzova, K.; Sisak, F.; Havlickova, H.; Babak, V.; Stejskal, K.; Zdrahal, Z.; Rychlik, I. Chicken innate immune response to oral infection with Salmonella enterica serovar Enteritidis. *Vet. Res.* **2013**, *44*, 37. [CrossRef]
160. Rychlik, I.; Elsheimer-Matulova, M.; Kyrova, K. Gene expression in the chicken caecum in response to infections with non-typhoid Salmonella. *Vet. Res.* **2014**, *45*, 119. [CrossRef]
161. Withanage, G.; Wigley, P.; Kaiser, P.; Mastroeni, P.; Brooks, H.; Powers, C.; Beal, R.; Barrow, P.; Maskell, D.; McConnell, I. Cytokine and chemokine responses associated with clearance of a primary Salmonella enterica serovar Typhimurium infection in the chicken and in protective immunity to rechallenge. *Infect. Immun.* **2005**, *73*, 5173–5182. [CrossRef] [PubMed]
162. Setta, A.; Barrow, P.; Kaiser, P.; Jones, M. Early immune dynamics following infection with Salmonella enterica serovars Enteritidis, Infantis, Pullorum and Gallinarum: Cytokine and chemokine gene expression profile and cellular changes of chicken cecal tonsils. *Comp. Immunol. Microbiol. Infect. Dis.* **2012**, *35*, 397–410. [CrossRef] [PubMed]
163. Weinberg, E.D. Nutritional immunity: Host's attempt to withhold iron from microbial invaders. *JAMA* **1975**, *231*, 39–41. [CrossRef] [PubMed]
164. Julien, L.A.; Fau, C.; Baron, F.; Bonnassie, S.; Guérin-Dubiard, C.; Nau, F.; Gautier, M.; Karatzas, K.A.; Jan, S.; Andrews, S.C. The three lipocalins of egg-white: Only Ex-FABP inhibits siderophore-dependent iron sequestration by Salmonella Enteritidis. *Front. Microbiol.* **2020**, *11*, 913. [CrossRef]
165. Giansanti, F.; Leboffe, L.; Pitari, G.; Ippoliti, R.; Antonini, G. Physiological roles of ovotransferrin. *Biochim. Biophys. Acta Gen. Subj.* **2012**, *1820*, 218–225. [CrossRef]
166. Hegenauer, J.; Saltman, P.; Nace, G. Iron (III)-phosphoprotein chelates: Stoichiometric equilibrium constant for interaction of iron (III) and phosphorylserine residues of phosvitin and casein. *Biochemistry* **1979**, *18*, 3865–3879. [CrossRef]
167. Denic, S.; Agarwal, M.M. Nutritional iron deficiency: An evolutionary perspective. *Nutrition* **2007**, *23*, 603–614. [CrossRef]
168. Muckenthaler, M.U.; Rivella, S.; Hentze, M.W.; Galy, B. A red carpet for iron metabolism. *Cell* **2017**, *168*, 344–361. [CrossRef]
169. Drakesmith, H.; Prentice, A.M. Hepcidin and the iron-infection axis. *Science* **2012**, *338*, 768–772. [CrossRef]
170. Hilton, K.B.; Lambert, L.A. Molecular evolution and characterization of hepcidin gene products in vertebrates. *Gene* **2008**, *415*, 40–48. [CrossRef]
171. Wessling-Resnick, M. Iron homeostasis and the inflammatory response. *Ann. Rev. Nutr.* **2010**, *30*, 105–122. [CrossRef] [PubMed]
172. Ganz, T. Hepcidin—a regulator of intestinal iron absorption and iron recycling by macrophages. *Best Pract. Res. Clin. Haematol.* **2005**, *18*, 171–182. [CrossRef] [PubMed]
173. Moreira, A.C.; Neves, J.V.; Silva, T.; Oliveira, P.; Gomes, M.S.; Rodrigues, P.N. Hepcidin-(in) dependent mechanisms of iron metabolism regulation during infection by Listeria and Salmonella. *Infect. Immun.* **2017**, *85*, e00353-17. [CrossRef] [PubMed]
174. Kim, D.-K.; Jeong, J.-H.; Lee, J.-M.; Kim, K.S.; Park, S.-H.; Kim, Y.D.; Koh, M.; Shin, M.; Jung, Y.S.; Kim, H.-S. Inverse agonist of estrogen-related receptor γ controls Salmonella typhimurium infection by modulating host iron homeostasis. *Nat. Med.* **2014**, *20*, 419–424. [CrossRef]
175. Willemetz, A.; Beatty, S.; Richer, E.; Rubio, A.; Auriac, A.; Milkereit, R.J.; Thibaudeau, O.; Vaulont, S.; Malo, D.; Canonne-Hergaux, F. Iron-and hepcidin-independent downregulation of the iron exporter ferroportin in macrophages during Salmonella infection. *Front. Immunol.* **2017**, *8*, 498. [CrossRef]

176. Hill, R.; Smith, I.; Mohammadi, H.; Licence, S. Altered absorption and regulation of iron in chicks with acute Salmonella gallinarum infection. *Res. Vet. Sci.* **1977**, *22*, 371–375. [CrossRef]
177. Ganz, T. Anemia of inflammation. *N. Engl. J. Med.* **2019**, *381*, 1148–1157. [CrossRef]
178. Canals, R.; Hammarlöf, D.L.; Kröger, C.; Owen, S.V.; Fong, W.Y.; Lacharme-Lora, L.; Zhu, X.; Wenner, N.; Carden, S.E.; Honeycutt, J. Adding function to the genome of African Salmonella Typhimurium ST313 strain D23580. *PLoS Biol.* **2019**, *17*, e3000059. [CrossRef]
179. Lokken, K.L.; Stull-Lane, A.R.; Poels, K.; Tsolis, R.M. Malaria parasite-mediated alteration of macrophage function and increased iron availability predispose to disseminated nontyphoidal Salmonella infection. *Infect. Immun.* **2018**, *86*, e00301-18. [CrossRef]
180. Allan, B.; Wheler, C.; Köster, W.; Sarfraz, M.; Potter, A.; Gerdts, V.; Dar, A. In Ovo Administration of Innate Immune Stimulants and Protection from Early Chick Mortalities due to Yolk Sac Infection. *Avian Dis.* **2018**, *62*, 316–321. [CrossRef]
181. Johnstone, T.C.; Nolan, E.M. Beyond iron: Non-classical biological functions of bacterial siderophores. *Dalton Trans.* **2015**, *44*, 6320–6339. [CrossRef] [PubMed]
182. Adler, C.; Corbalán, N.S.; Seyedsayamdost, M.R.; Pomares, M.F.; de Cristóbal, R.E.; Clardy, J.; Kolter, R.; Vincent, P.A. Catecholate siderophores protect bacteria from pyochelin toxicity. *PLoS ONE* **2012**, *7*, e46754. [CrossRef] [PubMed]
183. Adler, C.; Corbalan, N.S.; Peralta, D.R.; Pomares, M.F.; de Cristóbal, R.E.; Vincent, P.A. The alternative role of enterobactin as an oxidative stress protector allows Escherichia coli colony development. *PLoS ONE* **2014**, *9*, e84734. [CrossRef] [PubMed]
184. Singh, V.; San Yeoh, B.; Xiao, X.; Kumar, M.; Bachman, M.; Borregaard, N.; Joe, B.; Vijay-Kumar, M. Interplay between enterobactin, myeloperoxidase and lipocalin 2 regulates E. coli survival in the inflamed gut. *Nat. Commun.* **2015**, *6*, 1–11. [CrossRef] [PubMed]
185. Peralta, D.R.; Adler, C.; Corbalán, N.S.; Paz García, E.C.; Pomares, M.F.; Vincent, P.A. Enterobactin as part of the oxidative stress response repertoire. *PLoS ONE* **2016**, *11*, e0157799. [CrossRef]
186. Vazquez-Torres, A.; Jones-Carson, J.; Mastroeni, P.; Ischiropoulos, H.; Fang, F.C. Antimicrobial actions of the NADPH phagocyte oxidase and inducible nitric oxide synthase in experimental salmonellosis. I. Effects on microbial killing by activated peritoneal macrophages in vitro. *J. Exp. Med.* **2000**, *192*, 227–236. [CrossRef]
187. Stabler, J.; McCormick, T.; Powell, K.; Kogut, M. Avian heterophils and monocytes: Phagocytic and bactericidal activities against Salmonella enteritidis. *Vet. Microbiol.* **1994**, *38*, 293–305. [CrossRef]
188. Brooks, R.; Bounous, D.; Andreasen, C. Functional comparison of avian heterophils with human and canine neutrophils. *Comp. Haematol. Int.* **1996**, *6*, 153–159. [CrossRef]
189. Wigley, P.; Hulme, S.D.; Bumstead, N.; Barrow, P.A. In vivo and in vitro studies of genetic resistance to systemic salmonellosis in the chicken encoded by the SAL1 locus. *Microbes Infect.* **2002**, *4*, 1111–1120. [CrossRef]
190. Holden, V.I.; Breen, P.; Houle, S.; Dozois, C.M.; Bachman, M.A. Klebsiella pneumoniae siderophores induce inflammation, bacterial dissemination, and HIF-1α stabilization during pneumonia. *MBio* **2016**, *7*, e01397-16. [CrossRef]
191. Holden, V.I.; Lenio, S.; Kuick, R.; Ramakrishnan, S.K.; Shah, Y.M.; Bachman, M.A. Bacterial siderophores that evade or overwhelm lipocalin 2 induce hypoxia inducible factor 1α and proinflammatory cytokine secretion in cultured respiratory epithelial cells. *Infect. Immun.* **2014**, *82*, 3826–3836. [CrossRef] [PubMed]
192. Saha, P.; Xiao, X.; Yeoh, B.S.; Chen, Q.; Katkere, B.; Kirimanjeswara, G.S.; Vijay-Kumar, M. The bacterial siderophore enterobactin confers survival advantage to Salmonella in macrophages. *Gut Microbes* **2019**, *10*, 412–423. [CrossRef] [PubMed]
193. Lathrop, S.K.; Binder, K.A.; Starr, T.; Cooper, K.G.; Chong, A.; Carmody, A.B.; Steele-Mortimer, O. Replication of Salmonella enterica serovar Typhimurium in human monocyte-derived macrophages. *Infect. Immun.* **2015**, *83*, 2661–2671. [CrossRef] [PubMed]
194. Benoit, M.; Desnues, B.; Mege, J.-L. Macrophage polarization in bacterial infections. *J. Immunol.* **2008**, *181*, 3733–3739. [CrossRef]
195. Galván-Peña, S.; O'Neill, L.A. Metabolic reprograming in macrophage polarization. *Front. Immunol.* **2014**, *5*, 420.

12

Spheres of Influence: Insights into *Salmonella* Pathogenesis from Intestinal Organoids

Smriti Verma [1,2,*], Stefania Senger [1,2], Bobby J. Cherayil [1,2] and Christina S. Faherty [1,2]

[1] Mucosal Immunology and Biology Research Center, Division of Pediatric Gastroenterology and Nutrition, Massachusetts General Hospital, Charlestown Navy Yard, Boston, 02129 MA, USA; ssenger@mgh.harvard.edu (S.S.); cherayil@helix.mgh.harvard.edu (B.J.C.); csfaherty@mgh.harvard.edu (C.S.F.)

[2] Harvard Medical School, Boston, 02115 MA, USA

[*] Correspondence: sverma5@mgh.harvard.edu

Abstract: The molecular complexity of host-pathogen interactions remains poorly understood in many infectious diseases, particularly in humans due to the limited availability of reliable and specific experimental models. To bridge the gap between classical two-dimensional culture systems, which often involve transformed cell lines that may not have all the physiologic properties of primary cells, and in vivo animal studies, researchers have developed the organoid model system. Organoids are complex three-dimensional structures that are generated in vitro from primary cells and can recapitulate key in vivo properties of an organ such as structural organization, multicellularity, and function. In this review, we discuss how organoids have been deployed in exploring *Salmonella* infection in mice and humans. In addition, we summarize the recent advancements that hold promise to elevate our understanding of the interactions and crosstalk between multiple cell types and the microbiota with *Salmonella*. These models have the potential for improving clinical outcomes and future prophylactic and therapeutic intervention strategies.

Keywords: organoids; enteroids; *Salmonella*; host-pathogen interactions; model systems; infectious diseases; organotypic culture system

---

1. Introduction

Many basic life processes are conserved in all organisms, with similarities in molecular mechanisms often increasing as the phylogenetic distances decrease. This conservation enables investigation into various biological mechanisms and diseases, with the expectation that the knowledge gained from one system will provide insight into the workings of related organisms. The similarity between different organisms is particularly important for studying human biology and diseases, since human experimentation is typically unfeasible or unethical. However, several factors must be considered before employing an organism or derived cells as a model for humans, including ease of maintenance and reproducibility, amenability to genetic and molecular manipulations, and perhaps most importantly, similarity to the characteristics of the human biological process under investigation.

The mainstays of research for many decades have been the cell culture and animal model systems. Classically, the in vitro cell culture methodology involves either growing cell lines that are derived from tumors or are genetically transformed to allow continuous propagation, or culturing primary cells derived from the tissues of humans or experimental animals. Use of cell lines has a significant limitation in that the cells do not recapitulate "normal" cellular physiology. Primary cells closely represent the tissue of origin but are limited in availability, have a finite life-span in vitro without being transformed, and display variability arising from differences in donors. Conventional cell culture comprises growing cells (cell lines/primary cells) either in liquid suspension or as adherent, two dimensional (2D) monolayers on an impermeable solid surface. The cell culture model is also a reductionist approach since the model cannot account for dynamic and complex interactions that occur in vivo, particularly those that result from the interactions with multiple cell types. Although processes such as immune responses, cell signaling, or crosstalk with microbiota have been studied using cell culture models of various cell types either alone or in combination, the biggest disadvantage of this system is that the cells may not fully recapitulate in vivo phenotypes and behaviors. More complex model systems, such as *Caenorhabditis elegans*, *Danio rerio*, *Drosophila melanogaster*, mice, or primates provide a whole organism perspective and allow compensation for some of the limitations of cultured cells as the complexity of the models increase. However, these animal models resemble, but do not completely represent, all the conditions encountered in humans, an issue that is especially important in the understanding of disease and development [1]. Recently, many researchers have developed sophisticated, yet tractable, non-cancerous tissue culture models that bridge the gap between simple 2D cell culture and complex in vivo experiments. Such models are broadly known as organotypic culture systems, which can be composed of various types as detailed below. In general, these models consist of a three-dimensional (3D) organ-like structure that is made up of organ-specific differentiated cells of multiple lineages and that recapitulates the unique organizational and functional characteristics of the corresponding organ in vivo.

Historically, the term "organoid" referred to short-term in vitro cultures of tissues such as lung and intestine [2], or 3D cell aggregates such as spheroids. More recently, it has been applied to organized 3D structures generated in vitro from cells with a whole range of origins, such as tissue segments [3,4] and their derived adult stem cells (ASCs) [5,6], transformed cell lines [7], and pluripotent stem cells (PSCs) [8]. However, as research has progressed, the term "organoid" has taken on a more restricted meaning. Organoids have the following characteristics: (1) self-organization: individual cells arrange in vitro into a 3D structure that mimics the in vivo organ or tissue, (2) multicellularity: organoids are composed of multiple cell types typically found in the organ or tissue in equivalent proportions, 3) functionality: the organoid structure should be able to execute at least some of the organ- or tissue-specific functions, and 4) sustainability: organoids can propagate indefinitely without requiring transformation by maintaining a pool of progenitor cells. In 2012, the International Stem Cell Consortium [9] set guidelines for the nomenclature to be used to define the 3D structures generated in vitro depending on their origin and cellular composition. When referring to intestinal organotypic models, 3D structures that are composed of just epithelial cell types are generally known as "enteroids" if derived from the small intestinal epithelium, or "colonoids" if derived from colonic origin. The term "organoid" is usually reserved for 3D structures containing more than one cell lineage. However, it should be noted that these guidelines have not been uniformly adopted by the field. Many researchers commonly use "organoids" as a blanket term for 3D structures derived from ASCs, PSCs, or comprising transformed cell lines that resemble in vivo 3D architecture and physiology.

Methodologies have been adapted to develop organoids from various normal and cancerous mouse and human tissues including colon [6,10], stomach [11], liver [12–14], pancreas [15], and kidney [16] to name a few. These techniques have been well reviewed elsewhere [11,17–21]. For the purposes of this review, we will provide a historical context and examples of the different types of intestinal organoid models (Figure 1), followed by a discussion of the application of the models to the study of *Salmonella* pathogenesis.

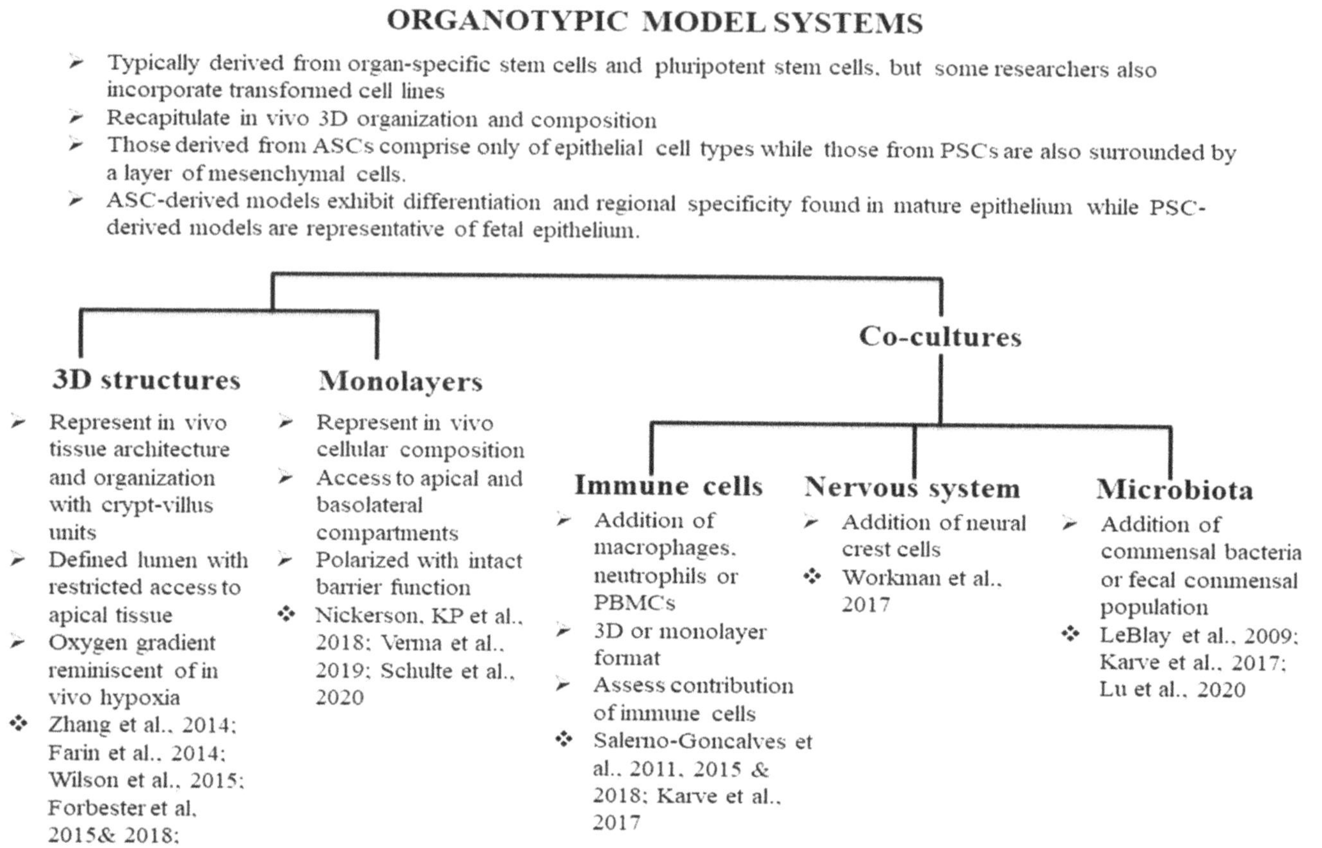

Figure 1. Use of organotypic models in *Salmonella* biology. We highlight studies that have utilized organotypic models to better understand *Salmonella* biology, as well as studies that do not directly pertain to *Salmonella* research but have the potential to be deployed for better understanding of the dynamics of host-*Salmonella* interactions.

2. Historical Background

The organoid model systems have been established on the basis of several studies that have contributed to various aspects of the technology [22]. One key advance was the development of cell culture methods that permitted cells to form 3D structures. Many of the non-physiological properties of cells in the conventional 2D cell cultures are believed to be due to the loss of 3D geometry [23]. Several techniques have been developed to deal with this problem, such as the hanging drop method [24], 3D micro-molds [25], and rotating wall vessel (RWV) bioreactors [26], a more advanced method that permits larger-scale production of 3D assemblies. Nickerson, CA et al. (2001) [26] utilized a RWV bioreactor developed by NASA that generates low shear and microgravity, allowing cells to remain in suspension to aggregate and grow three dimensionally. The authors were able to establish a 3D culture of Int-407 cells (derived from a normal fetal intestine but later shown to have HeLa cell contamination), thereby promoting cellular differentiation. The resulting 3D aggregates modeled human in vivo differentiation with well-defined cell-to-cell borders, tight junctions, apical-to-basal polarity, and microvilli development. These features were not present when the Int-407 cells were grown as conventional monolayer cultures. Thus, the study helped to demonstrate that 3D organization provides important physical and mechanical cues that facilitate organogenesis. A 3D platform is generally achieved by using matrices such as Matrigel, which consist of proteins typically found in the extracellular matrix (ECM). The ECM is the non-cellular component present within all tissues and organs, and consists mostly of collagen, enzymes, and glycoproteins to provide both structural and biochemical support to surrounding cells. ECMs have been shown to promote the maintenance of structural and functional characteristics of the tissue of origin [27]. The other major events that propelled the development of organoids were advancements in the understanding of stem cell properties and developmental biology of the intestine. The defining characteristics of stem cells—i.e., the capacity for clonal expansion and the ability to differentiate into daughter cells of multiple lineages—have been vital for the development of organoid technology. In fact, with the right cues daughter cells differentiate into multiple cell types and undergo two processes (1) cell sorting out—the formation of discrete domains by different cell types, and (2) spatially restricted lineage commitment, the specialization of function of a cell based on its position in the tissue architecture [28]. These processes result in complex 3D, self-propagating, multicellular, and functional structures [29]. The improved understanding of intestinal development helped define some of these cues. Studies have shown that different molecular gradients converge to create the micro-environment that shapes the intestinal epithelium. Epidermal growth factor (EGF) and Wingless-related integration site protein (Wnt) are highly active in the crypt and are necessary for proliferation, while bone morphogenetic protein (BMP) and Notch signaling pathways active in the villus control cell fate programming [30–32].

Another milestone in the field came in 2007 when Barker and colleagues [33] demonstrated in adult mice that intestinal crypt stem cells, which are responsible for proliferation and migration of the epithelial layer towards the villus tip, express the marker leucine-rich repeat containing G-protein coupled receptor 5 (Lgr5) [33]. Shortly thereafter, Ootani et al. [34] developed a long-term culture of primary mouse intestines using air-liquid interface methodology [34]. Fragments of neonatal mouse intestines containing epithelial and mesenchymal cells were cultured to generate cyst-like structures containing all major cell types found in an adult mouse intestine, including $Lgr5^+$ stem cells that the authors demonstrated could be modulated by Wnt signaling [34]. The next critical step occurred in 2009, when Sato and colleagues [5] realized the power of these organ-specific stem cells in 3D cultures by isolating intestinal crypts from adult mice. The authors demonstrated that a single $Lgr5^+$ cell could form 3D crypt-villus epithelial structures in the presence of appropriate cues, including an environmental signal from a lamin-rich 3D matrix (Matrigel) and a physiological signal in the form of growth factors (the Wnt agonist R-spondin1, EGF, and the BMP-inhibitor Noggin) [5]. The model recapitulated the physiology and organization of the mouse intestine; and when transplanted into mice, successfully reconstituted crypt-villus units [35,36]. Thus, the adult stem cells (ASCs) develop self-organized structures that consist of various types of intestinal epithelial cells. The authors referred to these structures as "organoids"; however, according to the guidelines set by the International Stem Cell Consortium [9], the model should be called "enteroids" since it was derived from the small intestinal epithelial cells.

Regardless of the definition, this work laid the groundwork for the utilization of pluripotent stem cells (PSCs), either derived from embryonic tissue or generated by inducing stemness in mature somatic cells (iPSCs) [37–40]. The latter offer the additional advantages that invasive procedures to isolate intestinal or colonic biopsies are not necessary and also iPSCs bypass ethical concerns regarding procurement of embryonic stem cells. The PSC-derived structures consist of epithelial cells surrounded by mesenchymal stromal cells and are referred to as "organoids". During embryonic development, the mesenchyme induces and specifies epithelial identity and differentiation, and is critical for the maintenance of tissue identity [41,42]. However, for interrogation of epithelial cell-specific functions, the mesenchymal cells may serve as a hindrance. Mithal and colleagues [43] have recently identified a directed differentiation protocol that generates mesenchyme-free human intestinal organoids (HIOs), which were employed to measure cystic fibrosis transmembrane conductance regulator (CFTR) gene function using cystic fibrosis patient-derived iPSC lines. The epithelial cells of organoids are not fully mature and resemble fetal epithelial cells when transcriptionally profiled [44]. The maturation of these organoids requires implantation in vivo, such as on the kidney capsule of immunocompromised mice [8,39,44,45]. The fetal-like nature of PSC-derived organoids presents an advantage as it allows for studies that would otherwise be difficult to conduct given the limited availability and ethical concerns surrounding the use of human fetal tissues. PSC-derived organoids follow a differentiation path observed during development [46] and take one to two months to develop, while tissue-specific ASCs develop organoids by a process that recapitulates tissue repair and is complete within weeks [20].

The epithelial cells derived from ASC (enteroids) represent adult-like mature epithelium. The cells of the enteroids also preserve characteristics of the tissue of origin including a diseased phenotype if derived from patients bearing an intestinal condition. These characteristics make enteroids from ASC a faithful model for intestinal diseases [47–49].

3. Intestinal Organoids/Enteroids

Intestinal enteroids derived from the intestinal stem cells develop multi-lobed structures (Figure 2) consisting of crypt-villus units, with a clearly defined proliferative, crypt-like zone and a large, non-proliferative differentiated zone surrounding proliferative areas [50]. To generate organoids, the pluripotent stem cells are first programmed towards endoderm development to form the epithelial tube that eventually gives rise to the foregut, midgut, and hindgut in response to a combination of anteriorizing and posteriorizing growth factors provided. Additional mesenchymal cells are also present and consist of myofibroblasts and smooth muscle cells surrounding the epithelial cells, presumably derived from remnant cells of mesodermal lineage after endoderm induction [20,51]. The epithelial cells reach homeostasis with a proliferative rate matching the rate of shedding of the cells at the edge of the monolayer. All major epithelial cell types are generated, including goblet cells, enteroendocrine cells, Paneth cells, antigen-sampling microfold cells (M cells), and columnar enterocytes that have a brush border of apical microvilli. The cells of the intestinal enteoroids are suitably polarized, and produce and secrete mucus from the apical surface. The cellular composition of the organoids/enteroids can be varied depending on the factors that are supplemented during the process of growth and differentiation [34]. Cell types not previously generated or maintained in traditional cell culture have been produced and/or characterized in organoids/enteroids, including the enteroendocrine cells and M cells [52,53]. In 2017, Haber and colleagues [54] profiled epithelial cells from both the mouse small intestine and crypt-derived enteroids generated from the mouse small intestine, with the aim of identifying novel subtypes and defining genetic signatures. As M cells are a scarce cell type comprising only 10% of the rare follicle associated epithelium, the authors did not detect M cells in the transcriptomes profiled from the mouse small intestines. However, small intestine-derived enteroids treated with growth factor Receptor Activator of Nuclear factor Kappa-B Ligand (RANKL) to generate M cells, displayed M cell specific signatures [54].

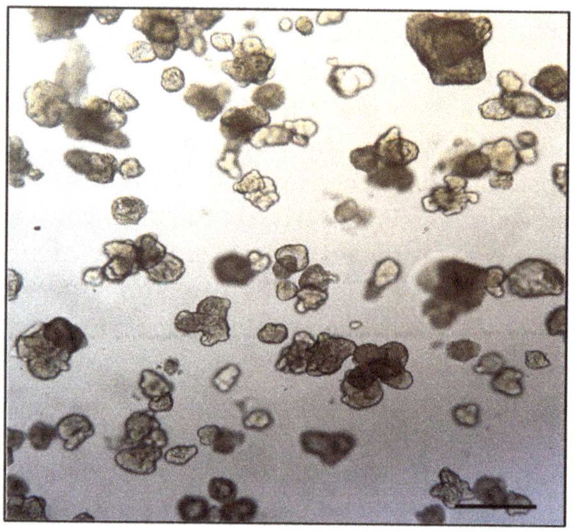

Figure 2. Bright field microphotograph depicting a representative field of human duodenum-derived enteroids in Matrigel. Each of the structures in the figure represents an enteroid at 8 days of culture, consisting of a 3D cellular aggregate organized into an epithelial monolayer resembling that of the small intestine. The apical surface of the monolayer faces the center of the enteroid while the basolateral surface faces the exterior. Bar scale indicates 1.0 mm; image from Stefania Senger, unpublished data.

A unique property of the enteroids is that the 3D structure of the tissue is not required for terminal cellular differentiation [55,56]. Thus, organoids/enteroids can be dissociated enzymatically and reseeded onto Transwells to generate short-term 2D monolayer cultures consisting of various differentiated epithelial cell types that can then be used for experimentation [55–58]. Moon and colleagues [55] established epithelial cell monolayers from cultured intestinal spheroids derived from the colon of mice. The differentiated monolayers displayed a robust transepithelial electrical resistance (TEER, a measure of barrier integrity) and the ability to transcytose secretory immunoglobulin A (sIgA) upon stimulation with microbial products [55]. The same group in another study (vanDussen et al., 2015) [56] adapted the technique to generate polarized 2D monolayers from human enteroids that were used to conduct adherence assays with enteropathogenic and diarrheagenic *Escherichia coli* [56]. The monolayers generated from enteroids maintain apical-to-basal polarity and barrier function while allowing easy access to the apical and basolateral compartments. The monolayers also maintain the genetic and functional phenotypes of the organoid/enteroids of origin [56] and can be manipulated to express a crypt-like or villus-like phenotype by changing media composition [49]. This system lends itself to many standard functional assays designed for 2D cells as well as to high throughput assays that cannot be easily performed on spherical enteroids/organoids, including but not limited to adhesion/invasion assays, transmigration assays, and inflammatory immune responses [49,51,55,56,59]. These monolayers can be cultured for up to three weeks (Stefania Senger, unpublished observations). Recent studies [60–62] have developed techniques to generate monolayers that exhibited compartmentalization of proliferative crypt-like domains and differentiated villus-like regions closely resembling in vivo distribution. Liu et al. [60] generated self-renewing 2D monolayers by plating intestinal stem cells on a thin layer (10 μM) of Matrigel coated onto glass sheets, while Wang et al. [63] relied on the presence of collagen hydrogels in tissue culture plates. Liu and colleagues [60] also altered the combination of growth factors added to the medium, such as addition of blebbistatin and removal of EGF to improve the survival and growth of the stem cell population. These models do not provide access to the basolateral side of the monolayers. To overcome this limitation, Altay and colleagues [62] cultured mouse-derived intestinal enteroids on Transwells coated with Matrigel that provided proper mechanical stiffness. The authors also boosted the proliferation of the stem cells by supplementing the culture medium for the basolateral compartment with conditioned medium from intestinal sub-epithelial myofibroblasts. The resulting monolayers possessed all cell types found in vivo as well as an effective barrier function. Thus, the 2D monolayers offer in vivo-like structural and functional characteristics with the convenience of the 2D format and should prove quite useful, particularly in studies interrogating effects on intestinal stem cells, including during *Salmonella* infection [64,65].

Overall, organoids/enteroids have several advantages. The models maintain the in vivo tissue architecture, cellular composition, and region-specific differentiation programming [28] while being genetically stable [66]. Organoids/enteroids are amenable to many of the established techniques of molecular analysis and manipulation, such as CRISPR/Cas9 technology [67], lentivirus transduction [42] single-cell RNA sequencing [53], and mass spectrometry [68] to name a few. Organoids/enteroids have been utilized for improving the basic understanding of tissue homeostasis, organogenesis, and physiological functions [4,69]. The systems have also been used to model diseases [49,51], to study host-pathogen interactions [59,65,70,71] and cancer [72], and to test potential vaccines and drugs [73–75]. The organoids/enteroids are also used as new tools for personalized medicine, where patient-derived models can serve as platforms for testing treatment options. For example, Dekker and colleagues [76] utilized intestinal enteroids derived from patients with cystic fibrosis to assess the responsiveness to CFTR-modulating drugs. Several large repositories of organoids/enteroids from multiple patients have been established and can be a source of both healthy and diseased cells globally, providing researchers access to a varied genetic background to test their hypotheses [10]. The models even have the potential to be a source for transplantation [35]. Below, we will highlight the use of organoids/enteroids for studying *Salmonella* pathogenesis.

4. *Salmonella enterica*

The genus *Salmonella* is a major foodborne pathogen [77]. It comprises two species: *S. bongori* and *S. enterica*. Almost all *Salmonella* organisms that cause disease in humans and domestic animals are serovars belonging to *S. enterica subspecies enterica*. Broadly, the diseases caused by *Salmonella* in humans are of two kinds: 1) systemic febrile illness termed typhoid/enteric fever, and 2) an acute self-limiting gastroenteritis. The serovars that cause typhoid are referred to as typhoidal *Salmonella* and include *S. enterica subsp. enterica* serovar Typhi and *S. enterica subsp. enterica* serovar Paratyphi A, B, and C. *S.* Typhi causes approximately 76.3% of global enteric fever cases [78]. *S.* Typhi and *S.* Paratyphi are restricted to humans and higher primates, and clinical manifestations of the infection include sustained high fever, abdominal pain, headache, weakness, malaise, and transient diarrhea/constipation. Without appropriate and effective antibiotic therapy, the infection may lead to gastrointestinal bleeding, intestinal perforation, septic shock, and death [79,80]. The Non-Typhoidal *Salmonella* (NTS) serovars cause self-limiting gastroenteritis and include *S. enterica subsp. enterica* serovar Typhimurium and *S. enterica subsp. enterica* serovar Enteridis, which are the most prevalent clinical isolates, according to the World Health Organization (WHO). These pathogens are broader in host range and infect humans and animals such as poultry, cattle, reptiles, and amphibians. Infections with NTS typically involve self-limiting diarrhea, stomach cramps, headache, vomiting, and fever that resolve on their own; however, the infection can be severe in children and the elderly and can sometimes be fatal [81]. NTS serovars have been reported to cause an invasive infection similar to typhoid, particularly in sub-Saharan Africa, predominantly in children and HIV-positive adults, with several co-morbidities such as ongoing or recent malaria infection and malnutrition contributing to higher mortality [82–84]. *Salmonella* infections represent a considerable economic burden and public health concern in both developing and developed countries. The Center for Disease Control and Prevention (CDC), estimates that 1.35 million infections by *Salmonella* occur in the United States. NTS causes more than 93 million global infections per year, with 155,000 deaths [85]. A study examining the global burden of diseases, injuries, and risk factors in 2017 reported 14.3 million cases of enteric fever globally, with a case fatality of 0.95% resulting in approximately 135,000 deaths [78]. Children, elderly, and those residing in lower-income countries account for the greatest incidences [86,87].

Salmonella is acquired via contaminated food and water. Luminal bacteria invade M cells and absorptive enterocytes via a specialized apparatus called the type three secretion system (T3SS) [88] encoded on the *Salmonella* Pathogenicity Islands (SPIs) [89]. The T3SS injects bacterial proteins into host cells allowing the bacteria to essentially commandeer host cellular processes to induce cytoskeletal rearrangements that engulf the bacteria into specialized vesicles called the *Salmonella* containing vacuoles (SCVs) [90]. This invasion process, with subsequent translocation across the epithelium, is followed by the uptake of the bacteria by macrophages and dendritic cells in the intestinal sub-mucosa, where bacterial proteins interfere with phagolysosomal maturation and allow the bacteria to survive inside the cells [91–93]. NTS serovars undergo prolific growth in the intestine, while T3SS effectors induce fluid secretion and promote inflammation. Immune signaling via recognition of pathogen-associated molecular patterns such as lipopolysaccharide (LPS) and flagella also induce a robust inflammatory response, which actually provides *Salmonella* with a growth advantage over resident microflora [81,94–96]. The immune response eventually limits *Salmonella* growth; nevertheless, the short-term proliferation is sufficient to ensure propagation. Typhoidal *Salmonella* strains elicit a more attenuated inflammatory response in the intestine, especially in terms of limited neutrophil recruitment [79,97,98]. Bacteria migrate to the mesenteric lymph nodes (MLN) and systemically within the reticuloendothelial cells, and as free bacteria in the blood or lymph, to establish new foci of infection in the liver, spleen, bone marrow, and gallbladder [99]. At these new sites the bacteria replicate and re-enter the intestinal lumen via secretion in bile, promoting shedding of the bacteria to continue the cycle of new infections by contaminated food and water. In 3%–5% of cases, the bacteria can persist for long durations in the gallbladder, which serves as a reservoir of chronic infection [100].

Chronic infection with *Salmonella* has been found to be a risk factor for the development of malignant neoplasms, including gallbladder cancer [101,102] and colorectal cancer [102,103].

The emergence of multi-drug resistance to conventional antibiotics complicates the treatment of *Salmonella* infection [104–107]. Antibiotic treatment destroys the resident microflora, provides a niche for *Salmonella* to proliferate, and may lead to increased levels of bacterial shedding [108]. Additionally, bacterial populations that express an antibiotic-tolerant phenotype can evade treatment and persist, causing relapses of the infection as well as the evolution of bacterial virulence [109,110]. Asymptomatic carriers act as reservoirs, contribute to the continued propagation of the pathogen, and are particularly important for food safety considerations. Currently, there are no effective vaccines against gastrointestinal *Salmonella* infections. Several typhoid vaccines are available and licensed in many countries; however, robust protection is limited and has been associated with injection site reactions. Furthermore, the vaccines have not been widely adopted by public health programs [111]. With the significant aging populations in both developed and developing countries [112,113], more people are at risk for severe consequences of *Salmonella* infections. Advances in the mechanistic understanding of *Salmonella* infections will facilitate the development of improved control strategies, particularly, safe and effective vaccines. The broad conservation of host responses as well as the molecular machinery used by *Salmonella* strains during infection of various hosts, namely T3SSs encoded by SPI1 and SPI2 that enable invasion of epithelial cells and subsequent intracellular survival, allows several model systems to be applied for *Salmonella* research [114]. Each non-human model has pros and cons, and varies in the ability to recapitulate natural infection. Given the host-specific aspects of infection physiology, it is necessary to be cautious in applying the results from these model systems to human patients. Additionally, with *Salmonella* being an important tool to understand host physiology, metabolism, immune function, and interactions with microbes, human-specific investigations are valuable to the research community.

5. Model Systems to Study *Salmonella* Biology

Transformed cell lines such as Cos-1, MDCK, HeLa, HepG2, CaCo2, and T-84 have been used to carry out several fundamental studies on *Salmonella* pathogenicity, such as the identification of the T3SS and the SPIs [88,115]. However, these cells have the drawback noted earlier inthat the cells do not adequately represent the physiological characteristics of normal human tissue [116,117]. Explant tissue cultures have organotypic properties that can be vital for studies on development and physiology, but are limited by culturing difficulties and short life span [118,119]. Classically, animal models have offered solutions for several of these limitations, and have been used to corroborate data obtained from other model systems as well as to investigate the deeper molecular mechanism of infection. For example, *S.* Typhimurium is a natural pathogen of calves and causes a gastroenteritis with clinical and pathological manifestations similar to humans, namely diarrhea, anorexia, fever, localized infection, and neutrophil infiltration [120,121]. Meanwhile, the bovine ligated loop was instrumental in characterizing fluid accumulation and host inflammatory responses following *S.* Typhimurium infection. For example, mutants lacking the invasion proteins SipA, SopA, and SopD were shown to have little to no effect on the ability of *S.* Typhimurium to invade epithelial cells, but were shown to reduce the fluid accumulation and neutrophil immigration in bovine loops [122,123].

More importantly, the vast majority of studies on *Salmonella* pathogenesis have been conducted in the murine model, including studies for the development of new vaccines. This model has been useful in clarifying various aspects of in vivo *Salmonella* pathogenesis; however, it does have limitations with respect to its ability to faithfully reproduce all aspects of *Salmonella* infection in humans. *S.* Typhimurium causes two very different types of diseases in human and mice. In humans, the infection is localized, dominated by the infiltration of neutrophils and self-limiting. In mice, *S.* Typhimurium spreads systemically, with slow infiltration of mononuclear inflammatory cells and little or no localized intestinal tissue injury. The host responses involved are also dramatically different. Since the clinical manifestations and pathology of mice infected with *S.* Typhimurium resemble those observed in humans with *S.* Typhi infection, the model has been used as a surrogate to study typhoid pathogenesis [124]. A mouse model of *S.* Typhimurium-induced enterocolitis has been developed and involves pre-treatment of mice with a single dose of streptomycin. This procedure diminishes the colonization resistance by the commensal microbiota, allowing *Salmonella* to grow to high densities in the cecum and large intestine and trigger acute gastroenteritis [125]. Mouse models have also been developed to mimic chronic infections of *Salmonella* observed in certain carrier individuals, which typically involve infecting susceptible mice with avirulent strains, or sub-lethal doses of *S.* Typhimurium in resistant mice. Experimental interpretations from the mouse model may not translate to human disease. *S.* Typhi and *S.* Typhimurium share about 89% of their genes, with approximately 500 genes unique to *S.* Typhimurium and 600 genes unique to *S.* Typhi, including the genes encoding typhoid toxin and the immunoprotective capsule [126,127]. *S.* Typhi and *S.* Paratyphi also have pseudogenes as well as small sequence differences in genes encoding the T3SS apparatuses and related effectors that may have important implications in pathogenesis. It is possible that virulence factors that may have no role in *S.* Typhi-mediated infection in humans may be important for mouse infection by *S.* Typhimurium and vice versa. Finally, *S.* Typhi genes required for causing typhoid but absent in *S.* Typhimurium cannot be studied easily using the latter. Typhoid fever can be induced experimentally by oral infection in higher primates or human volunteers, but these studies come with their own set of difficulties and ethical objections. Researchers have attempted to compensate for the discrepancies by developing humanized mice, i.e., immunodeficient mice engrafted with human hematopoietic cells [128,129], but these models are cumbersome, expensive, and still do not guarantee that mouse-specific factors will not add complexities or variations to the data generated. In addition, host genetic background has been found to play a role in susceptibility to invasive NTS infections, a concept that borders on the realm of personalized medicine [130]. Thus, organoids offer a promising model to mechanistically study host-specific aspects of infection.

6. Organoids/Enteroids in *Salmonella* Biology

One of the earliest studies that utilized organotypic 3D structures to investigate *Salmonella* pathology was carried out by Nickerson, CA et al., in 2001 [26]. As described above, the authors generated 3D organotypic cultures by growing human embryonic intestinal cell line Int-407 in RWV bioreactors and subsequently infected the cells with *S.* Typhimurium. The resulting infection was quite different from what had previously been observed in monolayer cultures. There was minimal loss of structural integrity, lower ability of the bacteria to adhere to and invade epithelia, and lowered expression of cytokine in 3D Int-407 aggregates as compared to infected Int-407 monolayers. Since the authors observed that the 3D Int-407 aggregates more closely resembled in vivo characteristics (tissue organization, tight junctions, apical-to-basal polarity, microvilli development, expression of extracellular and basement membrane proteins, and greater M cell glycosylation pattern), the authors concluded that the infection phenotypes observed in the 3D aggregates were likely representative of an in vivo infection. This study laid the groundwork for the use of 3D organotypic cultures to study *Salmonella* biology. The following section will highlight research performed in both mouse and human models that has improved our understanding of *Salmonella* pathogenesis (Figure 3).

6.1. Mouse-Derived Models

Following the establishment of protocols to generate crypt-derived mouse intestinal enteroids (referred to as organoids by the authors) by Sato et al., Zhang and colleagues [65] in 2014 utilized the system to analyze interaction of *S.* Typhimurium with epithelial cells. The authors visualized bacterial infection, while also observing bacterial-induced disruption of tight junctions, activation of the nuclear factor kappa-light-chain-enhancer of activated B cells (NF-kB)-mediated inflammatory response, and a decrease in the stem cell marker Lgr5. The authors noted that these observations were similar to findings in animal models. The caveat to this study is that the *Salmonella* were not delivered into the lumen of the enteroids, the location of the initial contact of bacteria with epithelial cells in vivo; instead, the bacteria were added to the medium and came in contact with the enteroids basolaterally. Nevertheless, this study established mouse-derived enteroids as a model system for studying *Salmonella* infection biology.

Since this initial study, enteroids have been used to interrogate various aspects of *Salmonella* pathology, including investigating cell types that were previously not accessible to study in vitro. Farin and colleagues [131], in a 2014 study, used mouse intestinal enteroids to study the control of Paneth cell (PC) degranulation in response to bacteria or bacterial molecules such as LPS. The authors found that PC degranulation did not occur upon stimulation with microbial molecules or *Salmonella*, but was induced by a novel mechanism requiring only the presence of recombinant interferon gamma (IFN-γ) [131]. In another study, Wilson and colleagues [132] interrogated the antimicrobial role of Paneth cell α-defensin peptides. The authors developed small intestinal epithelial enteroids from both wild-type mice or mice mutated for α-defensin production (*Mmp7*$^{-/-}$ mice, MMP7 is a matrix metalloprotease that is required to generate bactericidally active α-defensins in mice [133]), and infected the enteroids with *S.* Typhimurium by microinjecting the bacteria directly into the lumen. The absence of mature α-defensins reduced the intra-luminal bacterial killing, which could be partially restored by expression of the human defensin HD5 [132]. This study demonstrated the contribution of α-defensins to the innate immune response to *Salmonella*, which previously had been a challenge to examine since most of the earlier experimental systems inadequately recapitulated in vivo cellular processes [134].

Salmonella has been suggested to contribute to the development of cancer by epidemiological studies [102]. Scanu and colleague [135] probed this phenomenon in a 2015 study using the case of gallbladder cancer (GBC). The authors derived gallbladder enteroids from mice carrying mutations that inactivate p53 and are known to be found in GBC patients in India, where the disease is prevalent. When exposed to wild-type *S.* Typhimurium, single cells derived from the gallbladder enteroids carrying these predisposing mutations generated new enteroids that exhibited growth factor independence, which is one of the hallmarks of transformation, and had histopathological features consistent with neoplastic transformation, thus establishing a direct association between *Salmonella* and cancer. To delve into the mechanism of this transformation, the authors looked at the *Salmonella* T3SS-mediated activation of AKT or mitogen-activated protein (MAP) kinase pathways, which have been shown to be elevated in human cancers. The signals activated by AKT and MAPK were found to be key in driving the cellular transformation and were sustained even after the eradication of the *Salmonella* infection. Studies have shown that AKT and MAPK pathways are activated by other bacteria and viruses that have been associated with various cancers [136–139]. Although the authors employed a murine gallbladder enteroid model and *S.* Typhimurium to study GBC, the authors proposed that the AKT and MAPK pathways are activated by both *S.* Typhimurium and *S.* Typhi serovars, and contribute to development of cancer that is associated with chronic *S.* Typhi infection in humans. Chronic infection by *Salmonella* has also been found to be a risk factor for developing cancers in the ascending and transverse colon [103]. However, detailed mechanistic studies of *Salmonella*-associated colon carcinogenesis need to be carried out and organoid model systems may prove to be extremely useful for this purpose.

Finally, another important aspect of *Salmonella* is the interaction of the pathogen with the host microbiome. Lu and colleagues [140] recently demonstrated that *Lactobacillus acidophilus*, a well-established probiotic bacterium, can alleviate damage caused by *S.* Typhimurium. Earlier studies had shown that *L. acidophilus* can inhibit adhesion of *Salmonella* to CaCo2 cells [141]. In this study, the authors extended the mechanism of protection to include the effects on the host. *L. acidophilus* altered the differentiation of epithelial cells in crypt-derived enteroids by impeding the *Salmonella*-mediated expansion of Paneth cells [131], thus maintaining homeostasis and appropriate epithelial composition during the infection. This study not only improved our understanding of the role of *L. acidophilus* in protecting the epithelial lining, but also demonstrated the ability to include microbiota-specific analyses to study *Salmonella* infection with enteroids/organoids.

6.2. *Human-Derived Models*

The potential to gain significant insight into *Salmonella* pathogenesis is particularly relevant in relation to the use of human-specific organoids, especially since these models possess human genetic specificities absent in mice. Studies have interrogated the usefulness of intestinal enteroids/organoids derived from human ASCs or PSCs to understand complex interactions between the epithelium and *Salmonella*. In 2015 Forbester and colleagues [70] used RNA sequencing to examine the epithelial transcriptional signature following injection of *S.* Typhimurium into the lumen of organoids derived from human induced PSCs (hiPSCs). The analysis showed significant up-regulation of genes for cytokine-mediated signaling, NF-κB activation, angiogenesis, and chemotaxis. Enhanced release of pro-inflammatory cytokines IL-8, IL-6, and TNF-α was also confirmed. The findings were consistent with prior studies in animal and mouse organoid models, thus establishing the human organoids as a viable infection model for *Salmonella*. The study also demonstrated that a noninvasive mutant strain (deficient in *invA* gene) could be used in the model to examine *Salmonella* pathogenicity and the functionality of defined mutants [70]. Furthermore, the authors generated an RNA sequencing data set following basolateral administration of *Salmonella* to the organoids. Interestingly, 49 of the 100 most highly upregulated genes were also significantly induced in the data set obtained by microinjecting the bacteria for apical infection. The data provide credence to the results of the Zhang and colleagues study [65], which documented similar patterns of gene expression upon basolateral administration of *Salmonella* to mouse organoids as had been observed earlier in literature with other model systems. Thus, the hiPSC organoids maintain a conserved response to *Salmonella* infection and provide a human-specific model for pathogenesis studies.

A subsequent study further demonstrated the validity of hiPSCs as a model to study human-specific responses to *Salmonella* infection. Using the same model system, the role of the cytokine IL-22 in priming intestinal epithelial cells towards a more effective response to *S.* Typhimurium was also explored [142]. The study showed that IL-22 pre-treated hiPSC-derived organoids increased phagolysosomal fusion leading to enhanced antimicrobial activity. Thus, this study confirmed earlier observations made in mouse organoids [143].

The fidelity of organoid-derived data in representing human disease was further demonstrated in 2018 by Nickerson, KP and colleagues [71], who compared infection of human tissue biopsies and human intestinal enteroid-derived monolayers seeded on a 2D Transwell system, and observed that the enteroid-derived epithelial monolayers recapitulated *S.* Typhi infection observations made in the tissue biopsy model. The authors also carried out transcriptional profiling of both the host tissue and the bacteria in order to determine early critical interactions. Infection with *S.* Typhi significantly down-regulated several host genes, including those involved in activation of the mucosal immune response, bacterial clearance, and cytoskeletal rearrangement. Interestingly in this model, a down regulation of SPI1 genes in *S.* Typhi was observed. This work demonstrated that *S.* Typhi reduces intestinal inflammation by limiting the induction of pathogen-induced processes through the regulation of virulence gene expression, which is a characteristic feature of human infection with *S.* Typhi. Transmission electron microscopic comparisons of the tissues and human organoid-derived epithelial monolayers showed that the monolayers reproduced the cytoskeletal arrangements, microvilli destruction, and vesicle-bound bacteria observed in tissues. There were no changes observed in paracellular permeability, increased death of host cells, or bacterial association with M cells, suggesting divergence from *S.* Typhimurium infection in mice. This study highlights the ability of organoids to compare human-specific responses to each *Salmonella* serovar, which is important in the context of translational capacity for developing prophylactic or therapeutic intervention strategies against *S.* Typhimurium versus *S.* Typhi infections.

Despite the multiple advantages of the organoids as an experimental system, the technology is still in its infancy and has certain limitations. The complex structure of the organoids poses a practical limitation in accessing the internal luminal compartment. Researchers have used microinjections to access the apical epithelium. This approach may preserve the internal microenvironment, but is resource-intensive, may not allow synchronous exposure and suffers from variability in volume that can be injected due to heterogeneity of the organoid/enteroid sizes. In addition, the lumen of 3D organoid/enteroid accumulates cellular debris, which may bind bacteria or hamper interactions with the apical membranes. As noted above (in Section 3), researchers have turned to organoid/enteroid-derived 2D monolayers to better access the apical side of the model and enable more efficient, user-friendly analyses in a multiple-well plate format. However, this modification can limit the number of processes that can be interrogated, especially when considering the lack of 3D structure. Interestingly, Co and colleagues [144] demonstrated in a recent study that the polarity of human enteroids could be reversed such that the apical surface faced the medium and was readily accessible. The enteroids released mucus and extruded cells outwards into the culture medium rather than having the cells embedded in the basement membrane. Using enteroids with reversed polarity, the authors showed that *S.* Typhimurium invades and induces actin ruffles more efficiently at the apical surface compared to the basolateral surface. The authors observed a more diffuse process of epithelial invasion rather than invasion only or predominantly at the M cells [144], which confirmed the *S.* Typhi observations by Nickerson, KP et al. [71].

Current organoid/enteroid models are devoid of muscles, innervation, vascularization, and immune cells. There are a couple of approaches being carried out to increase the complexity of organoid models, including co-culturing techniques. In 2011, Salerno-Goncalves and colleagues [7] generated an organotypic model using the human ileococal adenocarcinoma cell line HCT-8 and adding primary endothelial cells, fibroblasts, and peripheral blood mononuclear cells (PBMCs), which they used in a 2019 study to probe the crosstalk between these cell types during infection with *S.* Typhi, *S.* Paratyphi A, or *S.* Paratyphi B [145]. An ECM composed of collagen-I enriched with other gastrointestinal basement proteins was embedded with the fibroblasts and epithelial cells, and transferred to a RWV bioreactor containing epithelial cells. Under low microgravity and low shear conditions, the HCT-8 cells behaved as multi-potent progenitor cells and gave rise to multiple cell types, including absorptive enterocytes, goblet cells, and M cells. After one to two weeks, PBMCs were added to the system. The co-culture model was then infected with the various *Salmonella* serovars to compare responses to the three strains. The authors found that the presence of the immune cells in the model resulted in secretion of the cytokines IL-1β and CCL3, while secretion of cytokines IL-6 and TNF-α was enhanced. Using depletion experiments, the authors showed that macrophages were the PBMC cell type responsible for the enhanced secretion of IL-6 and TNF-α. The authors further used the Transwell system to show that supernatants from organotypic models built with whole or macrophage-depleted PBMCs infected with the three *Salmonella* strains varied in their ability to elicit transmigration of macrophages and neutrophils [145]. Interestingly, the two immune cells displayed crosstalk during infections with *S.* Paratyphi A and *S.* Paratyphi B, such that the presence of macrophages in the co-culture reduced neutrophil migration as compared to the system built without macrophages [145]. This study illustrates that co-cultures can aid in probing the contribution of immune cells to *Salmonella* infection at the mucosal surface. Finally, this model has also been used to assess the inflammatory response to several candidate *S.* Typhi vaccine strains in comparison to the response elicited by the oral vaccine strain Ty21a strain and its parent wild-type Ty2 stain [146]. Salerno-Goncalves and colleagues [146] found that specific changes to the genetic makeup of the candidate vaccine strains (in the form of deletions of specific metabolic genes) elicited host changes in intestinal permeability, inflammatory cytokine secretion, as well as activation of innate immunity pathways. Higgins and colleagues [73] also used the model to test the inflammatory response of an *S.* Typhimurium vaccine strain that they generated. These studies highlight the usefulness of co-cultured organoid/enteroid models in assessing important factors to be considered while designing vaccines.

Schulte and colleagues [147] generated a co-culture system of human intestinal epithelial cell line (Caco-2), primary human microvascular endothelial cells, primary intestinal collagen scaffold, and PBMCs in a Transwell set up. Using GFP-labeled *S.* Typhimurium, microscopy, and flow cytometry, the authors demonstrated that the bacteria can be found in epithelial but not endothelial cells, thus modeling the epithelium-restricted infection of humans with *S.* Typhimurium. These findings are in contrast to those of Spadoni and colleagues [99] in the mouse model of *S.* Typhimurium infections where a breach of the gut-vascular barrier by the bacteria was observed. The endothelial cells respond to the infection process by bringing about changes in transcription of various genes and releasing the phagocyte chemoattractant IL-8. Such models, ideally with enteroid/organoid-derived cells replacing cell lines where used, should prove to be extremely useful and versatile in interrogating the role of different immune cells, vasculature, and the related crosstalk with epithelial cells during infection with *Salmonella,* especially for *S.* Typhi, where the bacteria spread systemically both as free bacteria and within reticuloendothelial cells [148].

7. Future Directions

Currently, researchers have little or no control over how cells self-organize into organoids. The physical environment of the enteroids/organoids in the form of the 3D scaffold provides cues such as adhesive ligands and stiffness. The current ECMs are derived from animals, are poorly defined, may show batch to batch variation that can lead to heterogeneous growth and differentiation between the organoids generated at different times, and are not mechanically pliable after plating. Thus, improvements to the 3D scaffolds are expected to yield better consistency, which would facilitate mechanistic infection studies and even provide a better platform for clinical applications. Some recent work [149] has focused on using chemically defined 3D scaffolds to improve the uniformity of the environmental cues for growth and differentiation. Indeed, a better defined and mechanically dynamic matrix would increase the potential of organoid technologies for therapeutic development (also reviewed in [150] and [151]).

Another important requirement is the further characterization of organoids/enteroids to ensure that the models faithfully represent the in vivo human physiology so that in vitro analyses with the system will be relevant for subsequent clinical development. Recent work in brain organoids has shown that important differences exist in the expression profiles between cells derived from organoids as compared to human brain cells [130]. Similar studies must be carried out in intestinal organoid/enteroid models, and indeed in all organoid models, to ensure fidelity of representation.

The enteric nervous system (ENS) carries out important functions in the gastrointestinal tract, such as motility and contractility, regulation of blood flow, maintenance of epithelial barrier, and fluid exchange [7]. Future investigations of the role of the ENS in *Salmonella* infection will be critical to our mechanistic understanding of the pathogen. Recent studies have shown that the neurons in the gut also protect against *S.* Typhimurium infections [152,153]. For example, Lai and colleagues [153] demonstrated that the pain-sensing neurons that lie beneath Peyer's patches in the gastrointestinal tracts of mice, become activated and release the neuropeptide calcitonin gene-related peptide (CGRP) upon detecting *S.* Typhimurium. This process results in a decreased number of M cells while increasing the levels of segmented filamentous bacteria (SFB) that can protect against *Salmonella* infection [153]. In light of studies like this, it becomes essential to probe and understand the interaction of *Salmonella* with the ENS. To facilitate analyses with the ENS, researchers have developed an ENS-HIO model. Workman and colleagues [154] generated vagal-like neural crest cells (NCCs, the precursors of ENS) from PSCs and incorporated them into human intestinal organoids via direct co-culture. The NCCs subsequently differentiated into multiple cell types including neurons and glia. The authors demonstrated that the neurons were functional by observing a response to oscillations in calcium. The ENS-HIO was then transplanted into mice and displayed contractile activity. Given the recent findings of the role of neurons in potential protection against *Salmonella* infection, this model has tremendous promise to further our understanding of the dynamics of the ENS-*Salmonella* interaction.

Methods to incorporate the microbiome into organoid-based models are essential to future *Salmonella* research. It is well known that *Salmonella* must successfully compete with the resident microflora in order to infect the intestinal epithelium, and several competitive mechanisms deployed by *Salmonella* have been elucidated [155]. Most often, microbiome studies are carried out in germ-free or humanized mice; however, there are significant differences between the composition of the microbiota and host physiology when using these animals as a model of humans. The healthy gut contains several anaerobic bacteria in the lumen given the decreasing oxygen gradient that extends from the anaerobic lumen to the hypoxic epithelium. Despite the complexities of microbiota interactions and oxygen levels, a few studies have made progress in incorporating the microbiota into organoid models or reproducing anaerobic environments such as the 2020 study by Lu et al., described above [140]. Karve and colleagues [156] in a 2017 study incubated induced human intestinal organoids (iHIOs) with human neutrophils to model innate cellular responses to commensal and pathogenic *Escherichia coli* in which neutrophil recruitment was monitored by microscopy. The authors were able to culture commensal *E. coli*, despite the fact that the bacterial strain is a facultative anaerobe. Greater recruitment of the neutrophils occurred when the organoids had been injected with pathogenic bacteria as compared to saline or commensal bacteria. In another study by Leslie and colleagues [157], the authors demonstrated that anaerobic *Clostridium difficile* could remain viable for at least 12h when injected into the lumen of HIOs, indicating the reproducibility of the appropriate oxygen levels in the model. Finally, LeBlay and colleagues [158] have devised a specialized bioreactor for cultivation of human intestinal microbiota that will enable researchers to grow a wide range of commensal bacteria for analyses. The authors immobilized fecal microbiota from a two year old child in gel beads and cultured under anaerobic conditions with continuous flow of medium containing chyme. The bacteria grew as biofilms and formed stable populations. *S.* Typhimurium also immobilized onto beads was added to the reactor to simulate gut infection in children. This step was followed by addition of two concentrations of amoxicillin, and the effects of the treatment on the microbial composition and the metabolites generated were analyzed. The authors observed a strong disturbance in the microbial composition upon antibiotic treatment, with *Bifidobateria* significantly decreasing in numbers while *C. cocoides-E.rectales* group strongly increased. S. Typhimurium levels were also strongly decreased upon amoxicillin treatment, but returned to previous levels upon interruption of the antibiotic treatment. Antibiotic treatment also resulted in a decrease in the concentration of the metabolites acetate and butyrate, which remained at lower levels even on the withdrawal of antibiotic treatment. Indeed, these studies show that the incorporation of the microbiota into human-specific organoid systems will allow mechanistic studies investigating the crosstalk between host physiology, microbiota, and *Salmonella* pathogenicity.

8. Conclusions

Infections caused by *S. enterica* remain a major health concern world-wide. Models used to study the disease pathology so far have provided valuable advancements. However, there remains a disconnect between what works at the bench versus at the bedside, particularly in the case of vaccines. The development of organoids/enteroids offers a tremendous opportunity to bridge this gap by bringing human-specific factors into the research models (Figure 3).

Gastrointestinal organoid and enteroid models have been shown to capture the cellularity, organization, and complexity of the intestine in vivo along with providing the flexibility of an in vitro system. These models have provided new and fundamental knowledge in human physiology, pathology and the molecular basis of host-microbe interactions. In addition, recent studies have seen efforts to build upon existing paradigms. Research is being conducted to improve the fidelity and reproducibility of the organoid model systems. Co-culture systems have been developed allowing the integration of various cell types, which allows us to better understand and interrogate the crosstalk between a wide-range of potential combinations of lineages in vivo. Most importantly, the integration of immune cell types is likely to help in understanding how *Salmonella* is viewed by and responds to immune processes, particularly at the mucosal epithelium that is the first site of contact and thus an important stage of the infection process for the development of vaccines. There have also been studies that have integrated the microbiota into the organoid model and future work may delve into the role of an individual's microbiota in *Salmonella* pathogenesis. Despite its potential, it is important to keep in mind certain limitations of organoid-based systems, the most significant being that the models have to be thoroughly characterized for their ability to represent in vivo conditions for appropriate translation into the clinic. The addition of multiple cell types into organoid co-cultures only recapitulates a part of the body i.e., the organ from which they are derived. The results of organoid co-cultures have to be complemented with whole organism studies and compared to human clinical findings.

We anticipate that the organoid and enteroid models will play key roles in future advancements in the understanding of *Salmonella* pathogenesis. Their use will facilitate research in drug development, host-microbe interactions, crosstalk between the host, microbiota and pathogens, and personalized medicine, and will contribute towards the development of successful vaccines for *Salmonella* Typhimurium and *Salmonella* Typhi.

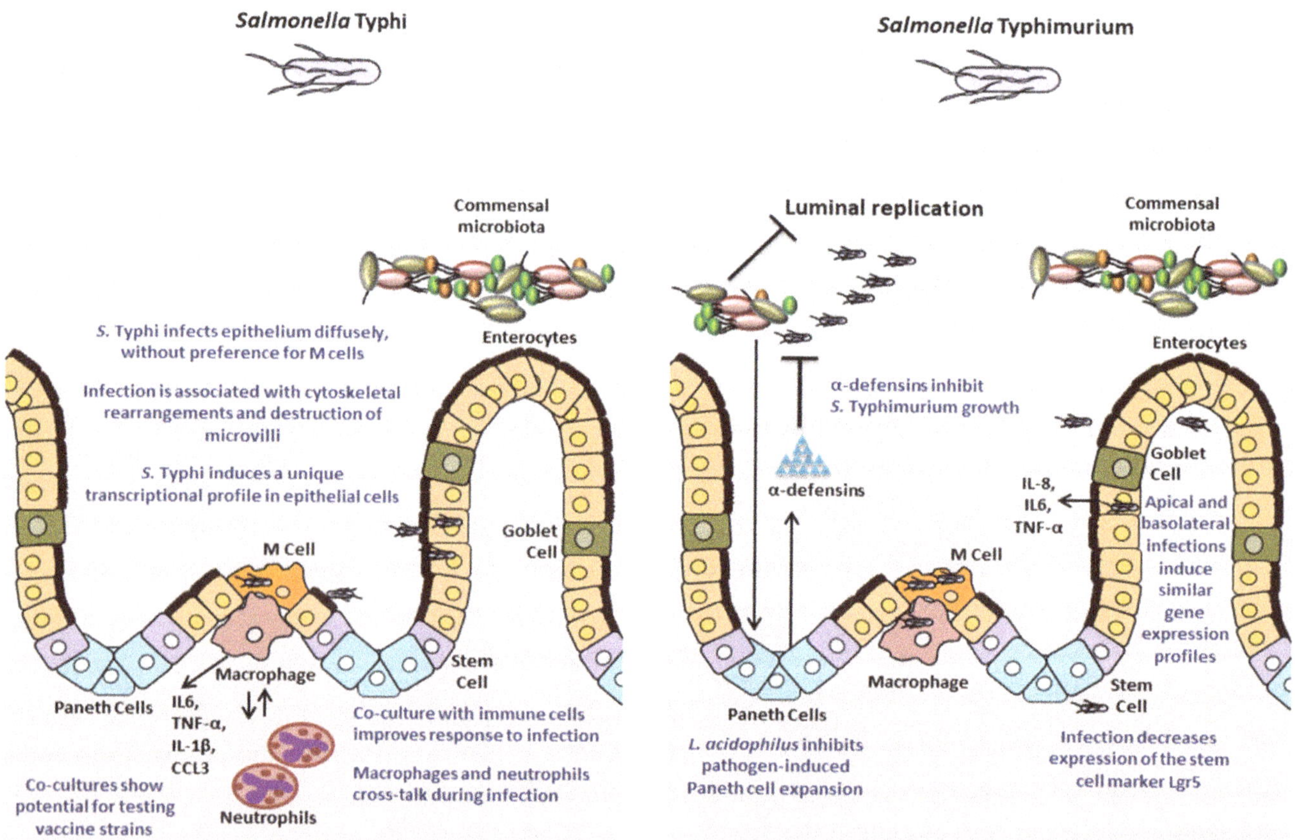

Figure 3. Insights into *Salmonella* pathogenesis from intestinal organoids/enteroids. The key findings for *S.* Typhi and *S.* Typhimurium are highlighted.

References

1. Mestas, J.; Hughes, C.C. Of mice and not men: Differences between mouse and human immunology. *J. Immunol.* **2004**, *172*, 2731–2738. [CrossRef]
2. Zimmermann, B. Lung organoid culture. *Differentiation* **1987**, *36*, 86–109. [CrossRef]
3. Sambuy, Y.; de Angelis, I. Formation of organoid structures and extracellular matrix production in an intestinal epithelial cell line during long-term in vitro culture. *Cell Differ.* **1986**, *19*, 139–147. [CrossRef]
4. Levy, E.; Delvin, E.E.; Ménard, D.; Beaulieu, J.-F. Functional development of human fetal gastrointestinal tract. *Adv. Struct. Saf. Stud.* **2009**, *550*, 205–224.

5. Sato, T.; Vries, R.G.; Snippert, H.J.; Van De Wetering, M.; Barker, N.; Stange, D.; Van Es, J.H.; Abo, A.; Kujala, P.; Peters, P.J.; et al. Single Lgr5 stem cells build crypt-villus structures in vitro without a mesenchymal niche. *Nature* **2009**, *459*, 262–265. [CrossRef] [PubMed]
6. Sato, T.; Stange, D.; Ferrante, M.; Vries, R.G.; Van Es, J.H.; Brink, S.V.D.; Van Houdt, W.J.; Pronk, A.; Van Gorp, J.M.; Siersema, P.D.; et al. Long-term expansion of epithelial organoids from human colon, adenoma, adenocarcinoma, and Barrett's epithelium. *Gastroenterology* **2011**, *141*, 1762–1772. [CrossRef]
7. Salerno-Gonçalves, R.; Fasano, A.; Sztein, M.B. Engineering of a multicellular organotypic model of the human intestinal mucosa. *Gastroenterology* **2011**, *141*, e18–e20. [CrossRef]
8. Finkbeiner, S.R.; Freeman, J.J.; Wieck, M.M.; El-Nachef, W.; Altheim, C.H.; Tsai, Y.-H.; Huang, S.; Dyal, R.; White, E.S.; Grikscheit, T.C.; et al. Generation of tissue-engineered small intestine using embryonic stem cell-derived human intestinal organoids. *Boil. Open* **2015**, *4*, 1462–1472. [CrossRef]
9. Stelzner, M.G.; Helmrath, M.; Dunn, J.C.Y.; Henning, S.J.; Houchen, C.W.; Kuo, C.; Lynch, J.; Li, L.; Magness, S.T.; Martin, M.G.; et al. A nomenclature for intestinal in vitro cultures. *Am. J. Physiol. Liver Physiol.* **2012**, *302*, G1359–G1363. [CrossRef]
10. Van De Wetering, M.; Francies, H.E.; Francis, J.M.; Bounova, G.; Iorio, F.; Pronk, A.; Van Houdt, W.; Van Gorp, J.; Taylor-Weiner, A.; Kester, L.; et al. Prospective derivation of a living organoid biobank of colorectal cancer patients. *Cell* **2015**, *161*, 933–945. [CrossRef]
11. Bartfeld, S.; Clevers, H. Organoids as model for infectious diseases: Culture of human and murine stomach organoids and microinjection of *Helicobacter pylori*. *J. Vis. Exp.* **2015**. [CrossRef] [PubMed]
12. Hu, H.; Gehart, H.; Artegiani, B.; Löpez-Iglesias, C.; Dekkers, F.; Basak, O.; Van Es, J.; Lopes, S.M.C.D.S.; Begthel, H.; Korving, J.; et al. Long-term expansion of functional mouse and human hepatocytes as 3D organoids. *Cell* **2018**, *175*, 1591–1606. [CrossRef] [PubMed]
13. Huch, M.; Gehart, H.; Van Boxtel, R.; Hamer, K.; Blokzijl, F.; Verstegen, M.M.; Ellis, E.; Van Wenum, M.; Fuchs, S.A.; De Ligt, J.; et al. Long-term culture of genome-stable bipotent stem cells from adult human liver. *Cell* **2014**, *160*, 299–312. [CrossRef] [PubMed]
14. Broutier, L.; Mastrogiovanni, G.; Verstegen, M.M.; Francies, H.E.; Gavarró, L.M.; Bradshaw, C.R.; Allen, G.E.; Arnes-Benito, R.; Sidorova, O.; Gaspersz, M.P.; et al. Human primary liver cancer–derived organoid cultures for disease modeling and drug screening. *Nature Med.* **2017**, *23*, 1424–1435. [CrossRef] [PubMed]
15. Boj, S.F.; Hwang, C.-I.; Baker, L.A.; Chio, I.I.C.; Engle, D.D.; Corbo, V.; Jager, M.; Ponz-Sarvise, M.; Tiriac, H.; Spector, M.S.; et al. Organoid models of human and mouse ductal pancreatic cancer. *Cell* **2014**, *160*, 324–338. [CrossRef] [PubMed]
16. Schutgens, F.; Rookmaaker, M.B.; Margaritis, T.; Rios, A.; Ammerlaan, C.; Jansen, J.; Gijzen, L.; Vormann, M.; Vonk, A.; Viveen, M.; et al. Tubuloids derived from human adult kidney and urine for personalized disease modeling. *Nat. Biotechnol.* **2019**, *37*, 303–313. [CrossRef] [PubMed]
17. Bartfeld, S.; Clevers, H. Stem cell-derived organoids and their application for medical research and patient treatment. *J. Mol. Med.* **2017**, *95*, 729–738. [CrossRef]
18. Dutta, D.; Heo, I.; Clevers, H. Disease modeling in stem cell-derived 3D organoid systems. *Trends Mol. Med.* **2017**, *23*, 393–410. [CrossRef]
19. Ho, B.X.; Pek, N.M.Q.; Soh, B.-S. Disease modeling using 3D organoids derived from human induced pluripotent stem cells. *Int. J. Mol. Sci.* **2018**, *19*, 936. [CrossRef]
20. Clevers, H. Modeling development and disease with organoids. *Cell* **2016**, *165*, 1586–1597. [CrossRef]
21. Kaushik, G.; Ponnusamy, M.P.; Batra, S.K. Concise Review: Current status of three-dimensional organoids as preclinical models. *Stem Cells* **2018**, *36*, 1329–1340. [CrossRef] [PubMed]
22. Simian, M.; Bissell, M.J. Organoids: A historical perspective of thinking in three dimensions. *J. Cell Boil.* **2016**, *216*, 31–40. [CrossRef]
23. Abbott, A. Biology's new dimension. *Nature* **2003**, *424*, 870–872. [CrossRef] [PubMed]
24. Kelm, J.M.; Fussenegger, M. Microscale tissue engineering using gravity-enforced cell assembly. *Trends Biotechnol.* **2004**, *22*, 195–202. [CrossRef] [PubMed]
25. Jafari, M.; Paknejad, Z.; Rad, M.R.; Motamedian, S.R.; Eghbal, M.J.; Nadjmi, N.; Khojasteh, A. Polymeric scaffolds in tissue engineering: A literature review. *J. Biomed. Mater. Res. Part B Appl. Biomater.* **2015**, *105*, 431–459. [CrossRef]

26. Nickerson, C.A.; Goodwin, T.J.; Terlonge, J.; Ott, C.M.; Buchanan, K.L.; Uicker, W.C.; Emami, K.; Leblanc, C.L.; Ramamurthy, R.; Clarke, M.S.; et al. Three-dimensional tissue assemblies: Novel models for the study of *Salmonella enterica* serovar Typhimurium pathogenesis. *Infect. Immun.* **2001**, *69*, 7106–7120. [CrossRef]
27. Frantz, C.; Stewart, K.M.; Weaver, V.M. The extracellular matrix at a glance. *J. Cell Sci.* **2010**, *123*, 4195–4200. [CrossRef]
28. Middendorp, S.; Schneeberger, K.; Wiegerinck, C.L.; Mokry, M.; Akkerman, R.D.L.; van Wijngaarden, S.; Clevers, H.; Nieuwenhuis, E.E.S. Adult stem cells in the small intestine are intrinsically programmed with their location-specific function. *Stem Cells* **2014**, *32*, 1083–1091. [CrossRef]
29. Lancaster, M.A.; Knoblich, J.A. Organogenesis in a dish: Modeling development and disease using organoid technologies. *Science* **2014**, *345*, 1247125. [CrossRef]
30. Crosnier, C.; Stamataki, D.; Lewis, J. Organizing cell renewal in the intestine: Stem cells, signals and combinatorial control. *Nat. Rev. Genet.* **2006**, *7*, 349–359. [CrossRef]
31. Barbara, P.D.S.; Brink, G.R.V.D.; Roberts, U.J. Development and differentiation of the intestinal epithelium. *Cell. Mol. Life Sci.* **2003**, *60*, 1322–1332. [CrossRef] [PubMed]
32. Vanuytsel, T.; Senger, S.; Fasano, A.; Shea-Donohue, T. Major signaling pathways in intestinal stem cells. *Biochim. Biophys. Acta Gen. Subj.* **2012**, *1830*, 2410–2426. [CrossRef] [PubMed]
33. Barker, N.; Van Es, J.H.; Kuipers, J.; Kujala, P.; Born, M.V.D.; Cozijnsen, M.; Haegebarth, A.; Korving, J.; Begthel, H.; Peters, P.J.; et al. Identification of stem cells in small intestine and colon by marker gene Lgr5. *Nature* **2007**, *449*, 1003–1007. [CrossRef]
34. Ootani, A.; Li, X.; Sangiorgi, E.; Ho, Q.T.; Ueno, H.; Toda, S.; Sugihara, H.; Fujimoto, K.; Weissman, I.L.; Capecchi, M.R.; et al. Sustained in vitro intestinal epithelial culture within a Wnt-dependent stem cell niche. *Nat. Med.* **2009**, *15*, 701–706. [CrossRef] [PubMed]
35. Yui, S.; Nakamura, T.; Sato, T.; Nemoto, Y.; Mizutani, T.; Zheng, X.; Ichinose, S.; Nagaishi, T.; Okamoto, R.; Tsuchiya, K.; et al. Functional engraftment of colon epithelium expanded in vitro from a single adult Lgr5+ stem cell. *Nat. Med.* **2012**, *18*, 618–623. [CrossRef] [PubMed]
36. Fukuda, M.; Mizutani, T.; Mochizuki, W.; Matsumoto, T.; Nozaki, K.; Sakamaki, Y.; Ichinose, S.; Okada, Y.; Tanaka, T.; Watanabe, M.; et al. Small intestinal stem cell identity is maintained with functional Paneth cells in heterotopically grafted epithelium onto the colon. *Genes Dev.* **2014**, *28*, 1752–1757. [CrossRef] [PubMed]
37. Spence, J.R.; Mayhew, C.N.; Rankin, S.A.; Kuhar, M.F.; Vallance, J.E.; Tolle, K.; Hoskins, E.E.; Kalinichenko, V.V.; Wells, S.I.; Zorn, A.M.; et al. Directed differentiation of human pluripotent stem cells into intestinal tissue in vitro. *Nature* **2010**, *470*, 105–109. [CrossRef] [PubMed]
38. McCracken, K.W.; Howell, J.C.; Wells, J.; Spence, J.R. Generating human intestinal tissue from pluripotent stem cells in vitro. *Nat. Protoc.* **2011**, *6*, 1920–1928. [CrossRef]
39. Watson, C.L.; Mahé, M.M.; Múnera, J.; Howell, J.C.; Sundaram, N.; Poling, H.M.; Schweitzer, J.I.; Vallance, J.E.; Mayhew, C.N.; Sun, Y.; et al. An in vivo model of human small intestine using pluripotent stem cells. *Nat. Med.* **2014**, *20*, 1310–1314. [CrossRef]
40. Múnera, J.O.; Sundaram, N.; Rankin, S.A.; Hill, D.R.; Watson, C.; Mahe, M.; Vallance, J.E.; Shroyer, N.F.; Sinagoga, K.L.; Zarzoso-Lacoste, A.; et al. Differentiation of human pluripotent stem cells into colonic organoids via transient activation of BMP signaling. *Cell Stem Cell* **2017**, *21*, 51–64. [CrossRef]
41. Kedinger, M.; Haffen, K.; Simon-Assmann, P. Intestinal tissue and cell cultures. *Differentiation* **1987**, *36*, 71–85. [CrossRef] [PubMed]
42. Aboseif, S.; El-Sakka, A.I.; Young, P.; Cunha, G.R. Mesenchymal reprogramming of adult human epithelial differentiation. *Differentiation* **1999**, *65*, 113–118. [CrossRef] [PubMed]
43. Mithal, A.; Capilla, A.; Heinze, D.; Berical, A.; Villacorta-Martin, C.; Vedaie, M.; Jacob, A.; Abo, K.M.; Szymaniak, A.; Peasley, M.; et al. Generation of mesenchyme free intestinal organoids from human induced pluripotent stem cells. *Nat. Commun.* **2020**, *11*, 215. [CrossRef] [PubMed]
44. Finkbeiner, S.R.; Hill, D.R.; Altheim, C.H.; Dedhia, P.; Taylor, M.J.; Tsai, Y.-H.; Chin, A.M.; Mahé, M.M.; Watson, C.L.; Freeman, J.J.; et al. Transcriptome-wide analysis reveals hallmarks of human intestine development and maturation in vitro and in vivo. *Stem Cell Rep.* **2015**, *4*, 1140–1155. [CrossRef]
45. Aurora, M.; Spence, J.R. hPSC-derived lung and intestinal organoids as models of human fetal tissue. *Dev. Boil.* **2016**, *420*, 230–238. [CrossRef]
46. McCauley, H.; Wells, J. Pluripotent stem cell-derived organoids: Using principles of developmental biology to grow human tissues in a dish. *Development* **2017**, *144*, 958–962. [CrossRef]

47. Dotti, I.; Salas, A. Potential Use of human stem cell-derived intestinal organoids to study inflammatory bowel diseases. *Inflamm. Bowel Dis.* **2018**, *24*, 2501–2509.
48. Dotti, I.; Mora-Buch, R.; Ferrer-Picón, E.; Planell, N.; Jung, P.; Masamunt, M.C.; Leal, R.F.; De Carpi, J.M.; Llach, J.; Ordas, I.; et al. Alterations in the epithelial stem cell compartment could contribute to permanent changes in the mucosa of patients with ulcerative colitis. *Gut* **2016**, *66*, 2069–2079. [CrossRef]
49. Freire, R.; Ingano, L.; Serena, G.; Cetinbas, M.; Anselmo, A.; Sapone, A.; Sadreyev, R.I.; Fasano, A.; Senger, S. Human gut derived-organoids provide model to study gluten response and effects of microbiota-derived molecules in celiac disease. *Sci. Rep.* **2019**, *9*, 7029. [CrossRef]
50. Almeqdadi, M.; Mana, M.; Roper, J.; Yilmaz, Ö.H. Gut organoids: Mini-tissues in culture to study intestinal physiology and disease. *Am. J. Physiol. Physiol.* **2019**, *317*, C405–C419. [CrossRef]
51. Senger, S.; Ingano, L.; Freire, R.; Anselmo, A.; Zhu, W.; Sadreyev, R.; Walker, W.A.; Fasano, A. Human fetal-derived enterospheres provide insights on intestinal development and a novel model to study necrotizing enterocolitis (NEC). *Cell. Mol. Gastroenterol. Hepatol.* **2018**, *5*, 549–568. [CrossRef] [PubMed]
52. Rouch, J.D.; Scott, A.; Lei, N.Y.; Solorzano-Vargas, R.S.; Wang, J.; Hanson, E.M.; Kobayashi, M.; Lewis, M.; Stelzner, M.G.; Dunn, J.C.Y.; et al. Development of functional microfold (M) cells from intestinal stem cells in primary human enteroids. *PLoS ONE* **2016**, *11*, e0148216. [CrossRef] [PubMed]
53. Grün, M.; Lyubimova, A.; Kester, L.; Wiebrands, K.; Basak, O.; Sasaki, N.; Clevers, H.; Van Oudenaarden, A. Single-cell messenger RNA sequencing reveals rare intestinal cell types. *Nature* **2015**, *525*, 251–255. [CrossRef] [PubMed]
54. Haber, A.L.; Biton, M.; Rogel, N.; Herbst, R.H.; Shekhar, K.; Smillie, C.; Burgin, G.; DeLorey, T.; Howitt, M.R.; Katz, Y.; et al. A single-cell survey of the small intestinal epithelium. *Nature* **2017**, *551*, 333–339. [CrossRef]
55. Moon, C.; VanDussen, K.L.; Miyoshi, H.; Stappenbeck, T.S. Development of a primary mouse intestinal epithelial cell monolayer culture system to evaluate factors that modulate IgA transcytosis. *Mucosal Immunol.* **2013**, *7*, 818–828. [CrossRef]
56. VanDussen, K.L.; Marinshaw, J.M.; Shaikh, N.; Miyoshi, H.; Moon, C.; Tarr, P.I.; Ciorba, M.A.; Stappenbeck, T.S. Development of an enhanced human gastrointestinal epithelial culture system to facilitate patient-based assays. *Gut* **2014**, *64*, 911–920. [CrossRef]
57. Kozuka, K.; He, Y.; Koo-McCoy, S.; Kumaraswamy, P.; Nie, B.; Shaw, K.; Chan, P.; Leadbetter, M.; He, L.; Lewis, J.G.; et al. Development and characterization of a human and mouse intestinal epithelial cell monolayer platform. *Stem Cell Rep.* **2017**, *9*, 1976–1990. [CrossRef]
58. Hee, V.D.B.; Loonen, L.; Taverne, N.; Taverne-Thiele, J.; Smidt, H.; Wells, J.M. Optimized procedures for generating an enhanced, near physiological 2D culture system from porcine intestinal organoids. *Stem Cell Res.* **2018**, *28*, 165–171.
59. Verma, S.; Prescott, R.A.; Ingano, L.; Nickerson, K.P.; Hill, E.; Faherty, C.S.; Fasano, A.; Senger, S.; Cherayil, B.J. The YrbE phospholipid transporter of *Salmonella enterica* serovar Typhi regulates the expression of flagellin and influences motility, adhesion and induction of epithelial inflammatory responses. *Gut Microbes* **2019**, 1–13. [CrossRef]
60. Liu, Y.; Qi, Z.; Li, X.; Du, Y.; Chen, Y.-G. Monolayer culture of intestinal epithelium sustains Lgr5+ intestinal stem cells. *Cell Discov.* **2018**, *4*, 32. [CrossRef]
61. Thorne, C.A.; Chen, I.W.; Sanman, L.E.; Cobb, M.H.; Wu, L.F.; Altschuler, S.J. Enteroid monolayers reveal an autonomous WNT and BMP circuit controlling intestinal epithelial growth and organization. *Dev. Cell* **2018**, *44*, 624–633. [CrossRef]
62. Altay, G.; Larrañaga, E.; Tosi, S.; Barriga, F.M.; Batlle, E.; Fernández-Majada, V.; Martínez, E. Self-organized intestinal epithelial monolayers in crypt and villus-like domains show effective barrier function. *Sci. Rep.* **2019**, *9*. [CrossRef]
63. Wang, Y.; Disalvo, M.; Gunasekara, D.B.; Dutton, J.; Proctor, A.; Lebhar, M.S.; Williamson, I.A.; Speer, J.; Howard, R.L.; Smiddy, N.M.; et al. Self-renewing monolayer of primary colonic or rectal epithelial cells. *Cell. Mol. Gastroenterol. Hepatol.* **2017**, *4*, 165–182. [CrossRef] [PubMed]
64. Liu, X.; Lu, R.; Wu, S.; Sun, J. *Salmonella* regulation of intestinal stem cells through the Wnt/β-catenin pathway. *FEBS Lett.* **2010**, *584*, 911–916. [CrossRef]
65. Zhang, Y.; Wu, S.; Xia, Y.; Sun, J. *Salmonella*-infected crypt-derived intestinal organoid culture system for host–bacterial interactions. *Physiol. Rep.* **2014**, *2*, e12147. [CrossRef]

66. Sato, T.; Van Es, J.H.; Snippert, H.J.; Stange, D.; Vries, R.G.; Born, M.V.D.; Barker, N.; Shroyer, N.F.; Van De Wetering, M.; Clevers, H. Paneth cells constitute the niche for Lgr5 stem cells in intestinal crypts. *Nature* **2010**, *469*, 415–418. [CrossRef] [PubMed]
67. Drost, J.; Van Jaarsveld, R.; Ponsioen, B.; Zimberlin, C.; Van Boxtel, R.; Buijs, A.; Sachs, N.; Overmeer, R.M.; Offerhaus, G.J.; Begthel, H.; et al. Sequential cancer mutations in cultured human intestinal stem cells. *Nature* **2015**, *521*, 43–47. [CrossRef]
68. Williams, K.E.; Lemieux, G.A.; Hassis, M.E.; Olshen, A.B.; Fisher, S.J.; Werb, Z. Quantitative proteomic analyses of mammary organoids reveals distinct signatures after exposure to environmental chemicals. *Proc. Natl. Acad. Sci. USA* **2016**, *113*, E1343–E1351. [CrossRef]
69. Yilmaz, Ö.H.; Katajisto, P.; Lamming, D.W.; Gültekin, Y.; Bauer-Rowe, K.E.; Sengupta, S.; Birsoy, K.; Dursun, A.; Yilmaz, V.O.; Selig, M.; et al. mTORC1 in the Paneth cell niche couples intestinal stem-cell function to calorie intake. *Nature* **2012**, *486*, 490–495. [CrossRef] [PubMed]
70. Forbester, J.L.; Goulding, D.; Vallier, L.; Hannan, N.R.F.; Hale, C.; Pickard, D.; Mukhopadhyay, S.; Dougan, G. Interaction of *Salmonella enterica* serovar Typhimurium with intestinal organoids derived from human induced pluripotent stem cells. *Infect. Immun.* **2015**, *83*, 2926–2934. [CrossRef] [PubMed]
71. Nickerson, K.; Senger, S.; Zhang, Y.; Lima, R.; Patel, S.; Ingano, L.; Flavahan, W.; Kumar, D.; Fraser, C.; Faherty, C.S.; et al. *Salmonella* Typhi colonization provokes extensive transcriptional changes aimed at evading host mucosal immune defense during early infection of human intestinal tissue. *EBioMedicine* **2018**, *31*, 92–109. [CrossRef] [PubMed]
72. Onuma, K.; Ochiai, M.; Orihashi, K.; Takahashi, M.; Imai, T.; Nakagama, H.; Hippo, Y. Genetic reconstitution of tumorigenesis in primary intestinal cells. *Proc. Natl. Acad. Sci. USA* **2013**, *110*, 11127–11132. [CrossRef] [PubMed]
73. Higginson, E.E.; Ramachandran, G.; Panda, A.; Shipley, S.T.; Kriel, E.H.; DeTolla, L.J.; Lipsky, M.; Perkins, D.J.; Salerno-Gonçalves, R.; Sztein, M.B.; et al. Improved tolerability of a *Salmonella enterica* serovar Typhimurium live-attenuated vaccine strain achieved by balancing inflammatory potential with immunogenicity. *Infect. Immun.* **2018**, *86*, e00440-18. [CrossRef] [PubMed]
74. Roy, P.; Canet-Jourdan, C.; Annereau, M.; Zajac, O.; Gelli, M.; Broutin, S.; Mercier, L.; Paci, A.; Lemare, F.; Ducreux, M.; et al. Organoids as preclinical models to improve intraperitoneal chemotherapy effectiveness for colorectal cancer patients with peritoneal metastases: Preclinical models to improve HIPEC. *Int. J. Pharm.* **2017**, *531*, 143–152. [CrossRef] [PubMed]
75. Llanos-Chea, A.; Citorik, R.J.; Nickerson, K.P.; Ingano, L.; Serena, G.; Senger, S.; Lu, T.K.; Fasano, A.; Faherty, C.S. Bacteriophage therapy testing against *Shigella flexneri* in a novel human intestinal organoid-derived infection model. *J. Pediatr. Gastroenterol. Nutr.* **2019**, *68*, 509–516. [CrossRef]
76. Dekkers, J.F.; Wiegerinck, C.L.; De Jonge, H.R.; Bronsveld, I.; Janssens, H.M.; Groot, K.M.D.W.-D.; Brandsma, A.M.; De Jong, N.W.; Bijvelds, M.J.; Scholte, B.J.; et al. A functional CFTR assay using primary cystic fibrosis intestinal organoids. *Nat. Med.* **2013**, *19*, 939–945. [CrossRef]
77. Callejón, R.M.; Rodríguez-Naranjo, M.I.; Ubeda, C.; Hornedo-Ortega, R.; García-Parrilla, M.C.; Troncoso, A.M. Reported foodborne outbreaks due to fresh produce in the United States and European Union: Trends and causes. *Foodborne Pathog. Dis.* **2015**, *12*, 32–38. [CrossRef]
78. Stanaway, J.D.; Reiner, R.C.; Blacker, B.F.; Goldberg, E.M.; Khalil, I.A.; Troeger, C.E.; Andrews, J.R.; Bhutta, Z.A.; Crump, J.A.; Im, J.; et al. The global burden of typhoid and paratyphoid fevers: A systematic analysis for the global burden of disease study 2017. *Lancet Infect. Dis.* **2019**, *19*, 369–381. [CrossRef]
79. Tsolis, R.M.; Young, G.M.; Solnick, J.; Bäumler, A.J. From bench to bedside: Stealth of enteroinvasive pathogens. *Nat. Rev. Genet.* **2008**, *6*, 883–892. [CrossRef]
80. Parry, C.M.; Hein, T.T.; Dougan, G.; White, N.J.; Farrar, J.J. Typhoid fever. *N. Engl. J. Med.* **2002**, *347*, 1770–1782. [CrossRef]
81. Anderson, C.; Kendall, M.M. *Salmonella enterica* Serovar Typhimurium strategies for host adaptation. *Front. Microbiol.* **2017**, *8*, 1983. [CrossRef] [PubMed]
82. Feasey, N.; Dougan, G.; Kingsley, R.A.; Heyderman, R.S.; Gordon, M.A. Invasive non-typhoidal *Salmonella* disease: An emerging and neglected tropical disease in Africa. *Lancet* **2012**, *379*, 2489–2499. [CrossRef]
83. Dhanoa, A.; Fatt, Q.K. Non-typhoidal *Salmonella* bacteraemia: Epidemiology, clinical characteristics and its' association with severe immunosuppression. *Ann. Clin. Microbiol. Antimicrob.* **2009**, *8*, 15. [CrossRef]

84. Brent, A.; Oundo, J.O.; Mwangi, I.; Ochola, L.; Lowe, B.; Berkley, J.A. *Salmonella* bacteremia in Kenyan children. *Pediatr. Infect. Dis. J.* **2006**, *25*, 230–236. [CrossRef]
85. Majowicz, S.E.; Musto, J.; Scallan, E.; Angulo, F.J.; Kirk, M.D.; O'Brien, S.J.; Jones, T.F.; Fazil, A.; Hoekstra, R.M. The global burden of nontyphoidal *Salmonella* gastroenteritis. *Clin. Infect. Dis.* **2010**, *50*, 882–889. [CrossRef]
86. Antillon, M.; Warren, J.L.; Crawford, F.W.; Weinberger, D.M.; Kürüm, E.; Pak, G.D.; Marks, F.; Pitzer, V.E. The burden of typhoid fever in low- and middle-income countries: A meta-regression approach. *PLOS Negl. Trop. Dis.* **2017**, *11*, e0005376. [CrossRef]
87. DeRoeck, D.; Jódar, L.; Clemens, J. Putting typhoid vaccination on the global health agenda. *N. Engl. J. Med.* **2007**, *357*, 1069–1071. [CrossRef] [PubMed]
88. Galan, J.E.; Curtiss, R. Cloning and molecular characterization of genes whose products allow *Salmonella* Typhimurium to penetrate tissue culture cells. *Proc. Natl. Acad. Sci. USA* **1989**, *86*, 6383–6387. [CrossRef] [PubMed]
89. Tsolis, R.M.; Adams, L.G.; Ficht, T.A.; Bäumler, A.J. Contribution of *Salmonella* Typhimurium virulence factors to diarrheal disease in calves. *Infect. Immun.* **1999**, *67*, 4879–4885. [CrossRef]
90. Ibarra, J.A.; Steele-Mortimer, O. *Salmonella*—The ultimate insider. *Salmonella virulence factors that modulate intracellular survival. Cell. Microbiol.* **2009**, *11*, 1579–1586.
91. Finiay, B.B.; Falkow, S. *Salmonella* as an intracellular parasite. *Mol. Microbiol.* **1989**, *3*, 1833–1841. [CrossRef] [PubMed]
92. Richter-Dahlfors, A.; Buchan, A.; Finlay, B.B. Murine salmonellosis studied by confocal microscopy: *Salmonella* Typhimurium resides intracellularly inside macrophages and exerts a cytotoxic effect on phagocytes in vivo. *J. Exp. Med.* **1997**, *186*, 569–580. [CrossRef] [PubMed]
93. Swart, A.L.; Hensel, M. Interactions of *Salmonella enterica* with dendritic cells. *Virulence* **2012**, *3*, 660–667. [CrossRef] [PubMed]
94. Wu, J.; Sabag-Daigle, A.; Borton, M.A.; Kop, L.F.M.; Szkoda, B.E.; Kaiser, B.L.D.; Lindemann, S.R.; Renslow, R.S.; Wei, S.; Nicora, C.D.; et al. *Salmonella*-mediated inflammation eliminates competitors for fructose-asparagine in the gut. *Infect. Immun.* **2018**, *86*, e00945-17. [CrossRef]
95. Thiennimitr, P.; Winter, S.E.; Winter, M.G.; Xavier, M.N.; Tolstikov, V.; Huseby, U.L.; Sterzenbach, T.; Tsolis, R.M.; Roth, J.R.; Bäumler, A.J. Intestinal inflammation allows *Salmonella* to use ethanolamine to compete with the microbiota. *Proc. Natl. Acad. Sci. USA* **2011**, *108*, 17480–17485. [CrossRef]
96. Winter, S.E.; Thiennimitr, P.; Winter, M.G.; Butler, B.P.; Huseby, U.L.; Crawford, R.W.; Russell, J.M.; Bevins, C.L.; Adams, L.G.; Tsolis, R.M.; et al. Gut inflammation provides a respiratory electron acceptor for *Salmonella*. *Nature* **2010**, *467*, 426–429. [CrossRef]
97. Winter, S.E.; Winter, M.G.; Poon, V.; Keestra, A.M.; Sterzenbach, T.; Faber, F.; Costa, L.F.; Cassou, F.; Costa, E.A.; Alves, G.E.S.; et al. *Salmonella enterica* serovar Typhi conceals the invasion-associated type three secretion system from the innate immune system by gene regulation. *PLoS Pathog.* **2014**, *10*, e1004207. [CrossRef]
98. Wangdi, T.; Lee, C.-Y.; Spees, A.M.; Yu, C.; Kingsbury, D.D.; Winter, S.E.; Hastey, C.J.; Wilson, R.P.; Heinrich, V.; Bäumler, A.J. The Vi capsular polysaccharide enables *Salmonella enterica* serovar Typhi to evade microbe-guided neutrophil chemotaxis. *PLoS Pathog.* **2014**, *10*, e1004306. [CrossRef]
99. Spadoni, I.; Zagato, E.; Bertocchi, A.; Paolinelli, R.; Hot, E.; Di Sabatino, A.; Caprioli, F.; Bottiglieri, L.; Oldani, A.; Viale, G.; et al. A gut-vascular barrier controls the systemic dissemination of bacteria. *Science* **2015**, *350*, 830–834. [CrossRef]
100. Hornick, R.B.; Greisman, S.E.; Woodward, T.E.; DuPont, H.L.; Dawkins, A.T.; Snyder, M.J. Typhoid fever: Pathogenesis and immunologic control. *N. Engl. J. Med.* **1970**, *283*, 686–691. [CrossRef]
101. Shukla, V.; Singh, H.; Pandey, R.; Upadhyay, S.; Nath, G. Carcinoma of the Gallbladder—Is it a sequel of typhoid? *Dig. Dis. Sci.* **2000**, *45*, 900–903. [CrossRef] [PubMed]
102. Caygill, C.; Hill, M.; Braddick, M.; Sharp, J. Cancer mortality in chronic typhoid and paratyphoid carriers. *Lancet* **1994**, *343*, 83–84. [CrossRef]
103. Mughini-Gras, L.; Schaapveld, M.; Kramers, J.; Mooij, S.; Neefjes-Borst, E.A.; Van Pelt, W.; Neefjes, J. Increased colon cancer risk after severe *Salmonella* infection. *PLoS ONE* **2018**, *13*, e0189721. [CrossRef] [PubMed]
104. Connerton, I.F.; Wain, J.; Hien, T.T.; Ali, T.; Parry, C.; Chinh, N.T.; Vinh, H.; Ho, V.A.; Diep, T.S.; Day, N.P.J.; et al. Epidemic typhoid in Vietnam: Molecular typing of multiple-antibiotic-resistant *Salmonella enterica* serotype Typhi from four outbreaks. *J. Clin. Microbiol.* **2000**, *38*, 895–897. [CrossRef]

105. Molloy, A.; Nair, S.; Cooke, F.J.; Wain, J.; Farrington, M.; Lehner, P.J.; Torok, E. First report of *Salmonella enterica* serotype Paratyphi A azithromycin resistance leading to treatment failure. *J. Clin. Microbiol.* **2010**, *48*, 4655–4657. [CrossRef]
106. Rowe, B.; Ward, L.R.; Threlfall, E.J. Multidrug-resistant *Salmonella* Typhi: A worldwide epidemic. *Clin. Infect. Dis.* **1997**, *24*, S106–S109. [CrossRef]
107. Wang, X.; Biswas, S.; Paudyal, N.; Pan, H.; Li, X.; Fang, W.; Yue, M. Antibiotic resistance in *Salmonella* Typhimurium isolates recovered from the food chain through national antimicrobial resistance monitoring system between 1996 and 2016. *Front. Microbiol.* **2019**, *10*, 985. [CrossRef]
108. Gopinath, S.; Lichtman, J.; Bouley, N.M.; Elias, J.E.; Monack, D.M. Role of disease-associated tolerance in infectious superspreaders. *Proc. Natl. Acad. Sci. USA* **2014**, *111*, 15780–15785. [CrossRef]
109. Diard, M.; Sellin, M.E.; Dolowschiak, T.; Arnoldini, M.; Ackermann, M.; Hardt, W.-D. Antibiotic treatment selects for cooperative virulence of *Salmonella* Typhimurium. *Curr. Boil.* **2014**, *24*, 2000–2005. [CrossRef]
110. Wotzka, S.Y.; Nguyen, B.D.; Hardt, W.-D. *Salmonella* Typhimurium diarrhea reveals basic principles of enteropathogen infection and disease-promoted DNA exchange. *Cell Host Microbe* **2017**, *21*, 443–454. [CrossRef]
111. Acosta, C.J.; Galindo, C.; Deen, J.; Ochiai, R.; Lee, H.; Von Seidlein, L.; Carbis, R.; Clemens, J.; Ochiai, L. Vaccines against cholera, typhoid fever and shigellosis for developing countries. *Expert Opin. Boil. Ther.* **2004**, *4*, 1939–1951. [CrossRef] [PubMed]
112. Ageing United Nations. Available online: https://www.un.org/en/sections/issues-depth/ageing/ (accessed on 9 February 2020).
113. Featured Graphic: Many Countries' Populations Are Aging—Population Reference Bureau. Available online: https://www.prb.org/insight/featured-graphic-many-countries-populations-are-aging/ (accessed on 9 February 2020).
114. Verma, S.; Srikanth, C.V. Understanding the complexities of *Salmonella*-host crosstalk as revealed by in vivo model organisms. *IUBMB Life* **2015**, *67*, 482–497. [CrossRef] [PubMed]
115. Criss, A.K.; Ahlgren, D.M.; Jou, T.S.; McCormick, B.A.; Casanova, J.E. The GTPase Rac1 selectively regulates *Salmonella* invasion at the apical plasma membrane of polarized epithelial cells. *J. Cell Sci.* **2001**, *114*, 1331–1341.
116. Sun, H.; Chow, E.C.; Liu, S.; Du, Y.; Pang, K.S. The Caco-2 cell monolayer: Usefulness and limitations. *Expert Opin. Drug Metab. Toxicol.* **2008**, *4*, 395–411. [CrossRef] [PubMed]
117. Sambuy, Y.; De Angelis, I.; Ranaldi, G.; Scarino, M.L.; Stammati, A.; Zucco, F. The Caco-2 cell line as a model of the intestinal barrier: Influence of cell and culture-related factors on Caco-2 cell functional characteristics. *Cell Boil. Toxicol.* **2005**, *21*, 1–26. [CrossRef] [PubMed]
118. Grossmann, J. Progress on isolation and short-term ex-vivo culture of highly purified non-apoptotic human intestinal epithelial cells (IEC). *Eur. J. Cell Boil.* **2003**, *82*, 262–270. [CrossRef]
119. Aldhous, M.C.; Shmakov, A.N.; Bode, J.; Ghosh, S. Characterization of conditions for the primary culture of human small intestinal epithelial cells. *Clin. Exp. Immunol.* **2001**, *125*, 32–40. [CrossRef]
120. Santos, R.L.; Tsolis, R.M.; Zhang, S.; Ficht, T.A.; Bäumler, A.J.; Adams, L.G. *Salmonella*-induced cell death is not required for enteritis in calves. *Infect Immun.* **2001**, *69*, 4610–4617. [CrossRef]
121. Santos, R.D.L.; Zhang, S.; Tsolis, R.M.; Bäumler, A.J.; Adams, L.G. Morphologic and Molecular Characterization of *Salmonella* Typhimurium infection in neonatal calves. *Veter Pathol.* **2002**, *39*, 200–215. [CrossRef]
122. Jepson, M.A.; Kenny, B.; Leard, A.D. Role of sipA in the early stages of *Salmonella* Typhimurium entry into epithelial cells. *Cell Microbiol.* **2001**, *3*, 417–426. [CrossRef] [PubMed]
123. Zhang, S.; Santos, R.D.L.; Tsolis, R.M.; Stender, S.; Hardt, W.-D.; Bäumler, A.J.; Adams, L.G. The *Salmonella enterica* serotype Typhimurium effector proteins SipA, SopA, SopB, SopD, and SopE2 act in concert to induce diarrhea in calves. *Infect. Immun.* **2002**, *70*, 3843–3855. [CrossRef]
124. Santos, R.D.L.; Zhang, S.; Tsolis, R.M.; Kingsley, R.A.; Adams, L.G.; Bäumler, A.J. Animal models of *Salmonella* infections: Enteritis versus typhoid fever. *Microbes Infect.* **2001**, *3*, 1335–1344. [CrossRef]
125. Barthel, M.; Hapfelmeier, S.; Quintanilla-Martinez, L.; Kremer, M.; Rohde, M.; Hogardt, M.; Pfeffer, K.; Rüssmann, H.; Hardt, W.-D. Pretreatment of mice with streptomycin provides a *Salmonella enterica* serovar Typhimurium colitis model that allows analysis of both pathogen and host. *Infect. Immun.* **2003**, *71*, 2839–2858. [CrossRef] [PubMed]

126. Virlogeux-Payant, I.; Waxin, H.; Ecobichon, C.; Popoff, M.Y. Role of the viaB locus in synthesis, transport and expression of *Salmonella* Typhi Vi antigen. *Microbiology* **1995**, *141*, 3039–3047. [CrossRef] [PubMed]
127. Sabbagh, S.C.; Forest, C.G.; Lepage, C.; Leclerc, J.-M.; Daigle, F. So similar, yet so different: Uncovering distinctive features in the genomes of *Salmonella enterica* serovars Typhimurium and Typhi. *FEMS Microbiol. Lett.* **2010**, *305*, 1–13. [CrossRef] [PubMed]
128. Mian, M.F.; Pek, E.A.; Chenoweth, M.; Coombes, B.K.; Ashkar, A. Humanized mice for *Salmonella* Typhi infection: New tools for an old problem. *Virulence* **2011**, *2*, 248–252. [CrossRef] [PubMed]
129. Libby, S.J.; Brehm, M.A.; Greiner, D.L.; Shultz, L.D.; McClelland, M.; Smith, K.D.; Cookson, B.T.; Karlinsey, J.E.; Kinkel, T.L.; Porwollik, S.; et al. Humanized non-obese diabetic-scid IL2rγnull mice are susceptible to lethal *Salmonella* Typhi infection. *Proc. Natl. Acad. Sci. USA* **2010**, *107*, 15589–15594. [CrossRef]
130. Bhaduri, A.; Andrews, M.G.; Leon, W.M.; Jung, D.; Shin, D.; Allen, D.; Jung, D.; Schmunk, G.; Haeussler, M.; Salma, J.; et al. Cell stress in cortical organoids impairs molecular subtype specification. *Nature* **2020**, *578*, 142–148. [CrossRef]
131. Farin, H.F.; Karthaus, W.R.; Kujala, P.; Rakhshandehroo, M.; Schwank, G.; Vries, R.G.; Kalkhoven, E.; Nieuwenhuis, E.E.; Clevers, H. Paneth cell extrusion and release of antimicrobial products is directly controlled by immune cell–derived IFN-γ. *J. Exp. Med.* **2014**, *211*, 1393–1405. [CrossRef]
132. Wilson, S.S.; Tocchi, A.; Holly, M.K.; Parks, W.C.; Smith, J.G. A small intestinal organoid model of non-invasive enteric pathogen-epithelial cell interactions. *Mucosal Immunol.* **2014**, *8*, 352–361. [CrossRef]
133. Wilson, C.L.; Ouellette, A.J.; Satchell, D.P.; Ayabe, T.; López-Boado, Y.S.; Stratman, J.L.; Hultgren, S.J.; Matrisian, L.M.; Parks, W.C. Regulation of intestinal-defensin activation by the metalloproteinase Matrilysin in innate host defense. *Science* **1999**, *286*, 113–117. [CrossRef] [PubMed]
134. Bevins, C.L.; Salzman, N. Paneth cells, antimicrobial peptides and maintenance of intestinal homeostasis. *Nat. Rev. Genet.* **2011**, *9*, 356–368. [CrossRef] [PubMed]
135. Scanu, T.; Spaapen, R.M.; Bakker, J.M.; Pratap, C.B.; Wu, L.-E.; Hofland, I.; Broeks, A.; Shukla, V.K.; Kumar, M.; Janssen, H.; et al. *Salmonella* manipulation of host signaling pathways provokes cellular transformation associated with gallbladder carcinoma. *Cell Host Microbe* **2015**, *17*, 763–774. [CrossRef] [PubMed]
136. Kuo, S.-C.; Hu, Y.-W.; Liu, C.-J.; Lee, Y.-T.; Chen, Y.-T.; Chen, T.-L.; Chen, T.-J.; Fung, C.-P. Association between tuberculosis infections and non-pulmonary malignancies: A nationwide population-based study. *Br. J. Cancer* **2013**, *109*, 229–234. [CrossRef] [PubMed]
137. Zhan, P.; Suo, L.-J.; Qian, Q.; Shen, X.-K.; Qiu, L.-X.; Yu, L.; Song, Y. Chlamydia pneumoniae infection and lung cancer risk: A meta-analysis. *Eur. J. Cancer* **2011**, *47*, 742–747. [CrossRef] [PubMed]
138. Arnheim-Dahlström, L.; Andersson, K.; Luostarinen, T.; Thoresen, S.; Ögmundsdottír, H.; Tryggvadottir, L.; Wiklund, F.; Skare, G.B.; Eklund, C.; Sjölin, K.; et al. Prospective seroepidemiologic study of uman Papillomavirus and other risk factors in cervical cancer. *Cancer Epidemiol. Biomark. Prev.* **2011**, *20*, 2541–2550. [CrossRef] [PubMed]
139. Gagnaire, A.; Nadel, B.; Raoult, D.; Neefjes, J.; Gorvel, J. Collateral damage: Insights into bacterial mechanisms that predispose host cells to cancer. *Nat. Rev. Genet.* **2017**, *15*, 109–128. [CrossRef]
140. Lu, X.; Xie, S.; Ye, L.; Zhu, L.; Yu, Q. *Lactobacillus* protects against *S.* Typhimurium –induced intestinal inflammation by determining the fate of epithelial proliferation and differentiation. *Mol. Nutr. Food Res.* **2020**, *64*, e1900655. [CrossRef]
141. Li, P.; Yu, Q.; Ye, X.; Wang, Z.; Yang, Q. *Lactobacillus* S-layer protein inhibition of *Salmonella*-induced reorganization of the cytoskeleton and activation of MAPK signalling pathways in Caco-2 cells. *Microbiology* **2011**, *157*, 2639–2646. [CrossRef]
142. Forbester, J.L.; Lees, E.A.; Goulding, D.; Forrest, S.; Yeung, A.; Speak, A.O.; Clare, S.; Coomber, E.L.; Mukhopadhyay, S.; Kraiczy, J.; et al. Interleukin-22 promotes phagolysosomal fusion to induce protection against *Salmonella enterica* Typhimurium in human epithelial cells. *Proc. Natl. Acad. Sci. USA* **2018**, *115*, 10118–10123. [CrossRef]
143. Pham, T.A.N.; Clare, S.; Goulding, D.; Arasteh, J.M.; Stares, M.D.; Browne, H.P.; Keane, J.A.; Page, A.; Kumasaka, N.; Kane, L.; et al. Epithelial IL-22RA1-mediated fucosylation promotes intestinal colonization resistance to an opportunistic pathogen. *Cell Host Microbe* **2014**, *16*, 504–516. [CrossRef] [PubMed]
144. Co, J.Y.; Margalef-Català, M.; Li, X.; Mah, A.T.; Kuo, C.J.; Monack, D.M.; Amieva, M. Controlling epithelial polarity: A human enteroid model for host-pathogen interactions. *Cell Rep.* **2019**, *26*, 2509–2520. [CrossRef] [PubMed]

145. Salerno-Gonçalves, R.; Kayastha, D.; Fasano, A.; Levine, M.M.; Sztein, M.B. Crosstalk between leukocytes triggers differential immune responses against *Salmonella enterica* serovars Typhi and Paratyphi. *PLOS Negl. Trop. Dis.* **2019**, *13*, e0007650. [CrossRef] [PubMed]
146. Salerno-Gonçalves, R.; Galen, J.E.; Levine, M.M.; Fasano, A.; Sztein, M.B. Manipulation of *Salmonella* Typhi gene expression impacts innate cell responses in the human intestinal mucosa. *Front. Immunol.* **2018**, *9*, 2543. [CrossRef] [PubMed]
147. Schulte, L.N.; Schweinlin, M.; Westermann, A.J.; Janga, H.; Santos, S.C.; Appenzeller, S.; Walles, H.; Vogel, J.; Metzger, M. An advanced human intestinal coculture model reveals compartmentalized host and pathogen strategies during *Salmonella* infection. *mBio* **2020**, *11*, e03348-19. [CrossRef] [PubMed]
148. Dougan, G.; Baker, S. *Salmonella enterica* serovar Typhi and the pathogenesis of typhoid fever. *Annu. Rev. Microbiol.* **2014**, *68*, 317–336. [CrossRef]
149. Gjorevski, N.; Sachs, N.; Manfrin, A.; Giger, S.; Bragina, M.E.; Ordóñez-Morán, P.; Clevers, H.; Lutolf, M.P. Designer matrices for intestinal stem cell and organoid culture. *Nature* **2016**, *539*, 560–564. [CrossRef]
150. Holloway, E.M.; Capeling, M.M.; Spence, J.R. Biologically inspired approaches to enhance human organoid complexity. *Development* **2019**, *146*, dev166173. [CrossRef]
151. Dutton, J.S.; Hinman, S.S.; Kim, R.; Wang, Y.; Allbritton, N.L. Primary cell-derived intestinal models: Recapitulating physiology. *Trends Biotechnol.* **2019**, *37*, 744–760. [CrossRef]
152. Lai, N.Y.; Mills, K.; Chiu, I.M. Sensory neuron regulation of gastrointestinal inflammation and bacterial host defence. *J. Intern. Med.* **2017**, *282*, 5–23. [CrossRef]
153. Lai, N.Y.; Musser, M.A.; Pinho-Ribeiro, F.A.; Baral, P.; Jacobson, A.; Ma, P.; Potts, D.E.; Chen, Z.; Paik, D.; Soualhi, S.; et al. Gut-innervating nociceptor neurons regulate Peyer's patch Microfold cells and SFB levels to mediate *Salmonella* host defense. *Cell* **2020**, *180*, 33–49. [CrossRef] [PubMed]
154. Workman, M.J.; Mahé, M.M.; Trisno, S.; Poling, H.M.; Watson, C.L.; Sundaram, N.; Chang, C.-F.; Schiesser, J.; Aubert, P.; Stanley, E.G.; et al. Engineered human pluripotent-stem-cell-derived intestinal tissues with a functional enteric nervous system. *Nature Med.* **2016**, *23*, 49–59. [CrossRef] [PubMed]
155. Thiennimitr, P.; Winter, S.E.; Bäumler, A.J. *Salmonella*, the host and its microbiota. *Curr. Opin. Microbiol.* **2011**, *15*, 108–114. [CrossRef]
156. Karve, S.S.; Pradhan, S.; Ward, Y.V.; Weiss, A.A. Intestinal organoids model human responses to infection by commensal and Shiga toxin producing *Escherichia coli*. *PLoS ONE* **2017**, *12*, e0178966. [CrossRef] [PubMed]
157. Leslie, J.; Huang, S.; Opp, J.S.; Nagy, M.S.; Kobayashi, M.; Young, V.B.; Spence, J.R. Persistence and toxin production by *Clostridium difficile* within human intestinal organoids result in disruption of epithelial paracellular barrier function. *Infect. Immun.* **2014**, *83*, 138–145. [CrossRef] [PubMed]
158. Le Blay, G.; Rytka, J.; Zihler, A.; Lacroix, C. New in vitro colonic fermentation model for *Salmonella* infection in the child gut. *FEMS Microbiol. Ecol.* **2009**, *67*, 198–207. [CrossRef] [PubMed]

13

Metabolic Activation of CsgD in the Regulation of *Salmonella* Biofilms

Akosiererem S. Sokaribo [1,2], Elizabeth G. Hansen [1], Madeline McCarthy [1,2], Taseen S. Desin [2,3], Landon L. Waldner [1], Keith D. MacKenzie [4,5], George Mutwiri Jr. [1], Nancy J. Herman [1], Dakoda J. Herman [1], Yejun Wang [6] and Aaron P. White [1,2,*]

1 Vaccine and Infectious Disease Organization-International Vaccine Centre, University of Saskatchewan, Saskatoon, SK S7N 5E3, Canada; ats172@mail.usask.ca (A.S.S.); egh367@mail.usask.ca (E.G.H.); mcm876@mail.usask.ca (M.M.); landonwaldner@hotmail.com (L.L.W.); gmm777@mail.usask.ca (G.M.J.); nfairburn@msn.com (N.J.H.); dakoda.herman@mail.utoronto.ca (D.J.H.)

2 Department of Biochemistry, Microbiology and Immunology, University of Saskatchewan, Saskatoon, SK S7N 5E5, Canada; taseen.desin@usask.ca

3 Basic Sciences Department, King Saud bin Abdulaziz University for Health Sciences, Riyadh 11481, Saudi Arabia

4 Institute for Microbial Systems and Society, Faculty of Science, University of Regina, Regina, SK S4S 0A2, Canada; keith.mackenzie@uregina.ca

5 Department of Biology, University of Regina, Regina, SK S4S 0A2, Canada

6 Department of Cell Biology and Genetics, School of Basic Medicine, Shenzhen University Health Science, Shenzhen 518060, China; wangyj@szu.edu.cn

* Correspondence: aaron.white@usask.ca

Abstract: Among human food-borne pathogens, gastroenteritis-causing *Salmonella* strains have the most real-world impact. Like all pathogens, their success relies on efficient transmission. Biofilm formation, a specialized physiology characterized by multicellular aggregation and persistence, is proposed to play an important role in the *Salmonella* transmission cycle. In this manuscript, we used luciferase reporters to examine the expression of *csgD*, which encodes the master biofilm regulator. We observed that the CsgD-regulated biofilm system responds differently to regulatory inputs once it is activated. Notably, the CsgD system became unresponsive to repression by Cpx and H-NS in high osmolarity conditions and less responsive to the addition of amino acids. Temperature-mediated regulation of *csgD* on agar was altered by intracellular levels of RpoS and cyclic-di-GMP. In contrast, the addition of glucose repressed CsgD biofilms seemingly independent of other signals. Understanding the fine-tuned regulation of *csgD* can help us to piece together how regulation occurs in natural environments, knowing that all *Salmonella* strains face strong selection pressures both within and outside their hosts. Ultimately, we can use this information to better control *Salmonella* and develop strategies to break the transmission cycle.

Keywords: biofilm; *Salmonella*; CsgD; curli; cellulose; CpxR

---

1. Introduction

Salmonella enterica strains that cause gastroenteritis and typhoid fever were recently ranked first and second in terms of global disease impact (i.e., disability adjusted life years) among 22 of the most common food borne pathogens [1]. *S. enterica* strains are distributed within >2000 serovars, with yearly estimates of approximately 94 million cases of gastroenteritis [2] and 21 million cases of typhoid fever worldwide [3]. The serovars associated with typhoid fever (i.e., Typhi, Paratyphi and few others [4]) consist of human-restricted strains and are collectively referred to as typhoidal *Salmonella* (TS). The serovars associated with gastroenteritis (i.e., Typhimurium, Enteritidis and >1600 others) consist of host-generalist strains and are collectively referred to as nontyphoidal *Salmonella* (NTS) [5]. NTS outbreaks are relatively common occurrences and are often linked to the consumption of contaminated food produce, such as poultry [6,7], fruits, vegetables [8,9] and processed foods [10]. In general, NTS strains have a remarkable ability to persist and survive in harsh conditions, including extremes of drying and nutrient limitation [11–13].

The majority of NTS strains can form biofilms, a specialized physiology that is characterized by multicellular aggregation, long-term survival, and resistance. Biofilm formation has been linked to *Salmonella* persistence on food surfaces, plants, and other produce, and is thought to provide protection during food processing [14–16]. Aside from the food-borne aspects, biofilm formation is hypothesized to be an integral part of the life cycle of gastroenteritis-causing *Salmonella* strains, by ensuring long-term survival of cells as they cycle between hosts and the environment [14,17]. We have speculated that biofilms are connected to the host generalist lifestyle since the environment (soil and water) would be a common collecting point for multiple host species. In contrast, there is widespread loss of biofilm formation in TS strains and other more invasive strains, such as the specialized NTS strains associated with human bloodstream infections in sub-Saharan Africa [18,19], although TS produce alternative biofilms on gallstones inside human carriers [20]. There are multiple selection pressures acting on biofilm formation in diverse *Salmonella* strains. In short, biofilms are thought to represent the most dominant form of bacterial life on the planet and understanding the regulation of this specialized physiology is important.

Biofilm-forming strains of *S. enterica* can be identified by the production of distinct rdar (red, dry and rough) morphotype colonies when grown on agar-containing media supplemented with the dye Congo red. Cells within the colony are held together by curli fimbriae for short-range interactions and cellulose for long-range interactions [12,21,22]. In addition, other polymers are part of the extracellular biofilm matrix, including polysaccharides (i.e., O-Ag capsule, colanic acid and cellulose) proteins (i.e., BapA, curli, and flagella), lipopolysaccharides and DNA [8,23]. Curli, cellulose and the biofilm matrix impart survival and persistence properties on cells within the biofilm [12–14]. It is not known if the survival traits are specific to the polymers themselves or are emergent properties associated with cells entering a unique physiological state [24–26]. Perhaps the microenvironments generated within a biofilm are responsible for the adaptations, heterogeneity and cellular differentiation observed during biofilm formation [27,28].

In *Salmonella*, regulation of curli, cellulose and other polymers is coordinated through CsgD, the main transcriptional controller of biofilms. The activation of CsgD in vitro has been well-defined, with growth conditions of low osmolarity, lower temperatures and limiting nutrients necessary to activate *csgD* transcription [29]. Expression of *csgD* is repressed tightly at early stages of growth but is induced up to 370-fold when cells enter the stationary phase of growth [30]. The same general principles apply in *E. coli*, which shares the CsgD, curli, and cellulose biofilm components [31]. In the stationary phase of growth, cell density in the culture is high, nutrients become limiting and cells express the alternative sigma factor RpoS [32]. RpoS controls the general stress response [33] and selectively transcribes *csgD* [34,35]. The effects of osmolarity are mediated through the EnvZ/OmpR and CpxA/CpxR two-component signal transduction systems [36]. In low osmolarity, low levels of phosphorylated OmpR bind to a high-affinity binding site −50.5 bp upstream of the *csgD* transcription start sites, which activates *csgD* transcription [37]. In high osmolarity, transcription is repressed through binding of phosphorylated CpxR to multiple sites on the *csgD* promoter [36], as well as phosphorylated OmpR binding to a low-affinity site in the *csgD* promoter [38]. We realized that the complex regulatory network behind *csgD* activation [8] was even more dynamic when it was discovered that CsgD was produced in a bistable manner [39–41]. Biofilm cells are maintained in a CsgD-ON state due to a predicted feed-forward loop consisting of RpoS, CsgD and IraP, a protein that stabilizes RpoS [35,42]. The remaining single cells are in a CsgD-OFF state and express several important virulence factors [14]. The connection between persistence and virulence during biofilm formation brings into question the hierarchical regulation of this process, as well as determining how individual cells become activated and remain in their CsgD-ON or -OFF states.

The regulation of *Salmonella* biofilms is also strongly influenced by the intracellular levels of the second messenger, cyclic-di-GMP (c-di-GMP). It is synthesized from two guanosine 5′-triphosphate molecules by diguanylate cyclases (DGCs) and degraded by specific phosphodiesterases (PDEs). In general, high levels of c-di-GMP are associated with biofilm formation, sessility and persistence, and low levels of c-di-GMP are associated with motility and virulence [43]. The change in c-di-GMP levels in *S. enterica* is controlled by the enzymatic activity of 17 different DGCs and PDEs. For biofilms, the cellulose synthase enzyme, BcsA, is allosterically activated by c-di-GMP that is produced by AdrA, a DGC that is transcriptionally activated by CsgD. Expression of CsgD itself is influenced by c-di-GMP synthesis and breakdown by a network of DGC and PDE enzymes [44]. The importance of c-di-GMP regulation is underscored by the observation that *S. enterica* isolates that are defective in the production of DGCs are both avirulent and unable to form biofilms [45].

In this manuscript, we analyzed the regulation of *csgD* transcription and the activity of CsgD through activation of curli biosynthesis (*csgBAC*) and cellulose production (*adrA*). We examined the response to different environmental signals (i.e., temperature, osmolarity, nutrients) and discovered that there is a hierarchy of regulation. These environmental signals were selected because their effects on csgD expression before induction have been well established and we hypothesize that these conditions would be encountered during food processing and in both host and non-host environments. We established that the CsgD system responds differently or not at all to known regulatory inputs once it has been activated. This is similar to some dedicated, point of no return processes, such as sporulation in *Bacillus subtilis* [46]; however, we show that the CsgD system can be reversed by other signals, such as glucose. The implications for the *Salmonella* lifecycle are discussed.

2. Materials and Methods

2.1. Bacterial Strains, Media, and Growth Conditions

The bacterial strains used in this study are listed in Table 1. For standard growth, strains were inoculated from frozen stocks onto LB agar (lysogeny broth, 1% NaCl, 1.5% agar) supplemented with appropriate antibiotic (50 μg mL^{-1} kanamycin (Kan), or 5 μg mL^{-1} tetracycline (Tet)) and grown overnight at 37 °C. Isolated colonies were used to inoculate 5 mL LB broth and the culture was incubated for 18 h at 37 °C with agitation at 200 RPM.

Table 1. Strains and plasmids used in this study.

Strains or Plasmids	Genotype	Reference
Strains		
Salmonella enterica subsp. *enterica* serovar Typhimurium		
14028	Wild-type strain	ATCC
14028 Δ*cpxR*	Deletion of *cpxR*	This study
14028 Δ*iraP*	Deletion of *iraP*	This study
14028 Δ*rpoS*	Deletion of *rpoS*	[12]
Plasmids		
pCS26, pU220	Bacterial luciferase	[47]
pCS26-*stm1987*::*luxCDABE*	*stm1987* promoter	This study
pU220-*cpxP*::*luxCDABE*	*cpxP* promoter	This study
pU220-*csgD*::*luxCDABE*	*csgDEFG* promoter	[12]
pCS26-*csgB*::*luxCDABE*	*csgBAC* promoter	[12]
pCS26-*adrA*::*luxCDABE*	*adrA* promoter	[12]
pBR322		
pBR322/*stm1987*	*stm1987*^14028	This study
pBR322/*yhjH*	*yhjH*^14028	This study
pACYC184		
pACYC/*rpoS*	*rpoS*^14028	[48]

For analysis of colony morphology and gene expression, 4 μl of overnight culture was spotted on 1% tryptone agar supplemented with 0.2% freshly made glucose, 25 mM salt or 100 mM salt (agar supplemented with glucose were used within 24 h). Plates were incubated at 28 °C or 37 °C for two days. Visible and luminescence images were captured with a spectrum CT in vivo imaging system (PerkinElmer, Waltham, MA, USA).

2.2. *Generation of* S. typhimurium *14028 Mutant Strains*

Lambda red recombination [49] was used to generate Δ*cpxR* and Δ*iraP S.* Typhimurium mutant strains. Primers containing 50-nuclelotide sequences on either side of *cpxR* or *iraP* (Table 2) were used to amplify the *cat* gene from pKD3 using Phusion high-fidelity DNA polymerase (New England Bio-Labs, Ipswich, MA, USA). The PCR products were solution purified and electroporated into *S.* Typhimurium 14028 cells containing pKD46. Mutants were first selected by growth at 37 °C on LB agar supplemented with 10 μg ml^{-1} chloramphenicol (Cam) before streaking onto LB agar containing 34 μg ml^{-1} Cam. PCR primers upstream and downstream of *cpxR* or *iraP* (Table 2) were used to amplify sequence from the genome of mutant *S. typhimurium* 14028 strains and verify loss of the corresponding open reading frames. The ΔcpxR or Δ*iraP* mutations were moved into a clean *S. typhimurium* strain background with P22 phage [50]. The *cat* gene was resolved from the chromosome using pCP20 [49].

Table 2. Oligonucleotides used in this study.

Primer	Sequence (5′–3′) [a]	Purpose
cpxRko sense	AAGATGCGCGCGGTTAAACTTCCT ATCATGAAGCGGAAACCATCAGATA GGTGTAGGCTGGAGCTGCTTC	To amplify *cat* gene product from pKD3 to generate Δ*cpxR* strain by lambda red recombination
cpxRko antisense	CCTGTTAGTTGATGATGACC GAGAGCTGACTTCCCTGTTAAAAGA GCTCCCCTCCTTAGTTCCTATTCCG	
cpxR ver F	CCAGCATTAGCACCAGCGCC	To confirm the deletion of *cpxR* from *S. typhimurium* 14028
cpxR ver R	TCTGCCTCGGAGGTACGTAAACA	
cpxR1	GCCCTCGAGGTAACTTTGCGCATCGCTTG	To amplify the *cpxR* and *cpxP* promoter regions from *S. typhimurium* 14028
cpxR2	GCCGGATCCTTCATTGTTTACGTACCTCCG	
iraPko sense	GGCAGTGGTTCTTCATAGTG ATAACGTCACCCTGGAACTAATAAGG AAATGTGTAGGCTGTAGCTGCTTC	To amplify *cat* gene product from pKD3 to generate Δ*iraP* strain by lambda red recombination
iraPko antisense	TGTTATTTCATAAAAGTAA CGTTATAACAACTGTGTTGTTTTAA ATACGACCTCCTTAGTTCCTATTCCG	
iraPko-detect1	CAAAAAGCGAAAGGCCAATA	To confirm the deletion of *iraP* from *S. typhimurium* 14028
iraPko-detect2	TAGCACCATCCTTTTGTCAG	
STM14_2408for1	GATCCTCGAGAAATTCGCGGTGTTTCGCAC	To amplify the *stm1987* promoter region from *S. typhimurium* 14028
STM14_2408rev2	GATCGGATCCCTAACAGTGTTTCGTGCGGC	
STM1987forEco	GATCGAATTCAAACGGTGTTTCGCAC	To amplify *stm1987* with native promoter region from *S. typhimurium* 14028
STM1987revAatII	GATCGACGTCGGACTATTTCTTTTCCCGCT	
yhjHforEco	GATCGAATTCTTGACAAGTTTCGGGGGCTG	To amplify *yhjH* with native promoter region from *S. typhimurium* 14028
yhjHrevAatll	GATCGACGTCGTATTACGGGAACAGTCTGG	
pZE05	CCAGCTGGCAATTCCGA	Used to verify promoter fusions to *luxCDABE*
pZE06	AATCATCACTTTCGGGAA	

[a] Nucleotide sequences corresponding to restriction enzyme sites are underlined.

2.3. *Generation of Bacterial Luciferase Reporters and Other Plasmid Vectors*

Luciferase fusion reporter plasmids containing the promoters of *csgDEFG*, *csgBAC* and *adrA* have been previously described [12]. The *cpxP* reporter plasmid was generated to monitor the levels of CpxA/CpxR activation within the cell. The intergenic region containing the *cpxR* and *cpxP* promoter sequences was PCR amplified from *S.* Typhimurium 14028 using primers cpxR1 and cpxR2 (Table 2) and Phusion high-fidelity DNA polymerase (New England BioLabs, Ipswich, MA, USA). The resulting PCR product was purified, sequentially digested with *Xho*I and *Bam*HI, and ligated (in the *cpxP* direction) using T4 DNA ligase (New England BioLabs, Ipswich, MA, USA) into pU220 digested with *Xho*I and *Bam*HI. The *stm1987* luciferase reporter plasmid was generated similarly using primers STM14_2408for1 and STM14_2408rev2 (Table 2), with cloning into pCS26. PCR screening with primers pZE05 and pZE06 was used to verify the successful fusion of promoter regions to *luxCDABE*.

For plasmid-based overexpression of cyclic-di-GMP related enzymes, fragments containing *stm1987* and *yhjH* genes with their native promoters were PCR amplified from *S. typhimurium* 14028 gDNA using Phusion high-fidelity DNA polymerase and appropriate primers (Table 2). Resulting PCR products were purified, digested with *Eco*RI and *Aat*II, and ligated using T4 DNA ligase into *Eco*RI/*Aat*II-digested pBR322. The pACYC-*rpoS* plasmid vector has previously been described [48]. Reporter plasmids and overexpression plasmids were co-transformed into *S. typhimurium* strains by electroporation and selected by growth at 37 °C on LB agar supplemented with 50 μg mL^{-1} Kan (pCS26) and 10 μg mL^{-1} Tet (pBR322 or pACYC).

2.4. Luciferase Reporter Assays

96-well bioluminescence assays were performed with *S.* Typhimurium luciferase reporter strains. Overnight cultures were diluted 1 in 600 into individual wells of black, clear bottom 96-well plates (9520 Costar; Corning Life Sciences, Tewksbury, MA, USA) containing 150 μL of 1% tryptone broth supplemented with 50 μg mL^{-1} of kanamycin (Kan). When noted, media was supplemented before growth with NaCl (25,150 mM), sucrose (50,150 mM), $CuCl_2$ (1 mM), casamino acids (12%) or individual amino acids (15 mM) to the final concentrations as indicated. For the addition of media supplements during growth, cells were inoculated into 135 μL of media and grown for 18 h at 28 °C before supplements were added as 15 μL aliquots to the appropriate wells. This included glucose ranging from 25–150 mM. To minimize evaporation of the media during the assays, cultures were overlaid with 50 μL of mineral oil per well. Cultures were assayed for absorbance (600 nm, 0.1 s) and luminescence (1s; in counts per second (CPS)) every 30 min during growth at 28 °C with agitation in a Victor X3 multilabel plate reader (Perkin-Elmer, Waltham, MA, USA).

3. Results

3.1. Osmolarity Has No Effect Once csgD Transcription Is Activated

Osmolarity is a key regulatory factor for Salmonella biofilm formation in vitro [29,51]. In the presence of high concentrations of NaCl, *csgD* transcription is abolished [52]. In *E. coli*, this repression is mediated through the CpxA/R two-component system [37]. We performed transcription experiments with *S. enterica* serovar Typhimurium ATCC 14028 (i.e., *S. typhimurium* 14028). Consistent with *E. coli*, expression of *csgD* was highest in low osmolarity media (i.e., no salt) and reduced sequentially in media supplemented with increasing concentrations of NaCl (Figure 1A). Reduced *csgD* expression in media supplemented with 75 mM or more salt correlated with basal expression of *csgBAC* (curli biosynthesis) and *adrA* (cellulose biosynthesis) (Figure 1B,C). To gauge the activity of the CpxA/R system, and its potential role in repression, we monitored expression of *cpxP*, a known regulatory target of CpxR [53]. Expression of cpxP was highest in media supplemented with 150 mM NaCl (Figure 1D), which was inversely correlated with *csgD* expression levels. This was consistent with CpxR-mediated repression of *csgD* transcription.

Regulation of *csgD* expression via the CpxA/R system is thought to be a dynamic process involving surface-sensing and feedback during curli production [36,54]. Therefore, we performed experiments where salt was added to growing cultures after 18 h of growth, rather than being premixed into the media before growth. At 18 h of growth, *csgD* expression level is rapidly increasing and *csgBAC* and *adrA* expression are just beginning to increase [26]. Under these conditions, *csgD* expression did not change when increasing concentrations of salt were added during growth; the expression curves were nearly superimposable regardless of the amount of salt added (Figure 1E). Expression of *csgBAC* was also not inhibited by the addition of salt and was actually increased at high salt concentrations (Figure 1F). For *adrA*, mild repression was observed, but expression was well above background levels, even in the presence of 150 mM salt (Figure 1G). *cpxP* expression, on the other hand, was similar to the premixed experiments, with highest expression in the 150 mM salt media and lowest expression in non-supplemented media (Figure 1H). These results indicated that the Cpx system was activated by the addition of salt during growth but was no longer causing repression of *csgD* transcription and the downstream genes involved in curli and cellulose production.

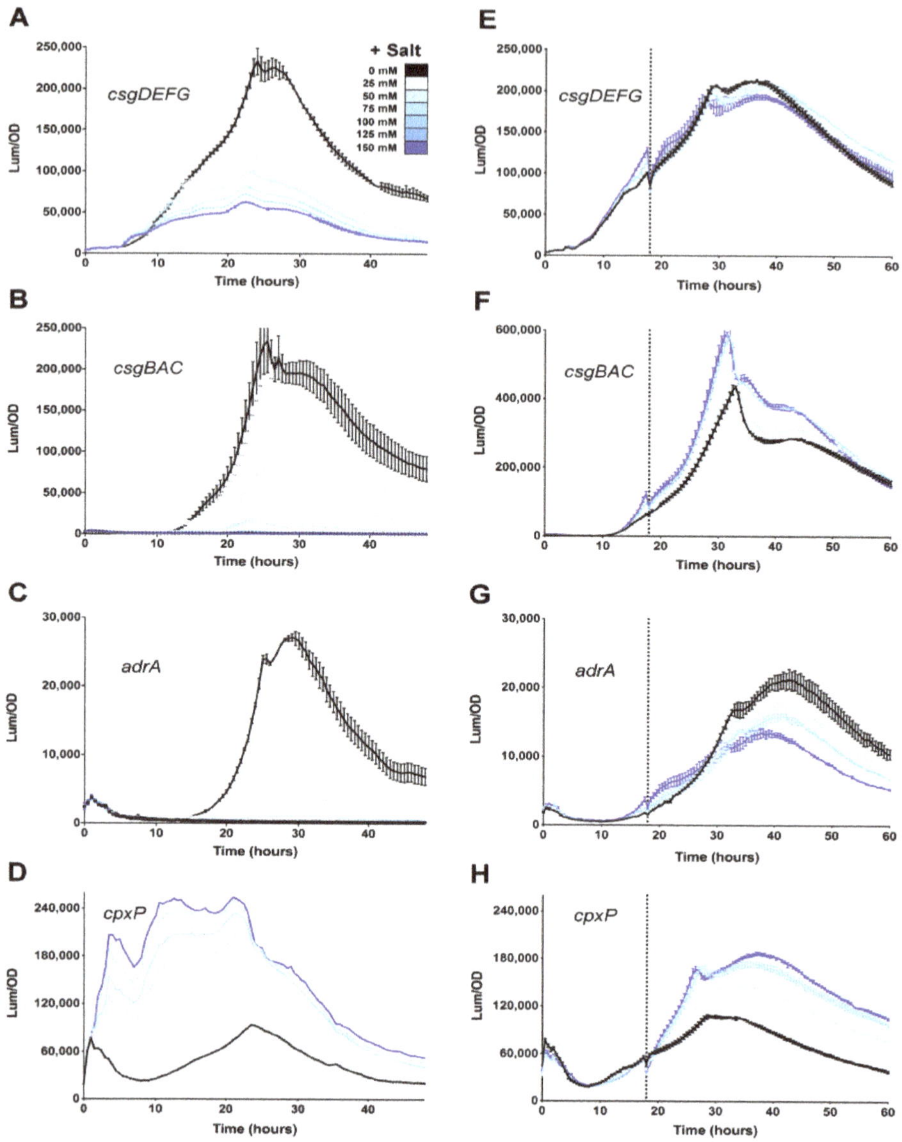

Figure 1. Response of the *Salmonella csgD* regulatory network to changes in osmolarity. *csgDEFG* (**A**,**E**), *csgBAC* (**B**,**F**), *adrA* (**C**,**G**), and *cpxP* (**D**,**H**) expression was measured in *S. typhimurium* 14028 during growth at 28 °C in media premixed with 25, 50, 75, 100, 125 or 150 mM salt (A–D) or with 50, 100, or 150 mM salt added during growth (E–H; vertical line shows the time of addition at 18 h). For each graph, luminescence (light counts per second) divided by the optical density at 600 nm (Lum/OD) was plotted as a function of time with each curve representing a single growth condition. The mean and standard deviations are plotted from experiments performed in triplicate (**A**–**C**, **E**–**H**) or from a single representative experiment (**D**).

3.2. Repressive Effect of CpxR on csgD Transcription Is Alleviated During Growth

To examine the effects of Cpx-mediated repression of *csgD* transcription in more detail, we monitored gene expression in a Δ*cpxR* mutant background. The Cpx system can be activated by high concentrations of metals and a variety of other signals, with each thought to represent a form of periplasmic stress [54,55]. Growth of *S. typhimurium* 14028 in media supplemented with 1 mM copper chloride resulted in activation of the Cpx system, as measured by an increase in *cpxP* expression (Figure 2A, + inducer). As expected, *cpxP* expression was off in the Δ*cpxR* strain background (Figure 2A, red line). In the presence of copper chloride, *csgD* expression reached high levels, similarly to when in the presence of non-supplemented media (Figure 2B). There was also a slight increase in the Δ*cpxR* strain, which was consistent with CpxR being a repressor of *csgD* transcription. This effect was more pronounced for *csgBAC*, as expression was approximately four times higher in the Δ*cpxR* strain (Figure 2C). We performed the same experiment with the addition of copper chloride after 18 h of growth. The Cpx system was activated normally, as shown by elevated *cpxP* expression levels in the presence of the inducer (Figure 2D). However, expression of *csgDEFG* and *csgBAC* was unchanged in the Δ*cpxR* mutant strain, showing no evidence of CpxR-mediated repression (Figure 2E,F). This indicated that once the *csgD* network was activated, the system was unresponsive to CpxR.

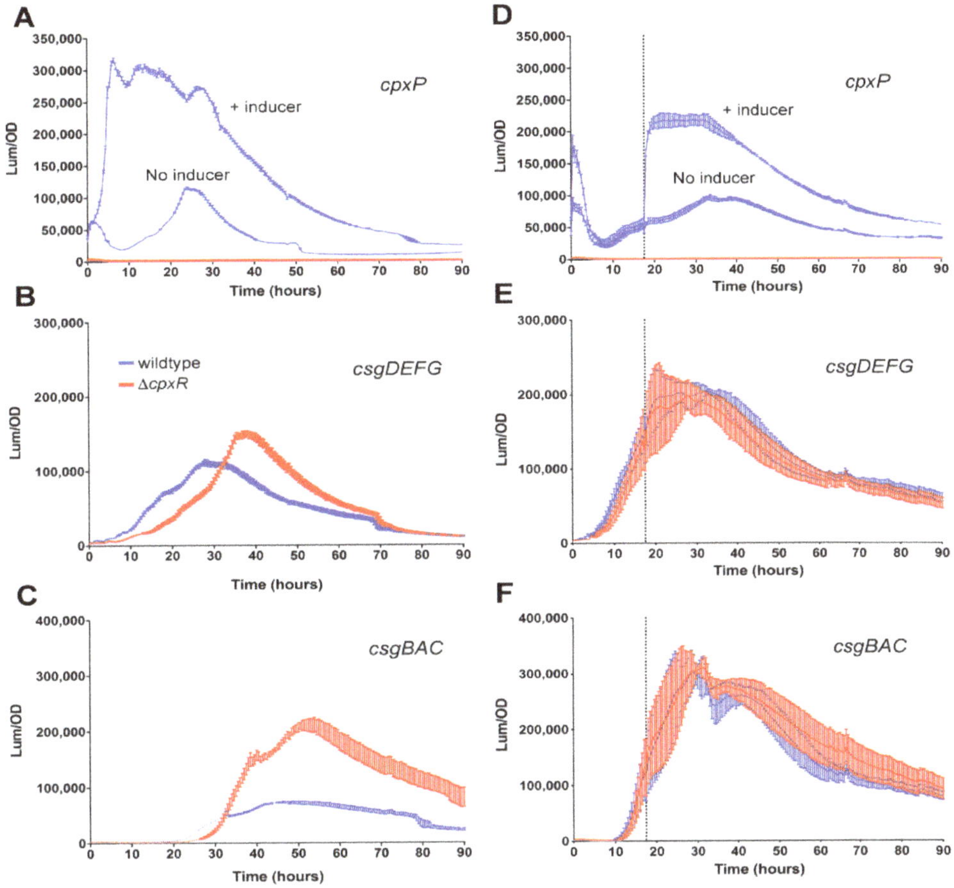

Figure 2. The Cpx system has no repressive effect on *csgD* transcription once the biofilm network is activated. Expression of *cpxP* (**A**,**D**), *csgDEFG* (**B**,**E**), and *csgBAC* (**C**,**F**) operons was measured during growth of *S. typhimurium* 14028 wild-type (blue) or Δ*cpxR* strains (red) at 28 °C in media supplemented with 1.0 mM $CuCl_2$ (+ inducer) added at the beginning of growth (**A**–**C**) or added after 18 h of growth (**D**–**F**; the vertical, dotted line represents the time of addition). For each graph, luminescence divided by the optical density at 600 nm (Lum/OD) was plotted as a function of time and each curve represents a single growth condition. The mean and standard deviations are plotted from three biological replicate experiments measured in triplicate.

We also measured biofilm gene expression after the addition of sucrose (Figure 3). In *E. coli*, sucrose has been shown to repress *csgD* transcription, due to the activity of H-NS [36]. Sucrose is also a cleaner measure of osmolarity because unlike salt, it does not result in a change of ionic strength. In general, the *csgDEFG*, *csgBAC* and *adrA* expression profiles were consistent with what was measured in response to salt addition. When sucrose was added to the media before growth, significant repression was observed for all three promoters (Figure 3A–C). However, when sucrose was added to growing cultures at 18 h, there was no repression measured (Figure 3E–G). The addition of sucrose had minimal effect on *cpxP* expression (Figure 3D,H), and, therefore, did not appear to engage the CpxR/A system, similar to what was observed in *E. coli* [36]. These results indicated that the *S. typhimurium csgD* biofilm network is not influenced by changes in osmolarity after it has been activated. Moreover, this appears to be a general effect that is not restricted to repression by the Cpx system.

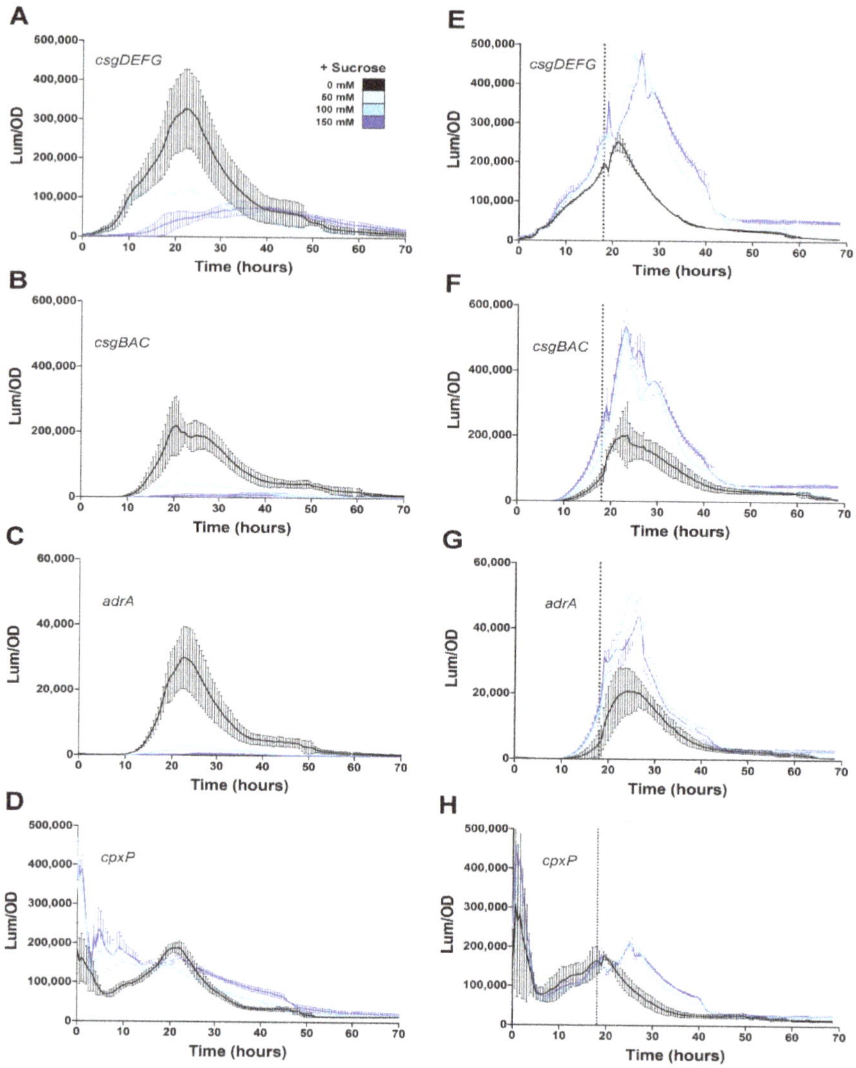

Figure 3. Effect of sucrose addition on the *Salmonella csgD* regulatory network. Expression of *csgDEFG* (**A**,**E**), *csgBAC* (**B**,**F**), *adrA* (**C**,**G**), and *cpxP* (**D**,**H**) operons was measured during growth of *S. typhimurium* 14028 at 28 °C in media premixed with 50, 100 or 150 mM sucrose (**A**–**D**) or with sucrose added during growth (**E**–**H**; vertical line represents the time of addition at 18 h). For each graph, luminescence (light counts per second) divided by the optical density at 600 nm (Lum/OD) is plotted as a function of time and each curve represents a single growth condition. The mean and standard deviations are plotted from three biological replicate experiments measured in triplicate.

3.3. Temperature and Glucose Repress csgD Expression

The idea that the biofilm system can become unresponsive to known regulatory inputs once it is activated fits with one of the hallmarks of a bistable gene expression system, in that a proportion of cells can remain activated even when the inducer is absent [56]. There are other bacterial physiologies, such as sporulation, where the cellular differentiation process is irreversible [46]. The *csgD* biofilm network has been shown to have bistable expression [40,42]. We wondered if the response we had observed with osmolarity was representative of a non-reversible system.

In most *Salmonella* and *E. coli* strains, *csgD* expression and biofilm formation is activated at temperatures below 30 °C and repressed at higher temperatures [52]. There are strains that produce biofilms at higher temperatures (i.e., 37 °C), but these typically possess single nucleotide polymorphisms in the *csgD* promoter region that allows for disregulated expression [50,52,57,58]. We tested whether increased temperature could shut off activated biofilm gene expression by first growing cells at 28 °C for 18 h and then shifting the temperature to 30, 32, 35, or 37 °C. At 30 °C or 32 °C, there was a measurable drop in *csgDEFG*, *csgBAC* and *adrA* expression, but it was still above background levels (Figure 4A–C). However, a temperature shift above 32 °C reduced gene expression to baseline levels (Figure 4A–C). This showed that high temperature was able to override the activation of *csgD* and biofilm related genes.

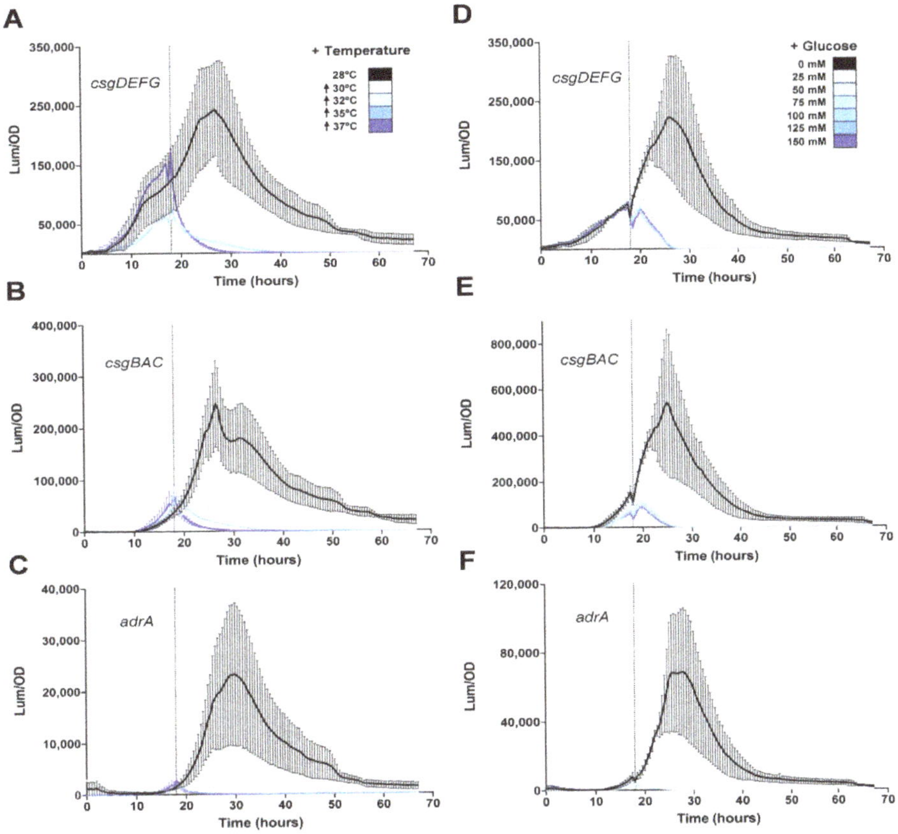

Figure 4. The *csgD* biofilm network in *Salmonella* is repressed by the addition of glucose or an increase in growth temperature. Expression of *csgDEFG* (**A**,**D**), *csgBAC* (**B**,**E**), and *adrA* (**C**,**F**) was measured during growth of *S. typhimurium* 14028 at 28 °C for 18 h prior to temperature shift (**A**–**C**) or the addition of 25, 50, 75, 100, 125, or 150 mM glucose (**D**–**F**). The vertical dotted line represents the time of temperature shift or glucose addition. For each graph, luminescence divided by the optical density at 600 nm (Lum/OD) is plotted as a function of time and each curve represents a single growth condition. The mean and standard deviations are plotted from three biological replicate experiments measured in triplicate.

Glucose is another powerful repressor of *csgD* expression and biofilm formation in vitro [26,59]. For *S. typhimurium*, the addition of glucose to growing cultures at 18 h rapidly abolished *csgDEFG* (Figure 4D), *csgBAC* (Figure 4E) and *adrA* (Figure 4F) expression, even at the lowest added concentration of 25 mM. We tested lower concentrations of glucose and found that in each case, *csgD* transcription was immediately repressed but was restored at later timepoints, presumably when all glucose was metabolized. This showed that glucose was a powerful repressive signal. Together, these experiments showed that activation of the *S.* Typhimurium *csgD* biofilm network is a reversible process and suggested the existence of a regulatory hierarchy.

3.4. Effect of Casamino Acids on Biofilm Formation

Expression of *csgD* is known to be activated once cells reach a critical density and nutrients start to run out [30]. Since 1% tryptone is primarily an amino acid-based media [60], we speculated that the addition of amino acids would reduce or delay expression of *csgD* and other biofilm genes. Casamino acids (CAA) are a complex mixture of amino acids and small peptides that are used for nutritional investigations of bacterial growth. The addition of CAA to the medium prior to *S.* Typhimurium growth reduced *csgDEFG* expression approximately 15-fold in the presence of 0.5, 1.0 or 2.0% CAA (Figure 5A). *csgBAC* and *adrA* expression dropped to near baseline levels when CAA was added at the beginning of growth (Figure 5B,C). The addition of CAA to growing *S. typhimurium* 14028 cultures also reduced the expression of all three promoters, but in a more dose-dependent manner. Expression of *csgDEFG* was reduced to ~75%, 50% and 25% of initial levels after the addition of 0.5% CAA, 1.0% CAA and 2% CAA, respectively (Figure 5D). Expression of *csgBAC* was reduced after the addition of 0.5% or 1.0% CAA, but the promoter was still considered active, whereas expression returned to baseline after the addition of 2.0% CAA (Figure 5E). *adrA* expression returned to near baseline levels, even with the addition of 0.5% CAA (Figure 5F). These experiments demonstrated that there is a metabolic feedback into *csgD* expression and that the system responds differently once it has been activated.

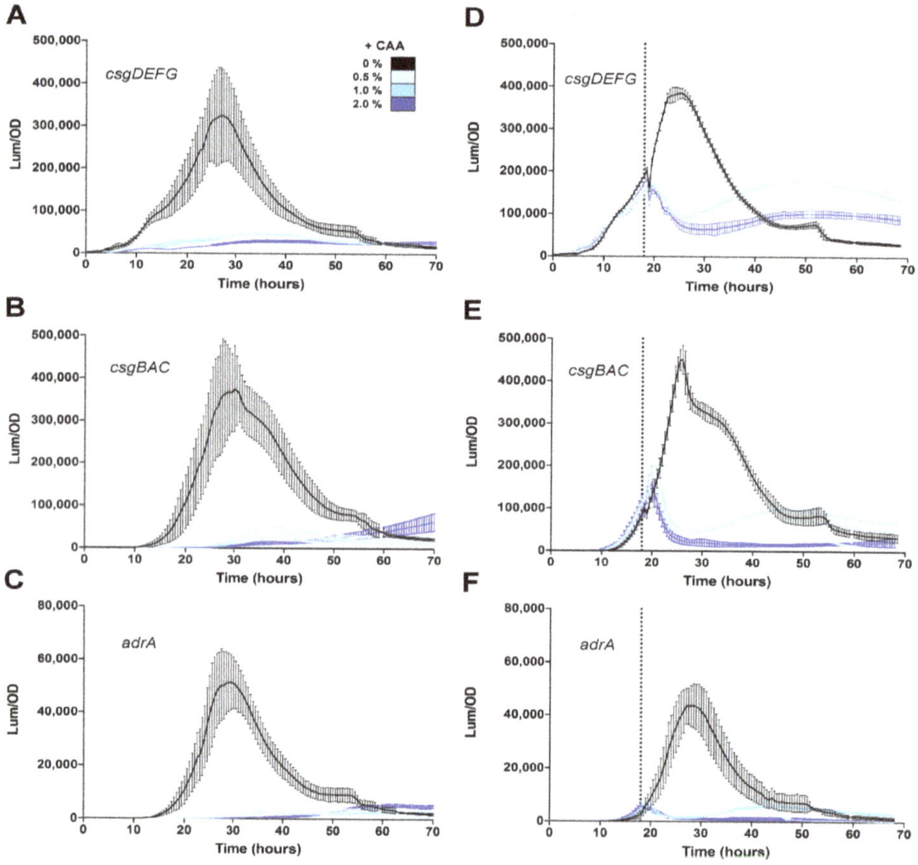

Figure 5. The *csgD* biofilm regulatory network in *Salmonella* is repressed by the addition of amino acids. Expression of *csgDEFG* (**A**,**D**), *csgBAC* (**B**,**E**), and *adrA* (**C**,**F**) was measured during growth of *S. typhimurium* 14028 at 28 °C in media premixed with 0.5%, 1.0% or 2.0% casamino acids (**A**–**C**) or in media where casamino acids were added during growth (D, E, F; the dotted line represents the time of addition at 18 h). For each graph, luminescence (light counts per second) divided by the optical density at 600 nm (Lum/OD) is plotted as a function of time and each curve represents a single growth condition. The mean and standard deviations are plotted from three biological replicate experiments measured in triplicate.

3.5. *Differing Effects of Individual Amino Acids on csgD Gene Expression*

We wanted to test how individual amino acids contributed to the repression of biofilm gene expression caused by CAA. We measured *csgBAC* expression i.e., curli production) as a proxy for biofilm formation and as readout for CsgD activity. Only Asn, Pro and Arg had a direct repressive effect on *csgBAC* expression when added individually (Figure 6A; blue bars). The expression curves were lower for the entirety of growth (Figure 6B). Six amino acids had no significant effect (Figure 6A, grey bars; examples in 6C) and seven amino acids caused an increase in expression (Figure 6A, pink bars). The addition of Gly and Thr yielded an approximately three-fold boost to *csgBAC* expression (Figure 6D), which was unexpected. These results indicated that the repression caused by CAA must have been due to the cumulative effect of multiple amino acids.

When individual amino acids were added to *S.* Typhimurium cultures after 18 h of growth, the effects on *csgBAC* expression were not predictable based on their previous groupings (Figure 6E; see color distribution). No amino acids caused a decrease in expression, and some that were repressive when added before growth (i.e., Arg, Pro), now caused a significant boost in expression (Figure 6E,F). Eight amino acids had no signficant difference from the water control (Figure 6G, Lys, Ser). Val, Ala, Gln and Thr led to increased *csgBAC* expression when added before or during growth, suggesting that these amino acids have a positive effect on curli fimbriae synthesis. Glycine, on the other hand, had no significant effect when added during growth (Figure 6H). Overall, we could not explain the differing effects of individual amino acids when added during growth. However, the results were consistent with our previous observation that the *S. typhimurium* biofilm network responds differently to regulatory inputs after the *csgD* network has been activated.

3.6. *Regulation of Rdar Morphotype on Agar-Containing Media*

In the bistable expression of CsgD, the proportion of cells in the "ON" state is thought to be maintained by a feed-forward loop consisting of RpoS, the stationary phase sigma factor that controls *csgD* transcription, IraP, a protein that stabilizes RpoS, and CsgD itself [35,42]. In addition, *csgD* expression and CsgD activity can be influenced by the bacterial secondary messenger, cyclic-di-GMP (c-di-GMP) [44]. We wanted to investigate how these additional regulatory components influenced metabolic control of the *S. typhimurium* biofilm regulatory network. Strains were grown at 28 °C or 37 °C on 1% tryptone agar, with different components added to the media. To modulate intracellular c-di-GMP levels, strains were transformed with plasmids over-expressing *stm1987*, encoding a DGC enzyme that generates c-di-GMP, or *yhjH*, encoding a PDE enzyme that breaks down c-di-GMP. To analyze the proposed feed-forward loop, we utilized a plasmid over-expressing RpoS and measured gene expression in Δ*rpoS* and Δ*iraP* strains. Each strain was transformed with a luciferase reporter plasmid so that we could visualize *csgBAC* expression.

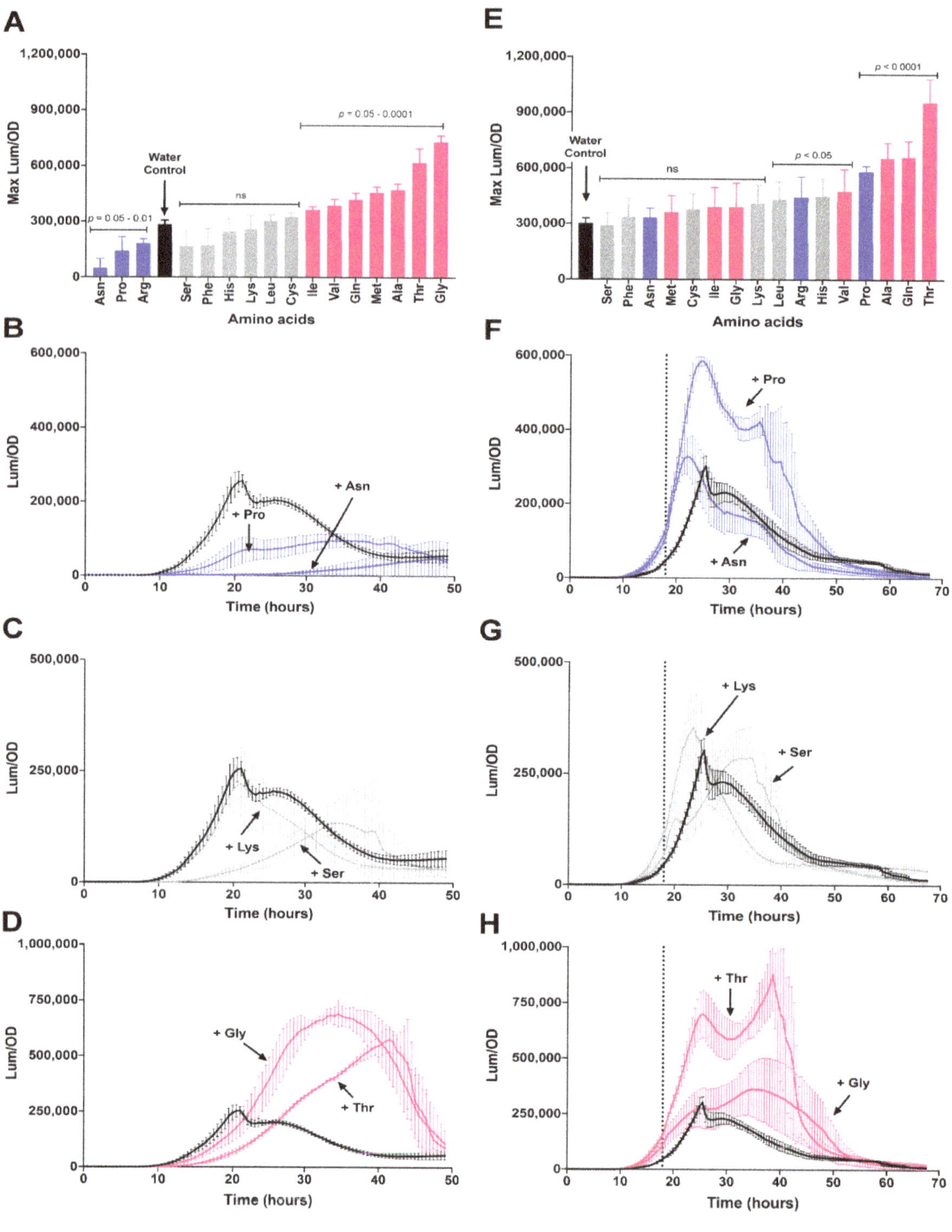

Figure 6. Individual amino acids have differing effects on the *csgD* biofilm regulatory network in *S. typhimurium* 14028. Maximum expression of the *csgBAC* operon (curli production) was recorded during growth of *S. typhimurium* 14028 at 28 °C in media premixed with 15 mM of individual amino acids (**A**) or in media where the amino acids were added after 18 h of growth. The maximum Lum/OD values after addition of each amino acid were statistically compared to a water control and amino acids were determined to have a repressive (blue), neutral (grey) or stimulatory effect (purple) on *csgB* expression (**A**). This color scheme was used to represent the same amino acids when they were added after 18 h of growth (**E**). Lum/OD values were plotted as a function of time corresponding to selected amino acids premixed into the media (**B**–**D**) or added at 18 h of growth (**F**–**H**; the dotted line represents the time of addition). For each curve, the mean and standard deviations are plotted from three biological replicate experiments measured in triplicate.

The vector-only *S*. Typhimurium 14028 control strain displayed robust light production at 28 °C, with faint *csgBAC* signals also observed in the presence of 25mM salt (Figure 7, vector). Over-expression of *rpoS* appeared to elevate *csgBAC* expression under most conditions, including in the presence of salt and at 37 °C (Figure 7, *rpoS*). The importance of RpoS was emphasized in that the Δ*rpoS* strain had no visible *csgBAC* expression under all tested conditions, unless it was co-transformed with pACYC/*rpoS* (Figure 7; 28 °C Δ*rpoS*). A strong stimulatory effect was also caused by over-expression of *stm1987*, which allowed for robust *csgBAC* expression and biofilm colony morphology under most conditions (Figure 7, *stm1987*). The strain transformed with pBR322/*stm1987* was the only one to have detectable *csgBAC* expression at 37 °C in the presence of 25 mM salt (Figure 7). This indicated that elevated levels of c-di-GMP may be enough to overcome temperature-based repression of *csgBAC*. Emphasizing the importance of c-di-GMP, the expression of *yhjH* was sufficient to abolish *csgBAC* expression at 28 °C (Figure 7, *yhjH*), as well as in all other tested conditions. In contrast, deletion of *iraP* appeared to have little effect on *csgBAC* expression, with only a mild reduction observed at 28 °C (Figure 7, *iraP*). Finally, the presence of glucose in the media abolished *csgBAC* expression in all strain and plasmid combinations (Figure 7, 0.2% Glc). This experiment indicated that increased levels of RpoS and c-di-GMP could partially overcome some *csgBAC* repression, and that glucose was perhaps the most powerful metabolic signal feeding into the *S. typhimurium csgD* regulatory network.

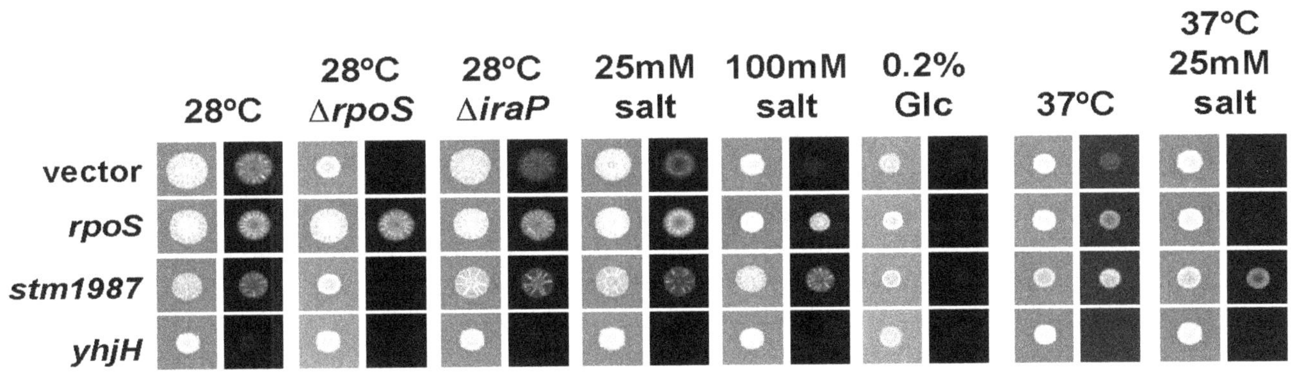

Figure 7. Visualization of *S. typhimurium* curli expression in response to changing growth conditions. *S. typhimurium* 14028 wild-type, Δ*rpoS* or Δ*iraP* reporter strains containing a *csgBAC* promoter–luciferase fusion were transformed with pBR322 (vector), pACYC/rpos (*rpoS*), pBR322/stm1987 (*stm1987*) or pBR322/yhjH (*yhjH*) plasmids. Cells were inoculated onto T agar or T agar supplemented with 0.2% glucose, 25 mM or 100 mM NaCl and grown at 28 °C or 37°C. Colony morphology (left column) and luminescence (right column) was recorded after 48 h growth. Control strains containing pACYC were also tested, but the *csgBAC* expression profiles were similar to strains transformed with pBR322; therefore, only the pBR322 pictures are shown.

4. Discussion

Biofilm formation is subject to tight and complex regulation through transcription factor CsgD. In *S*. Typhimurium, the intergenic region between divergent *csgDEFG* and *csgBAC* operons is among the longest non-coding region with 582 bp, which allows for a highly sophisticated signaling network. CsgD expression is regulated at the transcriptional, post transcriptional, translational and post translation level, in response to a variety of external and internal signals [8]. In this study we show that once activated, the CsgD biofilm network responds differently to metabolic inputs.

The ability of *S. enterica* strains to form biofilms is thought to be critical for the success of *Salmonella* as pathogens, particularly for gastroenteritis-causing strains [14]. With bistability of CsgD synthesis resulting in distinct cell types—multicellular aggregates associated with persistence (CsgD-ON), and single cells associated with virulence (CsgD-OFF) [42]—there is a need to have a flexible and dynamic response. We speculated that this phenotypic heterogeneity was a form of bet-hedging. A bet-hedging strategy ensures that at least one group of cells will be more adapted for a specific set of conditions that is encountered [61]. For some bacterial processes, such as sporulation, the advantage of the sporulating cell is obvious; however, for the non-sporulating cells, the advantage lies in being capable of more rapid growth when an influx of new nutrients occurs [62]. For *Salmonella*, there is a lot of energy devoted to generating the polymers associated with biofilm aggregates [26,63]; in the virulent, single cell group, synthesis of the type three secretion apparatus also requires a significant outlay of energy [64]. This type of population split makes the most sense in response to the unpredictability of transmission [65] or perhaps for modulating host–pathogen interactions, as observed for *Vibrio cholerae* [66]. We analyzed regulation before *csgD* activation, which has been tested before in *S. typhimurium* and *E. coli* and generally had the expected results, and compared this to regulation after *csgD* activation, which to our knowledge has not been tested before. We observed that *csgD* transcription and activation of downstream biofilm components was no longer repressed by increased osmolarity, and that the response to nutrient addition was also different, either as individual amino acids or a set of pooled amino acids. In contrast, the addition of glucose and temperatures above 32 °C rapidly repressed *csgD*, *csgB* and *adrA* expression even after induction. We approached these experiments from the point of view of biofilm formation as a developmental process [67,68], and our results show that CsgD biofilm formation is reversible, but can also be viewed as irreversible, depending on the signal. Our results, therefore, suggest the existence of a regulatory hierarchy among external signals that regulate biofilm formation.

For osmolarity, it has been well established that the optimal conditions for *csgD* expression and rdar biofilm formation in vitro include low osmolarity [51,52,69]. Key transcription factors have been identified (i.e., OmpR, CpxR, H-NS, MlrA and others) and binding within the *csgD* promoter region has been characterized [29,36,37,70,71]. Yet, there are still some intriguing aspects; for example, *S. enterica* biofilm cells produce high levels of osmoprotectants even when growing in low osmolarity conditions [26]. To explain the accumulation of osmoprotectants, we hypothesized that there could be high osmolarity microenvironments created within biofilms due to nutrient and ion trapping by the extracellular matrix [25,72]. The presence of hyperosmolar environments was recently observed with *E. coli* biofilms [73]. Our experiments show that once CsgD has activated downstream target genes (i.e., *csgBAC* (curli) and *adrA* (cellulose), transcription of all units becomes unresponsive to increases in osmolarity. This was specific to the CpxR/A two-component system in high salt conditions and by activating CpxR in ways that are not expected to significantly a change in osmolarity (i.e., metal stress) [55]. There has been some recent controversy about the role of CpxR in surface sensing or adhesion [74], but it is a well-established regulator of *csgD* [75]. The osmolarity effect was also general, as similar gene expression patterns were observed after the addition of sucrose, which was shown to repress *csgD* transcription in *E. coli* by acting through H-NS [36]. In our experiments, the CpxR/A system was not activated by the addition of sucrose, therefore, we assume that the same H-NS-mediated signaling occurs in *Salmonella*. To explain the results with *csgD*, it is possible that the presence of osmoprotectants produced early on during biofilm formation could mute the signaling effects associated with high external osmolarity [76]. Although we have shown that several osmoprotectant-associated genes are produced in time with *csgBAC* and *adrA* [26], we do not know the detailed time course for the appearance of the molecules themselves. The biological relevance for a lack of response to increased osmolarity is not clear, however, a recent paper described a real-world scenario where such a characteristic could be favored. Grinberg et al. 2019 [77] demonstrated that bacterial aggregates have enhanced survival on the surfaces of leaves in microdroplets that are not visible to the naked eye. As liquid evaporates from the leaf surfaces, solutes become concentrated and the microdroplets become hyperosmolar solutions. One could envision *S. enterica* biofilm aggregates surviving well in this scenario due to their stress-resistance adaptations and the altered *csgD* regulatory program identified here. We hypothesize that these microdroplets represent an environment where biofilms, and presumably biofilm-forming strains, would be favored over individual cells that do not aggregate together or strains that do not form biofilms.

Nutrient limitation was one of the first activating signals identified for *csgD* transcription [30,51]. In 1% tryptone or lysogeny broth, which are predominantly comprised of amino acids [60], *csgD* transcription occurs when cell density increases and cells start to run out of nutrients [8,63]. While this was initially attributed to phosphate and nitrogen depletion [30], we tested if supplementation with additional amino acids would delay or prevent activation of *csgD* transcription. When amino acids were added together (i.e., casamino acids), the transcription of *csgD* and downstream biofilm genes was delayed for almost the entire 70-h growth period, well after high cell densities were reached. When CAA were added during growth, *csgD* expression was shifted down in a dose-dependent manner. This showed that after induction, *csgD* expression was still responsive to negative regulation by CAA. The dose response could represent a subpopulation of *S. typhimurium* cells that retain metabolic flexibility [78] and are able to shift their metabolism away from biofilm formation. Based on the results with CAA, we predicted that individual amino acids might also have a repressive effect on biofilm formation. We measured the expression of the curli biosynthesis operon (i.e., *csgBAC*), a direct target of CsgD. Only Asn, Pro and Arg reduced *csgB* expression when added before growth, while Ile, Val, Gln, Met, Ala, Thr and Gly all increased expression. This indicated that the repression observed with CAA was the cumulative effect of the individual amino acids, as recently observed [79]. When added during growth, Leu, Arg, His, Val, Pro, Ala, Gln and Thr increased *csgB* expression, and no single amino acid decreased expression. This again showed that the CsgD biofilm network responds differently once it is activated. The production of sugars from gluconeogenesis is important for biofilm formation, as S. Typhimurium strains with mutations of *pckA* and *ppsA* are unable to form biofilms [26]. PckA and PpsA are important gluconeogenic enzymes required for the synthesis of phosphoenolpyruvate (PEP). Pck catalyzes the conversion of oxaloacetate to PEP [80], while Pps catalyzes the conversion of pyruvate to PEP. Ala, Gly and Thr are gluconeogenic amino acids that enter the gluconeogenic pathway through pyruvate [81]. In support of this, Ala and Thr increased *csgB* expression when introduced before and during growth. Gly also increased *csgB* expression when added before and during growth, but the change was not statistically significant. CsgD was shown to directly stimulate Gly biosynthesis during *E. coli* biofilm formation [82], presumably to ensure there is enough Gly supply to produce large quantities of the major curli subunit, CsgA (i.e., 16% Gly residues). Increased *csgB* expression in the presence of Ala, Gly and Thr is consistent with their conversion to pyruvate contributing to gluconeogenesis. For the aromatic amino acids, due to solubility and concentration problems, we only tested Phe, which had no significant effect on *csgB* expression. This was unfortunate since *S. enterica* strains defective in aromatic amino acid biosynthesis are unable to form biofilms [83], and tryptophan has been shown to have an important role in S. Typhimurium biofilms [84]. Tryptophan was also not present in CAA, as it is destroyed during the acid hydrolysis process [85]. More research is needed to understand the impact of individual amino acids on *csgD* expression.

Glucose was the most powerful external signal tested in our experiments. Under all growth conditions, the presence of exogenous glucose completely repressed the transcription of *csgD*, *csgB* and *adrA*. Expression of *csgD* was repressed in the presence of glucose even when *rpoS* was over-expressed from a plasmid or when levels of c-di-GMP were enhanced due to STM1987 activity. In the initial paper on carbon source foraging [86], the presence of glucose had a streamlining effect on the metabolism of *E. coli* when compared with growth on lower-quality carbon sources. This study was a genome-wide illustration of carbon catabolite repression [87], where growth on optimal carbon sources occurs first and genes for the metabolism of other carbon sources are repressed, usually acting through cyclic AMP (cAMP) and cAMP receptor proteins (CRP). Glucose had a repressive effect on biofilm formation in both S. Typhimurium and *E. coli* [12,59,79,88], however how the regulation is mediated is reported to be the opposite. High levels of cAMP repress *csgD* transcription in S. Typhimurium [79], but stimulate *csgD* transcription in *E. coli* [88]. It was also initially reported in S. Typhimurium that cAMP/CRP had no effect on *csgD* transcription [30]. It is hard to believe that the conserved divergent *csgDEFG* and *csgBAC* operons [89], biofilm networks and large intergenic region are capable of having opposite regulation in S. Typhimurium and *E. coli*. However, as pointed out by Hufnagel et al. [88], *E. coli* and

S. Typhimurium have different evolutionary histories, hence could have differing regulatory responses to glucose. Another important aspect of cAMP/CRP regulation and glucose metabolism pertains to the quality of nitrogen source available [90], making this complex regulatory network in need of further study. It should be noted that the repressive effect of glucose did not change according to whether *csgD* transcription was activated or not, which was in contrast to the other nutritional signals that we tested.

The effects of temperature and c-di-GMP on *csgD* transcription were also evaluated. Temperature was one of the first conditions identified to regulate biofilm formation [50,52]. Activation at temperatures below 30 °C is known to represent RpoS-dependent transcription of *csgD*. *S. enterica* strains with *csgD* promoter mutations can alleviate temperature-based repression by shifting transcription to be RpoD-dependent [51,52]. This may be a way for natural *rpoS* mutant strains to retain the ability to form biofilms, as there are always a few isolates within natural collections that display temperature-independent biofilm formation [12,21,50]. Temperature was able to shut off the biofilm network even after *csgD* was activated, proving that it is also a strong regulatory signal. *S. typhimurium* biofilm colonies were only formed at 37 °C if c-di-GMP levels were enhanced by *stm1987* overexpression, with partial restoration if *rpoS* was overexpressed. Although these conditions are somewhat artificial, the c-di-GMP regulatory principles could be an important observation. We recently discovered that curli can be synthesized by *S. typhimurium* during murine infections, with *csgD* transcription activated at 37 °C in vivo [91]. It is also of note that iron limitation [52] and exposure to bile [92] can alleviate temperature-based repression of *csgD* transcription. Finally, expression of the c-di-GMP-degrading enzyme, YhjH (or STM3611), was enough to repress *csgD* expression in all tested conditions, which is similar to previous observations [93,94].

5. Conclusions

We have started to dissect the external signal hierarchy that regulates *csgD* transcription and CsgD-mediated biofilm formation in *S. enterica*. Most significantly, we identified differences in the regulatory responses based on whether or not *csgD* was activated before being exposed to a signal. These findings are summarized in Figure 8A,B. We hypothesize that the differences upon activation are related to the bistable expression of CsgD [40,42], similar to dedicated processes in other bacterial species. Even seemingly well-understood processes, such as diauxie—the switching of *E. coli* growth between two carbon sources—is subject to heterogeneity, as one sub-population of cells ceases growth once glucose has been exhausted, while the other subpopulation begins to grow on the second carbon source without delay [78]. The diauxic behavior was originally interpreted as the whole population of cells stopping growth during a transition period before starting growth on the second carbon source [95]. We hypothesize that many of the *csgD* regulatory elements that we have examined here are consistent between *S.* Typhimurium and *E. coli* [41], with some notable differences. With respect to phenotypic heterogeneity, we may only fully understand biofilm regulation once we are able to examine the fate of individual cells [27].

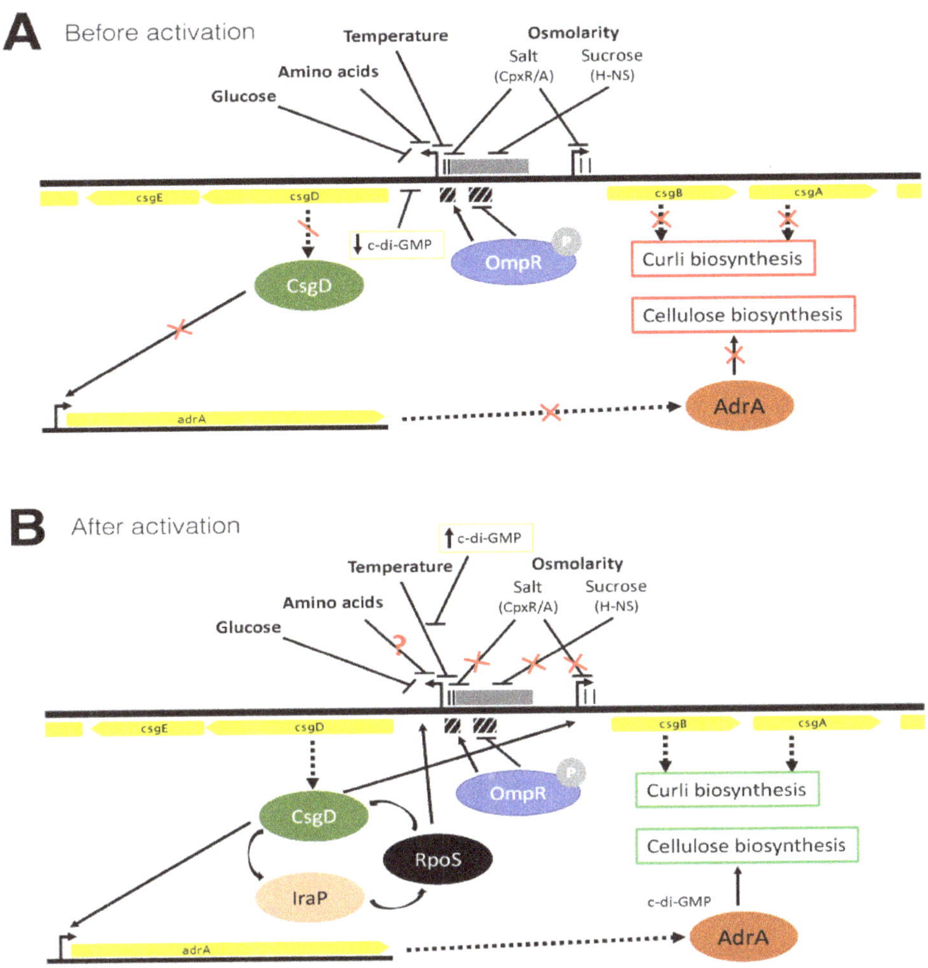

Figure 8. Graphical illustration of the CsgD regulatory principles identified in this manuscript. The divergent *csg* operons are shown (without *csgFG* and *csgC*) with the intergenic region highlighted by transcription factor binding sites that have been experimentally verified in *Salmonella* (CpxR—black bars; H-NS—grey box; OmpR—hatched boxes). Phosphorylated OmpR binds the proximal, high affinity site under conditions of low osmolarity, which activates *csgD* transcription, and binds the distal, low affinity sites under conditions of high osmolarity, which represses *csgD* transcription [38]. The different regulatory elements that we have tested are shown: glucose; amino acids; growth temperature; and osmolarity, with sodium chloride, which is known to act via the CpxR/A system [37], and sucrose, which is known to act via H-NS [36]. The *adrA* gene encodes a diguanylate cyclase, which produces cyclic-di-GMP and allosterically activates cellulose production. (**A**) Glucose (>25 mM), amino acids >0.5% casamino acids), temperature (>32 °C), salt and sucrose (> 25 mM) caused a reduction in *csgD* transcription and blocked transcription of *csgBAC* and *adrA*, preventing curli and cellulose biosynthesis. The effect of reduced c-di-GMP was tested by overexpression of the YhjH phosphodiesterase. The addition of individual amino acids was variable, with three leading to reduced *csgD* transcription (Asn, Pro, Arg), and seven leading to increased *csgD* transcription (Ile, Val, Gln, Met, Ala, Thr, Gly). **B**) When the same regulatory components were tested after 18 h of growth, the effects were different. We assume that by this time point, the CsgD-IraP-RpoS feed-forward loop [35] is activated, although deletion of *iraP* in our experiments had little effect. The addition of salt and sucrose had no effect on *csgD* transcription, and casamino acids were not as repressive. The effect of increased c-di-GMP was tested by overexpression of the diguanylate cyclase STM1987, which was able to relieve temperature-based repression of *csgD* transcription. The response to individual amino acids was again variable, however, none caused a reduction in *csgD* transcription and eight were stimulatory (Leu, Arg, His, Val, Pro, Ala, Gln, Thr). The question mark signifies that we do not fully understand the regulatory effects of individual amino acids.

Author Contributions: Conceptualization, A.P.W., L.L.W., Y.W.; methodology, A.P.W.; formal analysis, A.S.S., L.L.W., A.P.W.; investigation, A.S.S., E.G.H., M.M., T.S.D., L.L.W., K.D.M., G.M.J., N.J.H., D.J.H., Y.W.; resources, A.P.W.; data curation, A.S.S., A.P.W.; writing—original draft preparation, A.S.S., L.L.W., A.P.W.; writing—review and editing, A.P.W., A.S.S.; supervision, A.P.W.; project administration, A.P.W.; funding acquisition, A.P.W. All authors have read and agreed to the published version of the manuscript.

Acknowledgments: The authors would like to thank Tracy Raivio for helpful discussions about the Cpx system, Neil Rawlyk for assisting in experimental design and methodology, and Sylvia van den Hurk for use of her Victor multilable plate reader.

References

1. Kirk, M.D.; Pires, S.M.; Black, R.E.; Caipo, M.; Crump, J.A.; Devleesschauwer, B.; Döpfer, D.; Fazil, A.; Fischer-Walker, C.L.; Hald, T.; et al. Correction: World Health Organization Estimates of the Global and Regional Disease Burden of 22 Foodborne Bacterial, Protozoal, and Viral Diseases, 2010: A Data Synthesis. *PloS Med.* **2015**, *12*, e1001940. [CrossRef] [PubMed]
2. Majowicz, S.E.; Musto, J.; Scallan, E.; Angulo, F.J.; Kirk, M.; O'Brien, S.J.; Jones, T.F.; Fazil, A.; Hoekstra, R.M.; The International Collaboration on Enteric Disease "Burden of Illness" Studies. The Global Burden of Nontyphoidal *Salmonella* Gastroenteritis. *Clin. Infect. Dis.* **2010**, *50*, 882–889. [CrossRef] [PubMed]
3. Buckle, G.C.; Walker, C.L.F.; Black, R.E. Typhoid fever and paratyphoid fever: Systematic review to estimate global morbidity and mortality for 2010. *J. Glob. Health* **2012**, *2*, 010401. [CrossRef] [PubMed]
4. McClelland, M.; Sanderson, K.E.; Clifton, S.W.; Latreille, P.; Porwollik, S.; Sabo, A.; Meyer, R.; Bieri, T.; Ozersky, P.; McLellan, M.; et al. Comparison of genome degradation in Paratyphi A and Typhi, human-restricted serovars of *Salmonella* enterica that cause typhoid. *Nat. Genet.* **2004**, *36*, 1268–1274. [CrossRef]
5. Gal-Mor, O.; Boyle, E.C.; Grassl, G.A. Same species, different diseases: How and why typhoidal and non-typhoidal *Salmonella* enterica serovars differ. *Front. Microbiol.* **2014**, *5*, 391. [CrossRef]
6. Hassan, R.; Buuck, S.; Noveroske, D.; Medus, C.; Sorenson, A.; Laurent, J.; Rotstein, D.; Schlater, L.; Freiman, J.; Douris, A.; et al. Multistate Outbreak of *Salmonella* Infections Linked to Raw Turkey Products—United States, 2017–2019. *Morb. Mortal. Wkly. Rep.* **2019**, *68*, 1045–1049. [CrossRef]
7. Morton, V.K.; Kearney, A.; Coleman, S.; Viswanathan, M.; Chau, K.; Orr, A.; Hexemer, A. Outbreaks of *Salmonella* illness associated with frozen raw breaded chicken products in Canada, 2015–2019. *Epidemiol. Infect.* **2019**, *147*, e254. [CrossRef]
8. Steenackers, H.; Hermans, K.; Vanderleyden, J.; Keersmaecker, S.C.J.D. *Salmonella* biofilms: An overview on occurrence, structure, regulation and eradication. *Food Res. Int.* **2012**, *45*, 502–531. [CrossRef]
9. Proctor, M.E.; Hamacher, M.; Tortorello, M.L.; Archer, J.R.; Davis, J.P. Multistate Outbreak of *Salmonella* Serovar Muenchen Infections Associated with Alfalfa Sprouts Grown from Seeds Pretreated with Calcium Hypochlorite. *J. Clin. Microbiol.* **2001**, *39*, 3461–3465. [CrossRef]
10. Werber, D.; Dreesman, J.; Feil, F.; van Treeck, U.; Fell, G.; Ethelberg, S.; Hauri, A.M.; Roggentin, P.; Prager, R.; Fisher, I.S.; et al. International outbreak of *Salmonella* Oranienburg due to German chocolate. *BMC Infect. Dis.* **2005**, *5*, 7. [CrossRef] [PubMed]
11. Waldner, L.L.; MacKenzie, K.D.; Köster, W.; White, A.P. From Exit to Entry: Long-term Survival and Transmission of *Salmonella*. *Pathogens* **2012**, *1*, 128–155. [CrossRef] [PubMed]
12. White, A.P.; Gibson, D.L.; Kim, W.; Kay, W.W.; Surette, M.G. Thin Aggregative Fimbriae and Cellulose Enhance Long-Term Survival and Persistence of Salmonella. *J. Bacteriol.* **2006**, *188*, 3219–3227. [CrossRef] [PubMed]
13. Apel, D.; White, A.P.; Grassl, G.A.; Finlay, B.B.; Surette, M.G. Long-term survival of *Salmonella* enterica serovar Typhimurium reveals an infectious state that is underrepresented on laboratory media containing bile salts. *Appl. Environ. Microb.* **2009**, *75*, 4923–4925. [CrossRef] [PubMed]

14. MacKenzie, K.D.; Palmer, M.B.; Köster, W.L.; White, A.P. Examining the Link between Biofilm Formation and the Ability of Pathogenic *Salmonella* Strains to Colonize Multiple Host Species. *Front. Vet. Sci.* **2017**, *4*, 138. [CrossRef]
15. Finn, S.; Condell, O.; McClure, P.; Amézquita, A.; Fanning, S. Mechanisms of survival, responses and sources of *Salmonella* in low-moisture environments. *Front. Microbiol.* **2013**, *4*, 331. [CrossRef]
16. Galié, S.; García-Gutiérrez, C.; Miguélez, E.M.; Villar, C.J.; Lombó, F. Biofilms in the Food Industry: Health Aspects and Control Methods. *Front. Microbiol.* **2018**, *9*, 898. [CrossRef]
17. Winfield, M.D.; Groisman, E.A. Role of Nonhost Environments in the Lifestyles of Salmonella and Escherichia coli. *Appl. Environ. Microb.* **2003**, *69*, 3687–3694. [CrossRef]
18. Singletary, L.A.; Karlinsey, J.E.; Libby, S.J.; Mooney, J.P.; Lokken, K.L.; Tsolis, R.M.; Byndloss, M.X.; Hirao, L.A.; Gaulke, C.A.; Crawford, R.W.; et al. Loss of Multicellular Behavior in Epidemic African Nontyphoidal Salmonella enterica Serovar Typhimurium ST313 Strain D23580. *MBio* **2016**, *7*, e02265. [CrossRef]
19. MacKenzie, K.D.; Wang, Y.; Musicha, P.; Hansen, E.G.; Palmer, M.B.; Herman, D.J.; Feasey, N.A.; White, A.P. Parallel evolution leading to impaired biofilm formation in invasive *Salmonella* strains. *PloS Genet.* **2019**, *15*, e1008233. [CrossRef]
20. Crawford, R.W.; Rosales-Reyes, R.; Ramírez-Aguilar, M.; Chapa-Azuela, O.; Alpuche-Aranda, C.; Gunn, J.S. Gallstones play a significant role in *Salmonella* spp. gallbladder colonization and carriage. *Proc. Natl. Acad. Sci. USA* **2010**, *107*, 4353–4358. [CrossRef]
21. Römling, U.; Bokranz, W.; Rabsch, W.; Zogaj, X.; Nimtz, M.; Tschäpe, H. Occurrence and regulation of the multicellular morphotype in *Salmonella* serovars important in human disease. *Int. J. Med. Microbiol.* **2003**, *293*, 273–285. [CrossRef] [PubMed]
22. Romling, U.; Rohde, M.; Olsen, A.; Normark, S.; Reinkoster, J. AgfD, the checkpoint of multicellular and aggregative behaviour in *Salmonella* typhimurium regulates at least two independent pathways. *Mol. Microbiol.* **2000**, *36*, 10–23. [CrossRef] [PubMed]
23. Flemming, H.-C.; Wingender, J. The biofilm matrix. *Nat. Rev. Microbiol.* **2010**, *8*, 623–633. [CrossRef] [PubMed]
24. Dieltjens, L.; Appermans, K.; Lissens, M.; Lories, B.; Kim, W.; Van der Eycken, E.V.; Foster, K.R.; Steenackers, H.P. Inhibiting bacterial cooperation is an evolutionarily robust anti-biofilm strategy. *Nat. Commun.* **2020**, *11*, 107. [CrossRef]
25. Flemming, H.-C.; Wingender, J.; Szewzyk, U.; Steinberg, P.; Rice, S.A.; Kjelleberg, S. Biofilms: An emergent form of bacterial life. *Nat. Rev. Microbiol.* **2016**, *14*, 563–575. [CrossRef] [PubMed]
26. White, A.P.; Weljie, A.M.; Apel, D.; Zhang, P.; Shaykhutdinov, R.; Vogel, H.J.; Surette, M.G. A global metabolic shift is linked to *Salmonella* multicellular development. *PLoS ONE* **2010**, *5*, e11814. [CrossRef] [PubMed]
27. Ackermann, M. A functional perspective on phenotypic heterogeneity in microorganisms. *Nat. Rev. Microbiol.* **2015**, *13*, 497–508. [CrossRef]
28. Serra, D.O.; Richter, A.M.; Klauck, G.; Mika, F.; Hengge, R. Microanatomy at cellular resolution and spatial order of physiological differentiation in a bacterial biofilm. *MBio* **2013**, *4*, e00103-13. [CrossRef]
29. Gerstel, U.; Römling, U. The csgD promoter, a control unit for biofilm formation in *Salmonella* typhimurium. *Res. Microbiol.* **2003**, *154*, 659–667. [CrossRef]
30. Gerstel, U.; Romling, U. Oxygen tension and nutrient starvation are major signals that regulate agfD promoter activity and expression of the multicellular morphotype in *Salmonella* typhimurium. *Environ. Microbiol.* **2001**, *3*, 638–648. [CrossRef]
31. Beloin, C.; Roux, A.; Ghigo, J.-M. *Escherichia coli* biofilms. *Curr. Top. Microbiol.* **2008**, *322*, 249–289. [CrossRef]
32. Kolter, R.; Siegele, D.A.; Tormo, A. The Stationary Phase of The Bacterial Life Cycle. *Annu. Rev. Microbiol.* **1993**, *47*, 855–874. [CrossRef] [PubMed]
33. Hengge-Aronis, R. Signal Transduction and Regulatory Mechanisms Involved in Control of the σS (RpoS) Subunit of RNA Polymerase. *Microbiol. Mol. Biol. Rev.* **2002**, *66*, 373–395. [CrossRef]
34. Arnqvist, A.; Olsén, A.; Normark, S. σ^S-dependent growth-phase induction of the *csgBA* promoter in *Escherichia coli* can be achieved in vivo by σ^{70} in the absence of the nucleoid-associated protein H-NS. *Mol. Microbiol.* **1994**, *13*, 1021–1032. [CrossRef] [PubMed]
35. Gualdi, L.; Tagliabue, L.; Landini, P. Biofilm formation-gene expression relay system in *Escherichia coli*: Modulation of sigmaS-dependent gene expression by the CsgD regulatory protein via sigmaS protein stabilization. *J. Bacteriol.* **2007**, *189*, 8034–8043. [CrossRef] [PubMed]

36. Jubelin, G.; Vianney, A.; Beloin, C.; Ghigo, J.-M.; Lazzaroni, J.-C.; Lejeune, P.; Dorel, C. CpxR/OmpR Interplay Regulates Curli Gene Expression in Response to Osmolarity in *Escherichia coli*. *J. Bacteriol.* **2005**, *187*, 2038–2049. [CrossRef]
37. Prigent-Combaret, C.; Brombacher, E.; Vidal, O.; Ambert, A.; Lejeune, P.; Landini, P.; Dorel, C. Complex Regulatory Network Controls Initial Adhesion and Biofilm Formation in *Escherichia coli* via Regulation of the csgD Gene. *J. Bacteriol.* **2001**, *183*, 7213–7223. [CrossRef]
38. Gerstel, U.; Park, C.; Römling, U. Complex regulation of *csgD* promoter activity by global regulatory proteins: Regulation of *csgD* expression. *Mol. Microbiol.* **2004**, *49*, 639–654. [CrossRef]
39. White, A.P.; Gibson, D.L.; Grassl, G.A.; Kay, W.W.; Finlay, B.B.; Vallance, B.A.; Surette, M.G. Aggregation via the red, dry, and rough morphotype is not a virulence adaptation in *Salmonella* enterica serovar Typhimurium. *Infect. Immun.* **2008**, *76*, 1048–1058. [CrossRef]
40. Grantcharova, N.; Peters, V.; Monteiro, C.; Zakikhany, K.; Römling, U. Bistable expression of CsgD in biofilm development of *Salmonella* enterica serovar typhimurium. *J. Bacteriol.* **2009**, *192*, 456–466. [CrossRef]
41. DePas, W.H.; Hufnagel, D.A.; Lee, J.S.; Blanco, L.P.; Bernstein, H.C.; Fisher, S.T.; James, G.A.; Stewart, P.S.; Chapman, M.R. Iron induces bimodal population development by *Escherichia coli*. *Proc. Natl. Acad. Sci. USA* **2013**, *110*, 2629–2634. [CrossRef] [PubMed]
42. MacKenzie, K.D.; Wang, Y.; Shivak, D.J.; Wong, C.S.; Hoffman, L.J.L.; Lam, S.; Kröger, C.; Cameron, A.D.S.; Townsend, H.G.G.; Köster, W.; et al. Bistable expression of CsgD in *Salmonella* enterica serovar Typhimurium connects virulence to persistence. *Infect. Immun.* **2015**, *83*, 2312–2326. [CrossRef] [PubMed]
43. Römling, U.; Galperin, M.Y.; Gomelsky, M. Cyclic di-GMP: The first 25 years of a universal bacterial second messenger. *Microbiol. Mol. Biol. Rev. Mmbr* **2013**, *77*, 1–52. [CrossRef] [PubMed]
44. Ahmad, I.; Cimdins, A.; Beske, T.; Römling, U. Detailed analysis of c-di-GMP mediated regulation of *csgD* expression in *Salmonella* typhimurium. *Bmc Microbiol.* **2017**, *17*, 27. [CrossRef]
45. Solano, C.; García, B.; Latasa, C.; Toledo-Arana, A.; Zorraquino, V.; Valle, J.; Casals, J.; Pedroso, E.; Lasa, I. Genetic reductionist approach for dissecting individual roles of GGDEF proteins within the c-di-GMP signaling network in *Salmonella*. *Proc. Natl. Acad. Sci. USA* **2009**, *106*, 7997–8002. [CrossRef]
46. Dworkin, J.; Losick, R. Developmental Commitment in a Bacterium. *Cell* **2005**, *121*, 401–409. [CrossRef]
47. Bjarnason, J.; Southward, C.M.; Surette, M.G. Genomic Profiling of Iron-Responsive Genes in *Salmonella* enterica Serovar Typhimurium by High-Throughput Screening of a Random Promoter Library. *J. Bacteriol.* **2003**, *185*, 4973–4982. [CrossRef]
48. White, A.P.; Surette, M.G. Comparative Genetics of the rdar Morphotype in *Salmonella*. *J. Bacteriol.* **2006**, *188*, 8395–8406. [CrossRef]
49. Datsenko, K.A.; Wanner, B.L. One-step inactivation of chromosomal genes in *Escherichia coli* K-12 using PCR products. *Proc. Natl. Acad. Sci. USA* **2000**, *97*, 6640–6645. [CrossRef]
50. Maloy, S.R. *Experimental Techniques in Bacterial Genetics*; Jones & Bartlett Learning: Boston, MA, USA, 1990; p. 180.
51. Collinson, S.K.; Emödy, L.; Müller, K.H.; Trust, T.J.; Kay, W.W. Purification and characterization of thin, aggregative fimbriae from *Salmonella* enteritidis. *J. Bacteriol.* **1991**, *173*, 4773–4781. [CrossRef]
52. Romling, U.; Sierralta, W.D.; Eriksson, K.; Normark, S. Multicellular and aggregative behaviour of *Salmonella* typhimurium strains is controlled by mutations in the agfD promoter. *Mol. Microbiol.* **1998**, *28*, 249–264. [CrossRef] [PubMed]
53. Danese, P.N.; Silhavy, T.J. CpxP, a stress-combative member of the Cpx regulon. *J. Bacteriol.* **1998**, *180*, 831–839. [CrossRef] [PubMed]
54. Hunke, S.; Keller, R.; Müller, V.S. Signal integration by the Cpx-envelope stress system. *FEMS Microbiol. Lett.* **2011**, *326*, 12–22. [CrossRef] [PubMed]
55. Yamamoto, K.; Ishihama, A. Characterization of Copper-Inducible Promoters Regulated by CpxA/CpxR in *Escherichia coli*. *Biosci. Biotechnol. Biochem.* **2006**, *70*, 1688–1695. [CrossRef]
56. Novick, A.; Weiner, M. Enzyme induction as an all-or-none phenomenon. *Proc. Natl. Acad. Sci. USA* **1957**, *43*, 553–566. [CrossRef]
57. Uhlich, G.A.; Keen, J.E.; Elder, R.O. Mutations in the *csgD* promoter associated with variations in curli expression in certain strains of Escherichia coli O157:H7. *Appl. Environ. Microb.* **2001**, *67*, 2367–2370. [CrossRef]

58. Barnhart, M.M.; Chapman, M.R. Curli Biogenesis and Function. *Annu. Rev. Microbiol.* **2006**, *60*, 131–147. [CrossRef]
59. Jackson, D.W.; Simecka, J.W.; Romeo, T. Catabolite Repression of *Escherichia coli* Biofilm Formation. *J. Bacteriol.* **2002**, *184*, 3406–3410. [CrossRef]
60. Sezonov, G.; Joseleau-Petit, D.; D'Ari, R. *Escherichia coli* Physiology in Luria-Bertani Broth. *J. Bacteriol.* **2007**, *189*, 8746–8749. [CrossRef]
61. Veening, J.-W.; Smits, W.K.; Kuipers, O.P. Bistability, epigenetics, and bet-hedging in bacteria. *Annu. Rev. Microbiol.* **2008**, *62*, 193–210. [CrossRef]
62. Veening, J.-W.; Stewart, E.J.; Berngruber, T.W.; Taddei, F.; Kuipers, O.P.; Hamoen, L.W. Bet-hedging and epigenetic inheritance in bacterial cell development. *Proc. Natl. Acad. Sci. USA* **2008**, *105*, 4393–4398. [CrossRef] [PubMed]
63. Serra, D.O.; Hengge, R. Stress responses go three dimensional—The spatial order of physiological differentiation in bacterial macrocolony biofilms. *Environ. Microbiol.* **2014**, *16*, 1455–1471. [CrossRef] [PubMed]
64. Ali, S.S.; Soo, J.; Rao, C.; Leung, A.S.; Ngai, D.H.-M.; Ensminger, A.W.; Navarre, W.W. Silencing by H-NS potentiated the evolution of *Salmonella*. *Plos Pathog.* **2014**, *10*, e1004500. [CrossRef] [PubMed]
65. Monack, D.M. Salmonella persistence and transmission strategies. *Curr. Opin. Microbiol.* **2012**, *15*, 100–107. [CrossRef] [PubMed]
66. Silva, A.J.; Benitez, J.A. Vibrio cholerae Biofilms and Cholera Pathogenesis. *PloS Neglect. Trop. Dis.* **2016**, *10*, e0004330. [CrossRef]
67. Monds, R.D.; O'Toole, G.A. The developmental model of microbial biofilms: Ten years of a paradigm up for review. *Trends Microbiol.* **2009**, *17*, 73–87. [CrossRef]
68. Kragh, K.N.; Hutchison, J.B.; Melaugh, G.; Rodesney, C.; Roberts, A.E.L.; Irie, Y.; Jensen, P.Ø.; Diggle, S.P.; Allen, R.J.; Gordon, V.; et al. Role of Multicellular Aggregates in Biofilm Formation. *MBio* **2016**, *7*, e00237. [CrossRef]
69. Bokranz, W.; Wang, X.; Tschäpe, H.; Römling, U. Expression of cellulose and curli fimbriae by *Escherichia coli* isolated from the gastrointestinal tract. *J. Med. Microbiol.* **2005**, *54*, 1171–1182. [CrossRef]
70. Ogasawara, H.; Yamada, K.; Kori, A.; Yamamoto, K.; Ishihama, A. Regulation of the *Escherichia coli* csgD promoter: Interplay between five transcription factors. *Microbiol.* **2010**, *156*, 2470–2483. [CrossRef]
71. Brown, P.K.; Dozois, C.M.; Nickerson, C.A.; Zuppardo, A.; Terlonge, J.; Curtiss, R. MlrA, a novel regulator of curli (AgF) and extracellular matrix synthesis by *Escherichia coli* and *Salmonella* enterica serovar Typhimurium: Regulation of curli and aggregation by mlrA. *Mol. Microbiol.* **2001**, *41*, 349–363. [CrossRef]
72. Sutherland, I.W. Biofilm exopolysaccharides: A strong and sticky framework. *Microbiology* **2001**, *147*, 3–9. [CrossRef] [PubMed]
73. Szczesny, M.; Beloin, C.; Ghigo, J.-M. Increased Osmolarity in Biofilm Triggers RcsB-Dependent Lipid A Palmitoylation in *Escherichia coli*. *MBio* **2018**, *9*, e01415-18. [CrossRef] [PubMed]
74. Kimkes, T.E.P.; Heinemann, M. Reassessing the role of the *Escherichia coli* CpxAR system in sensing surface contact. *PLoS ONE* **2018**, *13*, e0207181. [CrossRef] [PubMed]
75. Raivio, T.L. Everything old is new again: An update on current research on the Cpx envelope stress response. *Biochim. Biophys. Acta* **2013**, *1843*, 1529–1541. [CrossRef]
76. Bremer, E.; Krämer, R. Responses of Microorganisms to Osmotic Stress. *Annu. Rev. Microbiol.* **2019**, *73*, 313–334. [CrossRef]
77. Grinberg, M.; Orevi, T.; Steinberg, S.; Kashtan, N. Bacterial survival in microscopic surface wetness. *Elife* **2019**, *8*, e48508. [CrossRef]
78. Solopova, A.; van Gestel, J.; Weissing, F.J.; Bachmann, H.; Teusink, B.; Kok, J.; Kuipers, O.P. Bet-hedging during bacterial diauxic shift. *Proc. Natl. Acad. Sci. USA* **2014**, *111*, 7427–7432. [CrossRef]
79. Paytubi, S.; Cansado, C.; Madrid, C.; Balsalobre, C. Nutrient Composition Promotes Switching between Pellicle and Bottom Biofilm in Salmonella. *Front. Microbiol.* **2017**, *8*, 2160. [CrossRef]
80. Sokaribo, A.; Novakovski, B.A.A.; Cotelesage, J.; White, A.P.; Sanders, D.; Goldie, H. Kinetic and structural analysis of *Escherichia coli* phosphoenolpyruvate carboxykinase mutants. *Biochim. Et Biophys. Acta Gen. Subj.* **2020**, *1864*, 129517. [CrossRef]

81. Lehninger, A.L.; Nelson, D.L.; Cox, M.M. *Lehninger principles of biochemistry*, 4th ed.; Worth Publishers: New York, NY, USA, 2000.
82. Chirwa, N.T.; Herrington, M.B. CsgD, a regulator of curli and cellulose synthesis, also regulates serine hydroxymethyltransferase synthesis in *Escherichia coli* K-12. *Microbiology* **2003**, *149*, 525–535. [CrossRef]
83. Malcova, M.; Karasova, D.; Rychlik, I. aroA and aroD mutations influence biofilm formation in *Salmonella* Enteritidis. *Fems Microbiol. Lett.* **2008**, *291*, 44–49. [CrossRef] [PubMed]
84. Hamilton, S.; Bongaerts, R.J.M.; Mulholland, F.; Cochrane, B.; Porter, J.; Lucchini, S.; Lappin-Scott, H.M.; Hinton, J.C.D. The transcriptional programme of *Salmonella* enterica serovar Typhimurium reveals a key role for tryptophan metabolism in biofilms. *BMC Genom.* **2009**, *10*, 599. [CrossRef] [PubMed]
85. Nolan, R. Amino Acids and Growth Factors in Vitamin-Free Casamino Acids. *Mycologia* **1971**, *63*, 1231–1234. [CrossRef] [PubMed]
86. Liu, M.; Durfee, T.; Cabrera, J.; Zhao, K.; Jin, D.; Blattner, F. Global Transcriptional Programs Reveal a Carbon Source Foraging Strategy by Escherichia coli. *J. Biol. Chem.* **2005**, *280*, 15921–15927. [CrossRef] [PubMed]
87. Görke, B.; Stülke, J. Carbon catabolite repression in bacteria: Many ways to make the most out of nutrients. *Nat. Rev. Microbiol.* **2008**, *6*, 613–624. [CrossRef]
88. Hufnagel, D.A.; Evans, M.L.; Greene, S.E.; Pinkner, J.S.; Hultgren, S.J.; Chapman, M.R. The Catabolite Repressor Protein-Cyclic AMP Complex Regulates csgD and Biofilm Formation in Uropathogenic *Escherichia coli*. *J. Bacteriol.* **2016**, *198*, 3329–3334. [CrossRef] [PubMed]
89. Römling, U.; Bian, Z.; Hammar, M.; Sierralta, W.D.; Normark, S. Curli Fibers Are Highly Conserved between *Salmonella* typhimurium and *Escherichia coli* with Respect to Operon Structure and Regulation. *J. Bacteriol.* **1998**, *180*, 722–731. [CrossRef]
90. Bren, A.; Park, J.O.; Towbin, B.D.; Dekel, E.; Rabinowitz, J.D.; Alon, U. Glucose becomes one of the worst carbon sources for *E. coli* on poor nitrogen sources due to suboptimal levels of cAMP. *Sci. Rep.* **2016**, *6*, 24834. [CrossRef]
91. Miller, A.L.; Pasternak, J.A.; Medeiros, N.J.; Nicastro, L.K.; Tursi, S.A.; Hansen, E.G.; Krochak, R.; Sokaribo, A.S.; MacKenzie, K.D.; Palmer, M.B.; et al. In vivo synthesis of bacterial amyloid curli contributes to joint inflammation during *S. typhimurium* infection. *Plos Pathog.* **2020**, *16*. [CrossRef]
92. González, J.F.; Tucker, L.; Fitch, J.; Wetzel, A.; White, P.; Gunn, J.S. Human Bile-Mediated Regulation of *Salmonella* Curli Fimbriae. *J. Bacteriol.* **2019**, *201*. [CrossRef]
93. Simm, R.; Lusch, A.; Kader, A.; Andersson, M.; Romling, U. Role of EAL-Containing Proteins in Multicellular Behavior of *Salmonella* enterica Serovar Typhimurium. *J. Bacteriol.* **2007**, *189*, 3613–3623. [CrossRef] [PubMed]
94. Kader, A.; Simm, R.; Gerstel, U.; Morr, M.; Romling, U. Hierarchical involvement of various GGDEF domain proteins in rdar morphotype development of *Salmonella* enterica serovar Typhimurium. *Mol. Microbiol.* **2006**, *60*, 602–616. [CrossRef] [PubMed]
95. Monod, J. The Growth of Bacterial Cultures. *Annu. Rev. Microbiol.* **1949**, *3*, 371–394. [CrossRef]

Permissions

All chapters in this book were first published by MDPI; hereby published with permission under the Creative Commons Attribution License or equivalent. Every chapter published in this book has been scrutinized by our experts. Their significance has been extensively debated. The topics covered herein carry significant findings which will fuel the growth of the discipline. They may even be implemented as practical applications or may be referred to as a beginning point for another development.

The contributors of this book come from diverse backgrounds, making this book a truly international effort. This book will bring forth new frontiers with its revolutionizing research information and detailed analysis of the nascent developments around the world.

We would like to thank all the contributing authors for lending their expertise to make the book truly unique. They have played a crucial role in the development of this book. Without their invaluable contributions this book wouldn't have been possible. They have made vital efforts to compile up to date information on the varied aspects of this subject to make this book a valuable addition to the collection of many professionals and students.

This book was conceptualized with the vision of imparting up-to-date information and advanced data in this field. To ensure the same, a matchless editorial board was set up. Every individual on the board went through rigorous rounds of assessment to prove their worth. After which they invested a large part of their time researching and compiling the most relevant data for our readers.

The editorial board has been involved in producing this book since its inception. They have spent rigorous hours researching and exploring the diverse topics which have resulted in the successful publishing of this book. They have passed on their knowledge of decades through this book. To expedite this challenging task, the publisher supported the team at every step. A small team of assistant editors was also appointed to further simplify the editing procedure and attain best results for the readers.

Apart from the editorial board, the designing team has also invested a significant amount of their time in understanding the subject and creating the most relevant covers. They scrutinized every image to scout for the most suitable representation of the subject and create an appropriate cover for the book.

The publishing team has been an ardent support to the editorial, designing and production team. Their endless efforts to recruit the best for this project, has resulted in the accomplishment of this book. They are a veteran in the field of academics and their pool of knowledge is as vast as their experience in printing. Their expertise and guidance has proved useful at every step. Their uncompromising quality standards have made this book an exceptional effort. Their encouragement from time to time has been an inspiration for everyone.

The publisher and the editorial board hope that this book will prove to be a valuable piece of knowledge for researchers, students, practitioners and scholars across the globe.

List of Contributors

Ricardo Álvarez
Microbiota-Host Interactions and Clostridia Research Group, Departamento de Ciencias Biológicas, Facultad de Ciencias de la Vida, Universidad Andres Bello, 8370186 Santiago, Chile

Fernando Díaz-Yáñez and Fernando Gil
Microbiota-Host Interactions and Clostridia Research Group, Departamento de Ciencias Biológicas, Facultad de Ciencias de la Vida, Universidad Andres Bello, 8370186 Santiago, Chile
ANID-Millennium Science Initiative Program-Millennium Nucleus in the Biology of the Intestinal Microbiota, 8370186 Santiago, Chile

Iván L. Calderón
Laboratorio de RNAs Bacterianos, Departamento de Ciencias Biológicas, Facultad de Ciencias de la Vida, Universidad Andres Bello, 8370186 Santiago, Chile

Juan A. Fuentes
Laboratorio de Genética y Patogénesis Bacteriana, Departamento de Ciencias Biológicas, Facultad de Ciencias de la Vida, Universidad Andres Bello, 8370186 Santiago, Chile

Caleb Wong de la Rosa, Chris R. Kerth and Thomas M. Taylor
Department of Animal Science, Texas A&M AgriLife Research, College Station, TX 77843-2471, USA

Kourtney A. Daniels
Department of Food Science and Technology, Texas A&M AgriLife Research, College Station, TX 77843-2253, USA

Rosana G. Moreira
Department of Biological and Agricultural Engineering, Texas A&M AgriLife Research, College Station, TX 77843-2117, USA

Bussarakam Chuppava, Volker Wilke, Clara Berenike Hartung, Josef Kamphues and Christian Visscher
Institute for Animal Nutrition, University of Veterinary Medicine Hannover, Foundation, Bischofsholer Damm 15, D-30173 Hanover, Germany

Amr Abd El-Wahab
Department of Nutrition and Nutritional Deficiency Diseases, Faculty of Veterinary Medicine, Mansoura University, Mansoura 35516, Egypt

Richard Grone and Andreas von Felde
KWS LOCHOW GmbH, Ferdinand von Lochowstrasse 5, D-29303 Bergen, Germany

Annah Lee and Cristiano Bortoluzzi
Department of Poultry Science, Texas A&M University, College Station, TX 77843, USA

Rachel Pilla
Department of Small Animal Clinical Sciences, Texas A&M University, College Station, TX 77843, USA

Michael H. Kogut
Food and Feed Safety Research Unit, United States Department of Agriculture/Agriculture Research Service, College Station, TX 77845, USA

Nicole A. Lerminiaux, Keith D. MacKenzie and Andrew D. S. Cameron
Department of Biology, Faculty of Science, University of Regina, Regina, SK S4S 0A2, Canada
Institute for Microbial Systems and Society, Faculty of Science, University of Regina, Regina, SK S4S 0A2, Canada

Qiaoyun Hu, Ruchika Dehinwal, Alexey V. Rakov, Nicholas Grams and Dieter M. Schifferli
Department of Pathobiology, University of Pennsylvania, School of Veterinary Medicine, Philadelphia, PA 19104, USA

Yanping Wu
Department of Pathobiology, University of Pennsylvania, School of Veterinary Medicine, Philadelphia, PA 19104, USA
College of Animal Science and Technology, College of Veterinary Medicine, Zhejiang Agriculture and Forestry University, Hangzhou 311300, China

Erin C. Clemens and Jennifer Hofmann
Department of Biology, Haverford College, Haverford, PA 19041, USA

Iruka N. Okeke
Department of Biology, Haverford College, Haverford, PA 19041, USA
Department of Pharmaceutical Microbiology, Faculty of Pharmacy, University of Ibadan, Ibadan 200284, Oyo State, Nigeria

Mark M. Hahn
Center for Microbial Pathogenesis, Abigail Wexner Research Institute at Nationwide Children's Hospital, Columbus, OH 43205, USA
Infectious Diseases Institute, The Ohio State University, Columbus, OH 43210, USA

John S. Gunn
Center for Microbial Pathogenesis, Abigail Wexner Research Institute at Nationwide Children's Hospital, Columbus, OH 43205, USA
Infectious Diseases Institute, The Ohio State University, Columbus, OH 43210, USA
Department of Pediatrics, College of Medicine, The Ohio State University, Columbus, OH 43210, USA

Satheesh Nair
Gastrointestinal Bacteria Reference Unit, Public Health England, Colindale, London NW9 5EQ, UK

Maria Fookes, Craig Corton and Nicholas R. Thomson
Wellcome Trust Sanger Institute, Hinxton, Cambridge CB10 1SA, UK

John Wain
Norwich Medical School, University of East Anglia, Norwich NR4 7UQ, UK
Microbes in the Food Chain, Quadram Institute, Norwich Research Park, Norwich NR4 7UQ, UK

Gemma C. Langridge
Microbes in the Food Chain, Quadram Institute, Norwich Research Park, Norwich NR4 7UQ, UK

Claudie Murret-Labarthe, Maud Kerhoas and Karine Dufresne
Département de microbiologie, infectiologie, immunologie, Université de Montréal, Montréal, QC H3T 1J4, Canada

Jean-Guillaume Emond-Rheault, Jérémie Hamel, Julie Jeukens, Luca Freschi, Irena Kukavica-Ibrulj, Brian Boyle and Roger C. Levesque
Institut de Biologie Intégrative et des Systèmes (IBIS), Université Laval, Québec, QC G1V 0A6, Canada

Sandeep Tamber
Health Canada, Bureau of Microbial Hazards, Ottawa, ON K1A 0K9, Canada

Danielle Malo
McGill Research Center on Complex Traits, McGill University, Montréal, QC H3G 0B1, Canada
Departments of Medicine and Human Genetics, McGill University, Montréal, QC H3G 0B1, Canada

Eelco Franz
Centre for Infectious Disease Control (CIb), National Institute for Public Health and the Environment (RIVM), 3720 BA Bilthoven, The Netherlands

Elton Burnett
Institute of Parasitology, McGill University, Montréal, QC H9X 3L9, Canada

France Daigle
Département de Microbiologie, Infectiologie et Immunologie, Université de Montréal, Montréal, QC H3T 1J4, Canada
Swine and poultry Infectious Diseases Research Center (CRIPA-FRQNT), Montréal, QC H3C 3J7, Canada

Gitanjali Arya
National Microbiology Laboratory, Public Health Agency of Canada, Guelph, ON N1G 3W4, Canada

Kenneth Sanderson
Department of Biological Sciences, University of Calgary, Calgary, AB T2N 1N4, Canada

Martin Wiedmann
Department of Food Science, Cornell University, Ithaca, NY 14853-7201, USA

Robin M. Slawson and Joel T. Weadge
Department of Biology, Wilfrid Laurier University, Waterloo, ON N2L 3C5, Canada

Roger Stephan
Institute for Food Safety and hygiene, University of Zürich, CH-8057 Zürich, Switzerland

Sadjia Bekal
Laboratoire de santé publique du Québec, Sainte-Anne-de-Bellevue, QC H9X 3R5, Canada

Samantha Gruenheid
Department of Microbiology & Immunology, McGill University, Montréal, QC H3G 0B1, Canada

Lawrence D. Goodridge
Food Science Department, University of Guelph, Guelph, ON N1G 2W1, Canada

Brenda Allan
Vaccine & Infectious Disease Organization-International Vaccine Centre, University of Saskatchewan, 120 Veterinary Rd., Saskatoon, SK S7N 5E3, Canada

Dinesh H. Wellawa and Wolfgang Köster
Vaccine & Infectious Disease Organization-International Vaccine Centre, University of Saskatchewan, 120 Veterinary Rd., Saskatoon, SK S7N 5E3, Canada
Department of Veterinary Microbiology, Western College of Veterinary Medicine, University of Saskatchewan, Saskatoon, SK S7N 5B4, Canada

Aaron P. White
Vaccine & Infectious Disease Organization-International Vaccine Centre, University of Saskatchewan, 120 Veterinary Rd., Saskatoon, SK S7N 5E3, Canada
Department of Veterinary Microbiology, Western College of Veterinary Medicine, University of Saskatchewan, Saskatoon, SK S7N 5B4, Canada
Department of Biochemistry, Microbiology and Immunology, University of Saskatchewan, Saskatoon, SK S7N 5E5, Canada

Smriti Verma, Stefania Senger, Bobby J. Cherayil and Christina S. Faherty
Mucosal Immunology and Biology Research Center, Division of Pediatric Gastroenterology and Nutrition, Massachusetts General Hospital, Charlestown Navy Yard, Boston, 02129 MA, USA
Harvard Medical School, Boston, 02115 MA, USA

Elizabeth G. Hansen, Landon L. Waldner, George Mutwiri Jr., Nancy J. Herman and Dakoda J. Herman
Vaccine and Infectious Disease Organization-International Vaccine Centre, University of Saskatchewan, Saskatoon, SK S7N 5E3, Canada

Akosiererem S. Sokaribo and Madeline McCarthy
Vaccine and Infectious Disease Organization-International Vaccine Centre, University of Saskatchewan, Saskatoon, SK S7N 5E3, Canada
Department of Biochemistry, Microbiology and Immunology, University of Saskatchewan, Saskatoon, SK S7N 5E5, Canada

Taseen S. Desin
Department of Biochemistry, Microbiology and Immunology, University of Saskatchewan, Saskatoon, SK S7N 5E5, Canada
Basic Sciences Department, King Saud bin Abdulaziz University for Health Sciences, Riyadh 11481, Saudi Arabia

Yejun Wang
Department of Cell Biology and Genetics, School of Basic Medicine, Shenzhen University Health Science, Shenzhen 518060, China

Index

A

Adhesin, 78-79, 85, 87-89, 91

Albumin, 159, 167-168

Alleles, 70, 76, 78-79, 81, 83-87, 89, 91

Allelic Exchange, 80, 90, 122-123

Allelic Variants, 78, 82, 86-88

Amino Acid, 2, 8-9, 11, 13-14, 59, 63, 78, 115, 150, 164, 211, 214, 217

Aminoglycoside, 123, 148, 151, 155

Antimicrobial Resistance, 28, 38, 41, 124, 138-139, 144, 152-155, 172-173, 200

Apical Surface, 184, 191

B

Bacteremia, 163, 165-168, 175, 178, 199

Bacterial Burden, 165, 168

Bacterial Strain, 80, 193

Basement Membrane, 188, 191

Biofilm, 92-108, 133, 203-205, 207, 209-218, 221-224

C

Cell Invasion, 78-79, 87, 89, 92, 125, 131

Cell Type, 12, 125, 184, 191

Cellular Differentiation, 182, 185, 204, 210

Cellulose, 92-94, 104-105, 203-205, 207, 216, 219-220, 223-224

Chelation, 81, 167-169

Chemotaxis, 93, 105, 109, 124, 134, 190, 199

Clinical Isolates, 75, 93-94, 98, 154, 186

Clinical Manifestation, 156

Comparative Genomics, 56-57, 68, 71, 113, 115, 153-154, 170, 173

Convergent Evolution, 109, 111-112, 117-118

Cytoskeletal Rearrangement, 190

D

Diarrhea, 155-156, 186-187, 200

E

Enteric Infection, 15, 39, 162, 168

Enterobacteriaceae, 47-53, 56-57, 63-64, 68-69, 71-72, 139, 142-143, 152-154, 160

Enteroids, 180-181, 183-185, 188-194, 197

Extracellular Polymeric Substance, 107

F

Ferritin, 168

Free Bacteria, 186, 192

G

Gastroenteritis, 1, 11, 41, 139, 156, 162-163, 174, 186-188, 199, 203-204, 215, 220

Gastrointestinal Tract, 14, 36, 42, 55, 162, 164, 168, 192, 194, 223

Genome Degradation, 111, 114-115, 118, 130, 220

Genomic Island, 56-57, 63, 65, 69-71, 74-75, 159-160, 173

Genomic Lesions, 111-118

Growth Factor, 79, 81, 89, 183-184, 189

H

Host Adaptation, 79, 88, 108, 111-112, 115, 118-120, 171, 173-174, 176, 198

Host Cell, 79, 86, 89, 92, 121, 125, 127, 129

Host Range, 79, 123, 168, 186

I

Immune Cell, 42, 52, 93, 99, 193, 201

Inflammatory Response, 42, 48, 51-53, 104, 159, 167, 178, 186, 188, 191

Innate Immunity, 92-93, 96, 105-106, 110, 191

Invasin, 78, 85, 87-89, 132

Iron Chelator, 160, 167

Iron Homeostasis, 156-157, 165, 167, 169-171, 178

Iron Transport, 66, 74, 77, 156, 160, 171-172

Iron-uptake System, 163, 167-168

L

Long-read Sequencing, 138-139, 144

M

Macrophage, 14, 58, 63, 70, 74, 89, 92, 95, 99-100, 104, 108-109, 124, 126, 169, 176, 179, 191

Microbiota, 1, 29, 36-37, 40-45, 48-55, 130, 180-181, 188-189, 193-194, 197, 199, 202

Microenvironment, 169, 190

Model Systems, 180-182, 187, 189-190, 193

Mono Glycosylated Enterobactin, 159

Multidrug Resistant, 154, 160, 162

N

Nucleotide Composition, 66-67

Nutritional Immunity, 167-168, 178

O

Organoids, 180-185, 188-190, 192-198, 201-202

P

Pathogenicity Island, 12, 15, 38, 56-58, 64, 71, 73-75, 77-78, 89, 91, 108, 120, 122, 132-133, 135-136, 159, 172

Phagocytic Cell, 99

Phenotype, 7, 41-42, 48, 51, 53, 64, 85, 96-97, 100, 102, 105, 110, 115, 125, 128-130, 162, 169, 184-185, 187

Phenotypic Heterogeneity, 215, 218, 221

Physiology, 13, 36, 38, 180-181, 183, 187, 192-193, 197, 202-204, 223

Plasmid, 5, 7, 59, 64, 68, 70, 73, 75, 79-82, 86, 88-89, 138-147, 149-155, 162, 172-173, 206-207, 213, 215, 217

R

Respiratory Burst, 109, 167, 169

S

Salmonella, 1-2, 9, 11-43, 45, 48-49, 51-59, 62-83, 85, 87-93, 95-101, 103-112, 114-122, 124, 126, 129-140, 142-146, 149-160, 162-182, 185-194, 196-205, 207-208, 210-212, 215-216, 219-224

Salmonella Enterica, 1, 13-17, 21-22, 25-26, 28, 39-43, 52-55, 58-59, 62, 73-76, 78, 88-93, 107-111, 119-122, 132-140, 151-156, 159, 163, 170, 172-179, 186, 196-203, 205, 220-224

Salmonellosis, 1, 28, 35, 37-38, 91, 110-111, 119, 137, 151, 153, 156-157, 162, 170, 174-176, 179, 199

Secretion System, 15, 56-57, 73, 75, 78, 91, 116, 122, 132, 135-136, 186, 199

Siderophores, 158-160, 162-163, 165-169, 172, 179

Spleen, 122, 165-168, 186

Systemic Infection, 2, 122, 134, 165-169, 177

T

Transcription Factor, 68, 76, 137, 215, 219

Transferrin, 81, 158, 162, 165, 167-168, 178

Two-component System, 87, 121, 134-136, 207, 216

Typhoid Fever, 92-93, 107, 110, 121-122, 132-133, 177, 188, 198-200, 202-203, 220

V

Virulence, 11, 13-15, 38-39, 54, 57, 64, 71-73, 75-80, 85, 87-89, 108-109, 121, 124-126, 129, 131-132, 134-139, 141, 143, 151, 153, 156, 160, 162-168, 172-177, 187-188, 190, 199-201, 204-205, 215, 222

Y

Yersiniabactin, 159-160, 162-163, 167, 169, 175

www.ingramcontent.com/pod-product-compliance
Lightning Source LLC
Chambersburg PA
CBHW081217180926
51613CB00003B/256